Mathematical Population Dynamics and Epidemiology in Temporal and Spatio-Temporal Domains

Mathematical Population Dynamics and Epidemiology in Temporal and Spatio-Temporal Domains

Harkaran Singh, PhD
Khalsa College of Engineering and Technology,
Amritsar–143001, Punjab, India

Joydip Dhar, PhD
ABV-Indian Institute of Information Technology and Management
Gwalior–474015, M.P., India

AAP | APPLE ACADEMIC PRESS

Apple Academic Press Inc.
3333 Mistwell Crescent
Oakville, ON L6L 0A2 Canada

Apple Academic Press Inc.
9 Spinnaker Way
Waretown, NJ 08758 USA

International Standard Book Number-13: 978-1-77188-671-0 (Hardcover)
International Standard Book Number-13: 978-1-351-25170-9 (eBook)

Library and Archives Canada Cataloguing in Publication

Singh, Harkaran, author
Mathematical population dynamics and epidemiology in temporal and spatio-temporal domains / Harkaran Singh, PhD, Joydip Dhar, PhD.
Includes bibliographical references and index.
Issued in print and electronic formats.
ISBN 978-1-77188-671-0 (hardcover).--ISBN 978-1-351-25170-9 (PDF)
1. Population biology--Mathematical models. 2. Ecology--Mathematical models. 3. Epidemiology--Mathematical models. 4. Biomathematics. I. Dhar, Joydip, author II. Title.
QH352.S56 2018 577.8'8 C2018-903438-6 C2018-903439-4

Library of Congress Cataloging-in-Publication Data

Names: Singh, Harkaran. | Dhar, Joydip.
Title: Mathematical population : dynamics and epidemiology in temporal and spatio-temporal domains / Harkaran Singh, PhD, Joydip Dhar, PhD.
Description: Toronto : New Jersey : Apple Academic Press, 2018. | Includes bibliographical references and index.
Identifiers: LCCN 2018026066 (print) | LCCN 2018029471 (ebook) | ISBN 9781351251709 (ebook) | ISBN 9781771886710 (hardcover : alk. paper)
Subjects: LCSH: Epidemiology--Statistical methods. | Epidemics--Mathematical models.
Classification: LCC RA652.2.M3 (ebook) | LCC RA652.2.M3 S56 2018 (print) | DDC 614.4072/7--dc23
LC record available at https://lccn.loc.gov/2018026066

Apple Academic Press also publishes its books in a variety of electronic formats. Some content that appears in print may not be available in electronic format. For information about Apple Academic Press products, visit our website at **www.appleacademicpress.com** and the CRC Press website at **www.crcpress.com**

Dedicated

To

Our Loving Daughters

Ekamjot Kaur

Eknoor Kaur

&

Juee Dhar

Contents

About the Authors

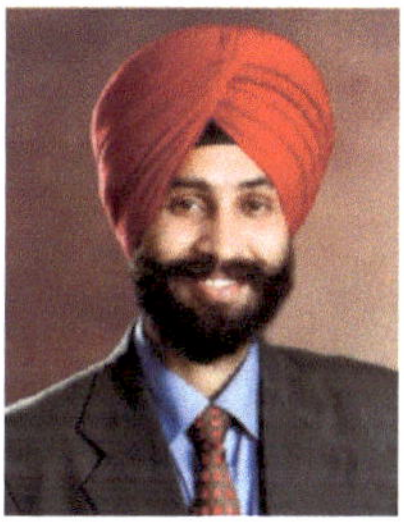

Harkaran Singh, PhD
Associate Professor, Khalsa College of Engineering and Technology, Amritsar, Punjab, India

Harkaran Singh, PhD, is an Associate Professor at Khalsa College of Engineering and Technology, Amritsar, India. He has 17 years of experience in teaching and 7 years of experience in research. He is a life member of the National Professional Society ISTE. He received an award for "Young Investigator from India and Southeast Asia" from the International Society of Infectious Diseases at the 17th International Congress on Infectious Diseases held at Hyderabad, India. He has published several research papers in peer-reviewed journals. He obtained his PhD degree in Mathematical Modeling in Population Biology from IKG-Punjab Technical University, Kapurthala, India.

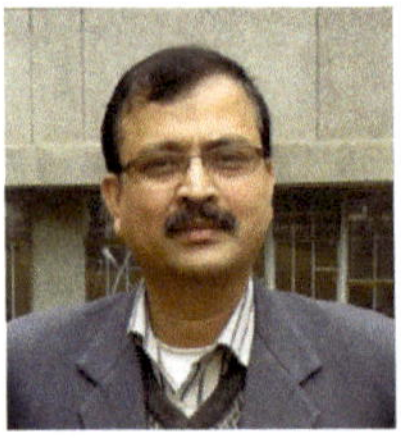

Joydip Dhar, PhD
Associate Professor, ABV-Indian Institute of Information Technology and Management, Madhya Pradesh, India

Joydip Dhar, PhD, is an Associate Professor at the ABV-Indian Institute of Information Technology and Management, Gwalior, India. He has been associated with the teaching profession and research for the past 21 years and has also published about 125 papers in his areas of interest and proficiency in internationally reputed journals. He has guided eight PhD students and several MTech and MBA theses. Currently eight students are pursuing PhDs under his guidance. Dr. Dhar has delivered more than 50 invited lectures at different universities and institutions in India and abroad, including the UK and Sweden. He has co-authored a research book and has conducted several conferences and short-term courses. A life member of many professional societies (ISTE, IMS, ISMMACS) and an annual member of the American Mathematical Society (AMS), Dr. Dhar has participated in the prestigious ACM-ICPC world finals as a mentor at Stockholm, Sweden 2009. He was the recipient of a Dewang Mehta National Education Award, among other awards. Recently, he attended a prestigious 8-day in-residence program for Inspired Teachers at Rashtrapati Bhavan, which is the highest recognition for any central government institution teacher.

List of Figures

List of Tables

List of Symbols

Parameter	Description
a	Intrinsic growth rate of prey
b	Predation rate of prey (Chapter 2), Predation rate of susceptible prey (Chapter 7)
b_0	Predation rate of infected prey
c	Growth rate of predator due to alternative resources
d	Death rate of predator (Model-1 in Chapter 2), Overcrowding of predator (Model-2 in Chapter 2, Chapter 7)
d_0	Death rate of the infective prey
h	Death rate of predator due to infected prey
k	Carrying capacity of the prey in a particular habitat
l	Half saturation constant
m	Maximum value which per capita reduction rate of predator can attend (Model-1 in Chapter 2), Conversion rate for a predator (Model-2 in Chapter 2, Chapter 3), Coefficient of media awareness (Chapter 9, 10, 11)
n	Measure of food quality that the prey provides for conversion into predator births
q	Extent to which alternatives are provided for the growth of the predator

Parameter	Description
α	Rate of infection of the premature individuals
β	Contact rate of infective prey with susceptible prey
γ	Birth rate of premature individuals
d_1	Death rates of premature individuals
d_2	Death rates of mature individuals
d_3	Death rates of infected individuals
β_1	Overcrowding rates of mature individuals
β_2	Overcrowding rates of infected individuals
τ_1	Maturation delay
τ_2	Latent period of infection
τ	Gestation delay for predator (Chapter 7), Latent period for of infection (Chapter 9)
Λ	Recruitment rate of susceptible
$\tilde{\delta}$	Disease-induced death rate
$\tilde{\beta}$	Transmission rate (in absence of NPIs through media awareness)
$1/\tilde{\mu}$	Average lifespan of individual
$1/\tilde{\sigma}$	Average time-span of infected individuals in exposed class
$1/\tilde{\gamma}$	Average length of infection of the infected individual
$\tilde{\omega}$	Rate at which susceptible individuals are vaccinated
$\tilde{q}$	Fraction of recovered individuals getting disease acquired immunity
$\tilde{\theta}$, $\tilde{\theta}_1$	Rate at which disease-induced immunity wanes
$\tilde{\theta}_2$	Rate at which vaccine-induced immunity wanes
$\tilde{\xi}_1$	Rate of recovery from exposed class due to pre-existing immunity or natural immunity
$\tilde{\xi}_2$	Rate at which exposed individuals are vaccinated

Parameter	Description
N_i	Population density in the i-th patch
$g_i(N_i)$	Growth rate function in the i-th patch
$p_i(N_i)$	Harvesting function in the i-th patch
K_i	Carrying capacity in the i-th patch
R_i	Density of the non-diffusing self-renewable supplementary resource in the i-th patch
β_i	Depletion rate of resource in the i-th patch
θ_i	Conversion rate of resource in the i-th patch
D_i, D_{1i}, D_{2i}	Diffusion Coefficient in the i-th patch
x_i, y_i	Population of two species competing for same resources in the i-th patch
$p_i(x_i)$	Interaction rates of x_i in the i-th patch
$q_i(y_i)$	Interaction rates of y_i in the i-th patch
C_i	Carrying capacity of the supplementary resource in the i-th patch
$g_i(x_i)$	Growth rates of x_i in the i-th patch
$f_i(y_i)$	Growth rates of y_i in the i-th patch

Preface

Mathematical Biosciences, also commonly known as Biomathematics, is an interdisciplinary subject. The link between mathematics and various biological sciences is mainly established throughout mathematical models. Modeling as such is very useful tool for understanding the behavior of a system. Different types of mathematical models have been developed to gain an insight into complex biological and ecological situations, and various mathematical techniques are employed to analyze these models.

Therefore, in this context, the study of population dynamics with special emphasis on the migration of population in a heterogeneous patchy habitat, the human and animal population, spreading of epidemic, etc. has become an important area of research in mathematical biology dealing with the survival of different species.

In this book, we have proposed 11 different models: (i) two models with different prey-predator interactions; (ii) four population models with diffusion in two patch environment; (iii) one prey-predator model with disease in the prey; and (iv) four epidemic models with different control strategies. The population in a particular region of study is divided into mutually exclusive compartments; also the movement of the population is instantaneous from one compartment to another in the models discussed in Chapters 2–6, 10, and 11; and the movement is delayed from one compartment to another in the models presented in Chapters 7–9. All the models are proposed in a homogeneous environment except the models proposed in Chapters 3–6.

Since population biology and epidemiology is a vast area of research and for basic understanding, people must read the phenomenon textbook on mathematical biology by J.D. Murray [1]. Our book presents some recent advancements in mathematical biology, generally accepted theoretical framework for a variety of situations from temporal to a spatiotemporal domain.

This book is suitable for the interdisciplinary researchers and policymakers; especially mathematical biologists, biologists, physicists, and epidemiologists. The book can be useful as textbook or reference book for graduate and postgraduate advanced level mathematical biology courses.

Authors are thankful to Dr. Harbax Singh Bhatti, Professor, B.B.S.B. Engineering College, Fatehgarh Sahib for their ever-supporting encouragement and valuable suggestions from time-to-time.

—Harkaran Singh, PhD
Joydip Dhar, PhD

Chapter 1

Introduction and Mathematical Preliminaries

1.1 Introduction

Mathematical biology, nowadays, is a well-known field, which is growing fast, being an interdisciplinary subject and undoubtedly, has been one of the most appealing applications of mathematics. The complexity of the biological sciences makes the interdisciplinary involvement essential. For the mathematicians, biology opens up numerous new branches, while, for the biologists, mathematical modeling offers another powerful research tool. Further, population biology and epidemiology is a fascinating domain of study in the field of biomathematics for today's researchers. The increasing study of realistic and practically useful mathematical models in population dynamics and epidemics is a reflection of their use in helping to understand the dynamic processes involved therein and in making practical predictions [1].

1.1.1 Population Dynamics

A population is a group of individuals who live together in the same habitat and are likely to interbreed. It may contain individuals of different ages, and the age of an individual is likely to change over time.

Further, the size of a population may grow or shrink depending on the biological and environmental parameters such as birth rates, death rates, immigration, and emigration. The study on these changes of age and size of a population is known as population dynamics. Some of the examples are population growth, population decline, and aging population. Also, for interpreting survey data and predicting pest outbreaks, a good understanding of population dynamics is very much useful [2–4].

1.1.2 Prey-Predator Interactions

The population dynamics of each species is affected when two or more species interact. There are three types of interactions among the species: (i) if the growth rate of one species is increasing and the others is decreasing, then they are in a prey-predator relationship; (ii) if the growth rate of each species is decreasing, then they are competing; and (iii) if the growth rate of each species is increasing, then they are in mutualism [5]. It is a well-known fact that the prey-predator interactions is a subject of great interest in the bio-mathematical literature starting with the pioneer work of Lotka [6] and Volterra [7], and the dynamic relationship between predator and prey living in the same environment will continue to be one of the important themes in mathematical ecology [8, 9]. A number of mathematicians, in the past, have studied prey-predator models and contributed to their development and even today's mathematicians are engaged in anticipating and understanding the diverse biological world of prey-predator systems [10–18].

1.1.3 Discrete Generations

A generation is the expected time from the birth of an individual to the birth of its first offspring. For a sexually mature individual of a population, if the remaining expected lifespan is less than or equal to one generation, then the population is said to have discrete generations. For many species, the population grows in discrete steps, however, the step lengths can vary depending on the type of species. It is a day for the fruit fly emergence from pupae; it can be a number of hours for the cells, while it can be considerably less for bacteria and viruses. For example, consider an insect that emerges from its egg in the spring, lays eggs in summer and dies in the autumn. The number of insects in the $(k+1)$-th generation depends only on the number of insects in the k-th generation (since no other generations have survived). If N_k denotes the population density in generation k then, we may write $N_{k+1} = f(N_k)$, k = 0,1,2, ..., which is mathematically a recursive relation. Discrete-time models are studied by the method of difference equations and are widely used in various bio-medical areas such as cancer growth, aging and genetics. Liu [19] investigated the existence of periodic solutions for discrete semi-ratio-dependent prey-predator model. Chen [20] proposed a discrete prey-predator system and obtained conditions for global stability of equilibrium for non-autonomous and periodic cases. Liao et al. [21] investigated a prey-predator discrete model and derived the conditions for the local asymptotic stability of equilibrium of the system. Further, a number of researchers have suggested that the discrete-time models have rich and complex dynamical behaviors [22–29].

1.1.4 Diffusion of Population

There is a natural tendency in the species living in a habitat to move or migrate towards better suited regions for resource, survival, and existence owing to several factors. Generally, the movement of the species from one place to other place occurs due to certain factors such as overcrowding, anticlimate, deforestation (industrialization), epidemic, predator chasing prey, fugitive strategies, and more importantly resource limitations [30–35].

This phenomenon of animal dispersion was investigated experimentally for the first time by taking the case of insects; the authors of Refs. [36, 37] have conducted experiments on the release of Drosophila flies and later some Japanese entomologists [38, 39], also made a few contributions to the concept of diffusion considering interactive forces between dispersing individuals in the form of density dependent dispersion. Various other experimental and mathematical studies have also been conducted on dispersion of Predator-Prey systems [40–44].

The classic theory of diffusion was founded more than one hundred years ago by the scientist A. Fick [45, 46]. According to Fick's law, the amount of matter transport in the x direction across a unit normal area in unit time is proportional to the gradient of the concentration, i.e.,

$J_x = -D\partial C/\partial x$, where C is the concentration of matter and D is the diffusivity. The minus sign indicates that diffusion occurs from higher concentration to lower concentration. Using this law, Fick's equation of diffusion can be obtained:

$$\frac{\partial C}{\partial t} = -\frac{\partial J_x}{\partial x} = \frac{\partial}{\partial x}\left(D\frac{\partial C}{\partial x}\right). \tag{1.1.1}$$

In population dynamics, where species interact and move about in a habitat or from one patch to another, the situation can best be described by continuous space-time interaction-migration models. Using Fick's Law of Diffusion, the governing equations for such models are generally of the form:

$$\frac{\partial N}{\partial t} = F(N) + D\nabla^2 N \tag{1.1.2}$$

here, N is an n-tuplet where each component represents the density of one species, F is a vector describing all reaction and interactions, D is a diffusion coefficient matrix and Δ is the Laplacian in spatial coordinates. Using the above equations, several population models with diffusion effect for single species and interacting populations for both homogeneous and heterogeneous environment, have been proposed and analyzed [41, 47–50]. Some wonderful examples of reaction-diffusion phenomenon in population dynamics can be seen in the books [5, 44, 51].

Some researchers have also studied the persistence, co-existence, and extinction in single species and the two species Lotka-Voltara reaction diffusion models [52–55] and the global stability in generalized Lotka-Voltara with diffusion [35, 47, 48] as well. Again, they studied the effects of dispersion on linear stability of interacting species in one dimension homogeneous finite habitat for Prey-Predator system taking dispersion coefficients to be equal and constant for both the species. Such dispersion is shown to have a stabilizing effect on the equilibrium state under non-homogeneous boundary conditions [48, 49]. Similar analysis has also been carried out by [56, 57] for competing species in case of homogeneous, finite, and semi-finite habitats. Interesting results regarding the effects of dispersive migration on the equilibrium states of above said habitats have been obtained. Since diffusion process in an ecosystem generally tends to maintain a uniform density of population in a habitat, this (diffusion), therefore, may be expected to play a general role of increasing stability in a system of mixed populations and resource. There is, of course, an important exception, known as diffusion induced instability and certainly not a rare case especially in Prey-Predator systems [44, 58].

1.1.5 Patchy Environment

Depending upon their environmental and ecological character, the real habitats are both homogeneous as well as heterogeneous. This heterogeneity can occur due to various geographical and topographical conditions. It can also be affected by seasonal climatic changes. In general in a habitat, patchiness, a type of heterogeneity, occurs due to discontinuous variations in geographical and ecological characteristics. In the case of forestry habitats, patchiness can arise due to industrialization, pollution and population [1, 44].

In real world situations, a particular habitat may be regarded as patchy if it's ecological characteristics are constants but different in each region. For instance, patchy distributions of plankton in sea and lakes are well documented [59, 60]. The factor, which helps maintain this patchiness, is still a subject of research. However, a few different possibilities that have been proposed are (a) food-chain association in prey-predator relationships, (b) behavioral reaction or association with temperature, salinity and nutrient distributions, (c) aggregative behavior for breeding and feeding, and (d) deforestation of the habitat caused by industrialization, pollution, and population growth.

In the last decade, a few researchers studied a single species diffusion model by assuming that the habitat consists of two or three patches and it has been shown that there exists a positive, monotonic, continuous non-uniform steady state solution that is linearly and non-linearly asymptotically stable under both reservoir and no-flux boundary conditions.

1.1.6 Epidemiology

Epidemics is the spread of an infectious disease to a large number of people in a particular region within a short period of time. Despite so many advances in the medical sciences, the communicable diseases significantly affect the human population when they occur. Actually, in the modern era, the spread of diseases are fast due to traveling of a huge population of the world from one place to another. Therefore, the study of the spread of diseases in human population is very important in these circumstances and this study is known as epidemiology. In fact, epidemiology is the science that focuses on the occurrence of disease in its broadest sense with the fundamental aim to understand, to control its causes, and the final eradication of the disease [61, 62]. A large number of scientists studied the disease models and contributed in making the effective control strategies to suppress the spread of epidemics in human population [63–85].

1.1.7 Eco-Epidemiology

It is a well-known fact that most of the ecological populations suffer from various infectious diseases and these diseases have a significant role in regulating the population sizes. The correlation between the disease and the population dynamics is a topic of significant interest, and the fusion of ecology and epidemiology is a comparatively new branch of study, known as eco-epidemiology. The mathematical study of such eco-epidemiological models have explored various unknown aspects of ecological populations [86, 87]. Hethcote et al. [88] discussed a prey-predator model with *Susceptible-Infected-Susceptible* infection in the prey and concluded that the predation on the more vulnerable prey can cause the disease to die out and it would remain endemic in the absence of the predators. Sinha et al. [89] studied a prey-predator model with infection in the prey and identified the thresholds when system persists and disease remains endemic. Mukhopadhyay et al. [90] modified a basic eco-epidemiological model by incorporating predator switching among susceptible and infected prey populations and analyzed the switching model in order to elucidate the role of switching on disease dynamics.

1.1.8 Stage-Structure

The dynamics of interacting species are affected by stage-structured population; for example, predator mostly prey on pre-mature population since the pre-mature prey is small in size and is physically weak. The rates of survival of species and reproduction almost always depend on age and size. Further, the children up to a certain age are affected mostly by the diseases like Rubella, Measles, Chickenpox, Polio, Mumps, etc. Therefore, in population as well as disease dynamics, the population can be divided into two major categories: pre-mature and mature stages; because the pre-mature population is more prone to the diseases than the mature population [91, 92]. Nisbet et al. [93] proposed the stage-structure models in terms of delay-differential equations in the situation where the processes of growth and development within a stage are distinct. Dyson et al. [94] investigated the instability and chaos in a nonlinear model of age and maturity structured population dynamics. Calsina et al. [95] studied an age-structured population model with two population groups, juveniles and adults, and obtained a complete description of the asymptotic behavior of the population dynamics and discussed the existence of a nontrivial equilibrium. Hence, stage-structure models are also important and one can think about better dynamics of reality by considering stage structured population [96, 97].

1.1.9 Time Delay

The time delay factor has a great importance in nature because growth is not instantaneous, it takes some time to perform and this time is called a time delay or time lag. For example, all species take some time to born a new offspring after mating and it is known as gestation delay; immature population takes a constant time to become mature and is called maturation delay. Another example is susceptible population that takes a constant time to become infective, when it comes in contact with an infected person and this constant time is known as latent period of infection. The inclusion of temporal delays in the models makes them more realistic and, therefore, in biological modeling, the delay models are becoming common and have been used for describing several aspects of the population dynamics and the disease dynamics [98–111].

1.1.10 Disease Acquired Immunity

Immunity acquired via infection gives protection to an individual from subsequent infection by the same or similar pathogens for some period of time and it is known as infection acquired immunity. For different diseases, the transition from complete to partial immunity can happen over different time scales; over days, a few weeks, over a month or a few years [112–114]. In literature, there are certain diseases like influenza for which immunity is developed for a very short period; even sometimes the period is negligible. The high proportion of susceptible population and short duration of immunity for influenza does all contribute to its rapid spread [115]. Influenza A (H1N1) viruses were spread in human population in 1957 and again in 2009. The disease burden in the elderly was relatively low due to pre-existing immunity in this age group. Actually, due to pre-existing immunity, a fraction of exposed population, instead of being infected, develops disease acquired a temporary immunity and hence joins the recovered class [116].

1.1.11 Vaccine Induced Immunity

The science of disease prevention in humans began with the initial understanding of immunity and the immune system starting with the discoveries of Metchnikoff [117], which is continuing to the present. With the recognition that specific infectious disease was caused by bacteria or virus, it became possible to develop vaccine to prevent the humans from that infectious disease [118–120]. The vaccination stimulates an individual's immune system to develop adaptive immunity against the pathogens and it is known as vaccine induced immunity. Quite often, the vaccine-induced immunity requires boosting after some period of time, as the vaccine effectiveness wanes due to absence of exposure to the disease. Hepatitis B vaccination gives only 10 to 15 years immunity, and after that the boost is required again in order for immunity to remain effective [121]. In the case of measles, the vaccinated individuals are less immune than those with naturally acquired immunity [122, 123]. Zaman et al. [124] studied the stability analysis of a SIR epidemic model and shown that an optimal control of the disease exists with the vaccination program. Curtiss [125] focused on infectious diseases and their prevention and control by development of vaccines with special emphasis on influenza. Development of anti-fungal drugs [126], anti-parasite drugs [127], and anti-viral drugs [128] and subsequent discoveries have contributed greatly to the control of infectious diseases in the developed world, but still, there are many infectious diseases for which no effective vaccine exists as yet.

1.1.12 Non-Pharmaceutical Interventions (NPIs) Through Media Awareness

To control the spread of communicable diseases, there are primarily two methods: one is pharmaceutical interventions and the other is non-pharmaceutical interventions (NPIs) [129]. NPIs are the actions apart from getting vaccinated and taking medicine that people and communities can take to slow the spread of communicable diseases. Pharmaceutical interventions (vaccines), to prevent the disease, may not be available in many areas of the world in sufficient quantities to make a significant contribution in suppressing the outbreak of infectious diseases [130, 131]. Also, most of the vaccines are too expensive for widespread use in the developing world [132]. So, it is very essential to carry out the studies on the control of the spreading of the communicable diseases with the help of NPIs. Media plays a very important role to aware the public for use of NPIs to control the epidemics. People are informed through media alert, which results in a decrease in the susceptibility as people try to protect themselves from being infected. There are two types of NPIs: personal and community. The personal NPIs are the everyday preventive actions one should always take to help keep oneself and others from getting sick, e.g., covering coughs and sneezes, washing hands often, using alcohol-based hand gel, staying home when sick, cleaning surfaces and objects routinely and using the face mask, etc. Community NPIs refer to the actions the communities might take to increase space among the people (social distancing) during a pandemic, e.g., closing schools temporarily, making sick leave policies more flexible, offering telework or remote-meeting options and postponing or canceling mass gatherings, etc. Many researchers have investigated the impact of NPIs through media awareness in controlling the diseases using mathematical modeling [133–142].

1.2 Mathematical Preliminaries

In this section, we introduce some of the mathematical theories and techniques, which are used to analyze the various models presented in this book.

1.2.1 Equilibria of Temporal System

Consider the following system of ordinary differential equations (ODEs):

$$\dot{x} = f(x;t;\mu);\ x \in U \subset R^n;\ t \in R^1;\ \text{and } \mu \in V \subset R^p, \tag{1.2.1}$$

where $\dot{x}$ is differentiation of x with respect to time t; U and V are open sets in R^n and R^p, respectively, and μ is a parameter. The right-hand side function, $f(x;t;\mu)$, of the equation (1.2.1) is called a *vector field.* ODEs, which explicitly depend on time, are called *non-autonomous*, while those that are not dependent on time are called *autonomous*.

Consider the following general autonomous system:

$$\dot{x} = f(x);\ x \in R^n. \tag{1.2.2}$$

Definition 1.2.1. *An equilibrium solution of the system (1.2.2) is given by* $x = \bar{x} \in R^n$; *where* $f(\bar{x}) = 0$. *The vector or point* $\bar{x}$ *is called an equilibrium point.*

Definition 1.2.2. *The Jacobian matrix of* f *at the equilibrium point* $\bar{x}$, *denoted by* $Df(\bar{x})$, *is the matrix of partial derivatives of* f *evaluated at* $\bar{x}$. *It is given by:*

$$J(\bar{x}) = \begin{bmatrix} \frac{\partial f_1}{\partial x_1}(\bar{x}) & \cdots\cdots\cdots & \frac{\partial f_1}{\partial x_n}(\bar{x}) \\ \cdots\cdots\cdots & \cdots\cdots\cdots & \cdots\cdots\cdots \\ \frac{\partial f_n}{\partial x_1}(\bar{x}) & \cdots\cdots\cdots & \frac{\partial f_n}{\partial x_n}(\bar{x}) \end{bmatrix}.$$

1.2.2 Nature of Roots

Consider the polynomial:

$$p(\lambda) = a_0\lambda^n + a_1\lambda^{n-1} + \ldots\ldots + a_{n-1}\lambda + a_n,\quad a_i \in R,\ a_0 \neq 0. \tag{1.2.3}$$

Theorem 1.2.1. *(Descartes' rule of signs) [143]. The equation* $p(\lambda) = 0$ *cannot have more positive roots than the changes of signs in* $p(\lambda)$, *and more negative roots than the changes of signs in* $p(-\lambda)$.

Routh-Hurwitz Criteria

An important criteria, which gives necessary and sufficient conditions for all of the roots of the characteristic polynomial (with real coefficients) to lie in the left half of the complex plane are known as Routh-Hurwitz criteria [144]. This criteria is used to determine the local asymptotic stability of an equilibrium for nonlinear systems of differential equations. The Routh-Hurwitz criteria is stated in the following theorem:

Theorem 1.2.2. *Given the polynomial,*

$$P(\lambda) = \lambda^n + a_1\lambda^{n-1} + \ldots + a_{n-1}\lambda + a_n, \quad a_i \in R, \quad i = 1,\, 2, \ldots, n$$

define n Hurwitz matrices for the characteristic polynomial $P(\lambda)$ as follows:

$$H_1 = (a_1), \; H_2 = \begin{pmatrix} a_1 & 1 \\ a_3 & a_2 \end{pmatrix}, \; H_3 = \begin{pmatrix} a_1 & 1 & 0 \\ a_3 & a_2 & a_1 \\ a_5 & a_4 & a_3 \end{pmatrix}$$

and

$$H_n = \begin{pmatrix} a_1 & 1 & 0 & 0 & \cdots & 0 \\ a_3 & a_2 & a_1 & 1 & \cdots & 0 \\ a_5 & a_4 & a_3 & a_2 & \cdots & 0 \\ \vdots & \vdots & \vdots & \vdots & \cdots & \vdots \\ 0 & 0 & 0 & 0 & \ddots & a_n \end{pmatrix},$$

where $a_j = 0$ if $j > n$. All of the roots of the polynomial $P(\lambda)$ are negative or have negative real part iff the determinants of all Hurwitz matrices are positive:

$$\det H_j > 0, \quad j = 1, 2, \ldots, n.$$

When $n = 2$, the Routh-Hurwitz criteria simplifies as

$$\det H_1 = a_1 > 0 \;\; and \;\; \det H_2 = det \begin{pmatrix} a_1 & 0 \\ 0 & a_2 \end{pmatrix} = a_1 a_2 > 0$$

or $a_1 > 0$ and $a_2 > 0$. For polynomials of degree $2, 3, 4, 5$, the Routh-Hurwitz criteria are summarized as follows:

$$n = 2: \;\; a_1 > 0 \;\; and \;\; a_2 > 0.$$

$$n = 3: \ a_1 > 0, \ a_3 > 0 \ \textit{and} \ a_1 a_2 > a_3.$$

$$n = 4: \ a_1 > 0, \ a_3 > 0, \ a_4 > 0 \ \textit{and} \ a_1 a_2 a_3 > a_3^2 + a_1^2 a_4 > 0.$$

$$n = 5: \ a_i > 0, \ i = 1,2,3,4,5, \ a_1 a_2 a_3 > a_3^2 + a_1^2 a_4 > 0 \ \textit{and}$$
$$(a_1 a_4 - a_5)(a_1 a_2 a_3 - a_3^2 - a_1^2 a_4) > a_5 (a_1 a_2 - a_3)^2 + a_1 a_5^2.$$

1.2.3 Stability of Equilibrium Points

Let $\bar{x}(t)$ be any solution of the general autonomous system (1.2.2). Then, $\bar{x}(t)$ is *stable* if solutions starting "close" to $\bar{x}(t)$ at a given time remain close to $\bar{x}(t)$ for all later times. It is *asymptotically-stable* if nearby solutions converge to $\bar{x}(t)$ as $t \to \infty$. A solution which is not stable is said to be unstable [145].

Theorem 1.2.3 (145). . *Suppose all the eigenvalues of $Df(\bar{x})$ have negative real parts, then the equilibrium solution $x = \bar{x}$ of the system (1.2.2) is asymptotically stable. The equilibrium $\bar{x}$ is unstable if at least one of the eigenvalues has positive real part.*

1.2.4 Lyapunov's Direct Method

Let $V : D \to R$ be a continuously differentiable function defined on the domain $D \subset R^n$ that contains the origin. The rate of change of V along the trajectories of the nonlinear autonomous system $\dot{x} = f(x)$, where $f : D \to R^n$ is a locally Lipschitz map from the domain $D \subset R^n$ to R^n, is given by

$$\dot{V}(x) = \sum_{i=1}^{n} \frac{\partial V}{\partial x_i} \frac{dx_i}{dt} = \left[\frac{\partial V}{\partial x_1} \frac{\partial V}{\partial x_2} \cdots\cdots \frac{\partial V}{\partial x_n} \right] \dot{x} = \frac{\partial V}{\partial x} f(x)$$

The main idea of the Lyapunov's theory is that if $\dot{V}(x)$ is negative along the trajectories of the system, the $V(x)$ will decrease as the time goes forward.

Theorem 1.2.4. *Let the origin $x = 0 \in D \subset R^n$ be an equilibrium point for $\dot{x} = f(x)$. Let $V : D \to R$ be a continuous differentiable function such that*

$$\begin{aligned} &V(0) = 0, \\ &V(x) > 0, \qquad \forall x \in D - \{0\} \\ &\dot{V}(x) \leq 0, \qquad \forall x \in D \end{aligned}$$

then, $x = 0$ is stable. Moreover, if

$$\dot{V}(x) \leq 0, \quad \forall x \in D - \{0\},$$

then $x = 0$ is asymptotically stable.

1.2.5 Bifurcation in Continuous System

Definition 1.2.3. *Consider the following system of ODEs:*

$$\dot{x} = f(x;\mu);\ x \in R;\ \mu \in R. \tag{1.2.4}$$

An equilibrium solution of (1.2.4) given by $(x;\mu) = (0;0)$ is said to undergo bifurcation at $\mu = 0$ if the flow for μ near zero and x near zero is not qualitatively the same as the flow near $x = 0$ at $\mu = 0$.

Theorem 1.2.5. *[146]. Consider the following general system of ODEs with a parameter ϕ*

$$\frac{dx}{dt} = f(x,\phi), f : R^n \times R, \text{ and } f \varepsilon C^2(R^n \times R). \tag{1.2.5}$$

Without loss of generality, it is assumed that 0 is an equilibrium for the system (1.2.5) for all values of the parameter ϕ, (i.e., $f(0,\phi) \equiv 0$ for all ϕ). Assume

A1: *$A = D_x f(0,0) = (\frac{\partial f_i}{\partial x_j},0,0)$ is the linearized matrix of the system (1.2.5) around the equilibrium point 0 with ϕ evaluated at 0, zero is a simple eigenvalue of A and all other eigenvalue of A have negative real parts;*

A2: *Matrix A has a nonnegative right eigenvector w and a left eigenvector v corresponding to the zero eigenvalue.*

Let f_k be the k-th component of f and

$$\mathbf{a} = \sum_{k,i,j=1}^{n} v_k w_i w_j \frac{\partial^2 f_k}{\partial x_i \partial x_j}(0,0),$$

$$\mathbf{b} = \sum_{k,i=1}^{n} v_k w_i \frac{\partial^2 f_k}{\partial x_i \partial \phi}(0,0).$$

Then the local dynamics of system (1.2.5) around 0 are totally determined by **a** *and* **b**, *as follows:*

i. $\mathbf{a} > 0, \mathbf{b} > 0$. *When $\phi < 0$ with $|\phi| \ll 1$, 0 is locally asymptotically stable, and their exists a positive unstable equilibrium; when $0 < \phi \ll 1$, 0 is unstable, and their exists a negative and locally asymptotically stable equilibrium.*

ii. $\mathbf{a} < 0, \mathbf{b} < 0$. *When $\phi < 0$ with $|\phi| \ll 1$, 0 is unstable; when $0 < \phi \ll 1$, 0 is locally asymptotically stable, and their exists a positive unstable equilibrium;*

iii. $\mathbf{a} > 0, \mathbf{b} < 0$. *When $\phi < 0$ with $|\phi| \ll 1$, 0 is unstable, and there exists a locally asymptotically stable negative equilibrium; when $0 < \phi \ll 1$, 0 is stable, and a positive unstable equilibrium appears;*

iv. $\mathbf{a} < 0, \mathbf{b} > 0$. *When ϕ changes from negative to positive, 0 changes its stability from stable to unstable. Correspondingly a negative unstable equilibrium becomes positive and locally asymptotically stable.*

Corollary 1.2.6. *When* **a** > 0 *and* **b** > 0, *the bifurcation at $\phi = 0$ is subcritical (backward).*

Hopf Bifurcation

The bifurcation is intimately linked to mathematical or biological threshold parameters like the spectral bound (or radius in discrete time) of the linearized system [147]. It refers to the branching of solutions at some critical value τ^* of parameter τ, causing a loss of structural stability. As τ varies, the dynamical system is stable for $\tau < \tau^*$, unstable for $\tau > \tau^*$, then at τ^*, there exists a switch of stability and bifurcation takes place. Hopf bifurcation arises when one pair of complex eigenvalues crosses the imaginary axis at nonzero speed. Suppose initially all eigenvalues of the linearized part $A(\tau) = D_x f(x,\tau)$ of $\dot{x} = f(x,\tau) : R^{n+1} \longrightarrow R^n$ lie in the open half plane and as τ varies, one and only pair $\lambda(\tau) = \alpha(\tau) \pm i\beta(\tau)$ crosses the imaginary axis at $\tau = \tau^*$, i.e., $\alpha(\tau^*) = 0 \neq \frac{d\alpha(\tau^*)}{d\tau}$ and $\beta \neq 0$, then near τ^*, the equilibrium bifurcates into a limit cycle. By convention, the crossing is from the left, i.e., $\frac{d\alpha(\tau^*)}{d\tau}$.

1.2.6 Euler's Scheme for Discretization

Consider the equation

$$\frac{dy}{dx} = f(x,y), y(x_0) = y_0,$$

and $y = g(x)$ be its solution. Let x_0, $x_1 = x_0 + h$, $x_2 = x_0 + 2h$,... be equidistant values of x.

In the small interval, a curve is approximately a straight line. This is the property used in the Euler's method. The equation of the tangent at $P_0(x_0,y_0)$ is

$$y - y_0 = \left(\frac{dy}{dx}\right)_{(x_0,y_0)} .(x - x_0)$$

$$y = y_0 + f(x_0,y_0).(x - x_0) \tag{1.2.6}$$

The value of y on the curve corresponding to $x = x_1$ is given by the value of y in (1.2.6) approximately.

Therefore, putting $x = x_1 = x_0 + h$ in (1.2.6), we have $y_1 = y_0 + hf(x_0,y_0)$. Similarly approximating the curve through $P_1(x_1,y_1)$ and tangent line is given by $y_2 = y_1 + hf(x_1,y_1)$.

Repeating this process, we have $y_{n+1} = y_n + hf(x_n,y_n)$, in general. This is called Euler's algorithm and interval h is called step size [148].

1.2.7 Stability of Fixed Points in Discrete System

Definition 1.2.4 (145). . *Consider the map $x \to g(x)$, where $x \in \Re^n$, then $x = \bar{x}$ is a fixed point of the map if $g(\bar{x}) = \bar{x}$.*

Definition 1.2.5 (145). . *Let $S \subset R^n$ be a set, then S is said to be invariant under the map $x \to g(x)$ if for any $x_0 \in S$ we have $g^n(x_0) \in S$ for all n.*

1.2.8 Center Manifold in Discrete System

Suppose that we have the map

$$x \to Ax + f(x,y) \tag{1.2.7}$$

$$y \to By + g(x,y), \quad (x,y) \in R^c \times R^s, \tag{1.2.8}$$

or

$$\begin{aligned} x_{n+1} &= Ax_n + f(x_n, y_n), \\ y_{n+1} &= By_n + g(x_n, y_n), \end{aligned}$$

where

$$\begin{aligned} f(0,0) &= 0, \quad Df(0,0) = 0, \\ g(0,0) &= 0, \quad Dg(0,0) = 0, \end{aligned}$$

and f and g are $C^r (r \geq 2)$ in some neighborhood of the origin, A is $c \times c$ matrix with eigenvalues of modulus one, and B is an matrix with eigenvalues of modulus less than one.

Evidently $(x,y) = (0,0)$ is a fixed point of (1.2.7)–(1.2.8), and we have the following theorem:

Theorem 1.2.7 (145). . *There exists a C^r center manifold for (1.2.7)–(1.2.8) which can be locally represented as a graph as follows:*

$$W^c(0) = \{(x,y) \in R^c \times R^s \mid y = h(x), \ |x| < \delta, \ h(0) = 0, \ Dh(0) = 0\}$$

for δ sufficiently small. Moreover, the dynamics of (1.2.7)–(1.2.8) restricted to the center manifold is, for u sufficiently small, given by c-dimensional map

$$u \to Au + f(u, h(u)), \quad u \in R^c. \tag{1.2.9}$$

Next we want to compute the center manifold as below:

$$y_{n+1} = h(x_{n+1}) = Bh(x_n) + g(x_n, h(x_n)),$$

or

$$N(h(x)) = h(Ax + f(x, h(x))) - Bh(x) - g(x, h(x)) = 0.$$

Theorem 1.2.8 (145). . *Suppose, the zero solution of (1.2.9) is stable (asymptotically stable) (unstable); then, the zero solution of (1.2.7) is stable (asymptotically stable) (unstable).*

1.2.9 Bifurcation in Discrete System

Flip Bifurcation

Bifurcations with eigen value –1 are associated with flip bifurcations, also referred as period doubling or subharmonic bifurcations.

Theorem 1.2.9 (11). . *Assume that $f : R^2 \to R$ is a C^r function jointly in both variables with $r \geq 3$, and that f satisfies the following conditions.*

(i) The point X_0 is a fixed point for $\mu = \mu_0$: $f(x_0, \mu_0) = x_0$.

(ii) The derivative of f_{μ_0} at x_0 is minus one: $f'_{\mu_0}(x_0) = -1$. Since this derivative is not equal to 1, there is a curve of fixed points $x(\mu)$ for μ near μ_0.

(iii) The derivative of $f'_{\mu}(x(\mu))$ with respect to μ. is nonzero (the derivative is varying along the family of fixed points):

$$\alpha = \left[\frac{\partial^2 f}{\partial \mu \partial x} + \left(\frac{1}{2}\right)\left(\frac{\partial f}{\partial \mu}\right)\left(\frac{\partial^2 f}{\partial x^2}\right)\right]\Big|_{(x_0,\mu_0)} \neq 0.$$

(iv) The graph of $f^2_{\mu_0}$ has nonzero cubic term in its tangency with the diagonal (the quadratic term is zero):

$$\beta = \left(\frac{1}{6}\frac{\partial^3 f}{\partial x^3}(x_0, \mu_0)\right) + \left(\frac{1}{2}\frac{\partial^2 f}{\partial x^2}(x_0, \mu_0)\right)^2 \neq 0.$$

Then there is a period doubling bifurcation at (x_0, μ_0). *More specifically, there is a differentiable curve of fixed points,* $x(\mu)$, *passing through* x_0 *at* μ_0, *and the stability of the fixed point changes at* μ_0. *(Which side of* μ_0 *is attracting depends on the sign of* α.*) There is also a differentiable curve* γ *passing through* (x_0, μ_0) *so that* $\gamma \setminus \{(x_o, \mu_0)\}$ *is the union of hyperbolic period 2 orbits. The curve* γ *is tangent to the line* $R \times \{\mu_0\}$ *at* (x_0, μ_0), *so* γ *is the graph of a function of* x, $\mu = m(x)$ *with* $m'(x_0) = 0$ *and* $m''(x_0) = -2\beta/\alpha \neq 0$. *The stability type of the period 2 orbit depends on the sign of* β: *if* $\beta > 0$ *then the period 2 orbit is attracting, and if* $\beta < 0$ *then the period 2 orbit is repelling.*

Hopf Bifurcation (Neimark-Sacker Bifurcation)

Hopf bifurcation occurs when pair of complex eigenvalues have absolute value one, but are not equal to $\pm$ 1.

Theorem 1.2.10. *[149]. Let* $f_\mu : R^2 \to R^2$ *be a one parameter family of mappings which has a smooth family of fixed points* $x(\mu)$ *at which eigen values are complex conjugates* $\lambda(\mu)$, $\bar{\lambda}(\mu)$. *Assume*

(H_1) $|\lambda(\mu_0)| = 1$, *but* $|\lambda^j(\mu_0)| = 1$ *for* $j = 1,2,3,4$.

(H_2) $\frac{d}{d\mu}(|\lambda(\mu_0)) = d \neq 0$.

Then there is a smooth change of coordinates h so that the expression of $hf_\mu h^{-1}$ *in polar coordinates has the form*

$$hf_\mu h^{-1}(r,\theta) = (r(1+d(\mu-\mu_0)+ar^2)+\theta+c+br^2)+higher\ order\ terms. \tag{1.2.10}$$

If, in addition

(H_3) $a \neq 0$.

Then there is a two-dimensional surface $\sum$ *(no necessarily infinite differentiable) in* $R^2 \times R$ *having quadratic tangency with the plane* $R^2 \times \mu_0$ *which is invariant for* f. *If* $\sum \cap (R^2 \times \mu)$ *is larger than a point, then it is a simple closed curve.*

A stability formula, giving an expression for the coefficient a in the normal form (1.2.10), can be derived. Assuming that the bifurcating system is of the form

$$\begin{pmatrix} x \\ y \end{pmatrix} \rightarrow \begin{pmatrix} cos(c) & -sin(c) \\ sin(c) & cos(c) \end{pmatrix} + \begin{pmatrix} f(x,y) \\ g(x,y) \end{pmatrix}, \qquad (1.2.11)$$

with eigen values $\lambda, \bar{\lambda} = e^{\pm ic}$, one obtains

$$a = -Re\left[\frac{(1-2\overline{\lambda})\overline{\lambda}^2}{1-\lambda}\varphi_{11}\varphi_{20}\right] - \frac{1}{2}\|\varphi_{11}\|^2 - \|\varphi_{02}\|^2 + Re(\overline{\lambda}\varphi_{21}), \qquad (1.2.12)$$

where

$$\varphi_{20} = \frac{1}{8}\left[(f_{xx} - f_{yy} + 2g_{xy}) + i(g_{xx} - g_{yy} - 2f_{xy})\right],$$

$$\varphi_{11} = \frac{1}{4}\left[(f_{xx} + f_{yy}) + i(g_{xx} + g_{yy})\right],$$

$$\varphi_{02} = \frac{1}{8}\left[(f_{xx} - f_{yy} - 2g_{xy}) + i(g_{xx} - g_{yy} + 2f_{xy})\right],$$

$$\varphi_{21} = \frac{1}{16}\left[(f_{xxx} + f_{xyy} + g_{xxy} + g_{yyy}) + i(g_{xxx} + g_{xyy} - f_{xxy} - f_{yyy})\right].$$

1.2.10 Next Generation Operator Method

The next generation operator method is popularly used to compute the reproduction number of disease transmission models [150, 151]. The formulation given in Ref. [151], for autonomous systems, is briefly described below.

Suppose the model, with non-negative initial conditions, can be expressed in the following form of autonomous system:

$$\dot{x}_i = f(x_i) = F_i(x) - V_i(x), i = 1, ..., n, \qquad (1.2.13)$$

where $V_i = V_i^- - V_i^+$. Here, $X_S = \{x \geq 0 | x_i = 0, i = 1, ..., m\}$ is defined as the disease-free states of the model and $x = (x_1, ..., x_n)^t, x_i \geq 0$ represents the number of individuals in each compartment of the model.

(A1) if x$\geq$ 0, then $F_i, V_i^-, V_i^+ \geq 0$ for $i = 1, ..., m$.

(A2) if $x_i = 0$, then $V_i^- = 0$. In particular, if x$\in X_S$ then $V_i^- = 0$ for $i = 1, ..., m$.

(A3) $F_i = 0$ if $i > m$.

(A4) if x$\in X_S$, then $F_i(x) = 0$ and $V_i^+(x) = 0$ for $i = 1, ..., m$.

(A5) if F(x) is set to zero, then all eigenvalues of $Df(x_0)$ have negative real part.

In the above, $F_i(x)$ presents the rate of emergence of infections in compartment i, $V_i^+(x)$ represents the rate of transfer of individuals into compartment i and $V_i^-(x)$ represents the rate of transfer of individuals out of compartment i [151].

Definition 1.2.6. *(M -Matrix). An $n \times n$ matrix A is an M -matrix if and only if every off-diagonal entry of A is non-positive and the diagonal entries are all positive.*

Lemma 1.2.11. *[151]. If $\bar{x}$ is a DFE of (1.2.13) and $f_i(x)$ satisfy (A1)-(A5), then the derivatives $DF(\bar{x})$ and $DV(\bar{x})$ are partitioned as*

$$DF(\bar{x}) = \begin{pmatrix} F & 0 \\ 0 & 0 \end{pmatrix}, DV(\bar{x}) = \begin{pmatrix} V & 0 \\ J_3 & J_4 \end{pmatrix},$$

where F and V are the $m \times m$ matrices defined by,

$$F = \left[\frac{\partial F_i}{\partial x_j}(\bar{x}) \right] \text{ and } V = \left[\frac{\partial V_i}{\partial x_j}(\bar{x}) \right] \text{with } 1 \le i, j \le m.$$

Furthermore, F is non-negative, V is a non-singular M-matrix and J_3, J_4 are matrices associated with the transition terms of the model, and all eigenvalues of J_4 have positive real parts.

Theorem 1.2.12. *[151]. Consider the disease transmission model given by (1.2.13) with $f(x)$ satisfying axioms (A1)–(A5). If $\bar{x}$ is a DFE of the model, then $\bar{x}$ is LAS if $\mathscr{R}_0 = \rho(FV^{-1}) < 1$ (where ρ is the spectral radius), but unstable if $\mathscr{R}_0 > 1$.*

1.2.11 Sensitivity Analysis

Sensitivity indices allow us to measure the relative change in a state variable when a parameter changes. For a system, the ratio of relative change in a variable to the relative change in a parameter is known as the normalized forward sensitivity index of the variable to that particular parameter. Chitnis et al. [152] have evaluated the sensitivity indices of the basic reproduction number and the endemic equilibrium to the model parameters. Further, sensitive analysis in epidemic models has been calculated by many researchers by Partial rank correlation coefficients method [134, 153–156].

For a system, the ratio of relative change in a variable to the relative change in a parameter is known as the normalized forward sensitivity index of the variable to that particular parameter [152]. When the variable is a differentiable function of the parameter, the sensitivity index may be alternatively defined using partial derivatives [152]. Let u be a function of parameter p, a small perturbation δ_p to the parameter p and the corresponding change in u as δ_u is given by

$$\delta_u = u(p+\delta_p) - u(p) = \frac{u(p+\delta_p) - u(p)}{\delta_p}.\delta_p \approx \delta_p \frac{\partial u}{\partial p}$$

Definition [73, 152]: The normalized forward sensitivity index of a variable, u, that depends on a parameter, p, is defined as:

$$\Upsilon_p^u = \frac{\partial u}{\partial p} \times \frac{p}{u}.$$

Estimation of highly sensitive parameter should be done very carefully, because a small variation in the parameter will lead to relatively large quantitative change. On the other hand, a less sensitive parameter does not require as much effort to estimate, since a small variation in that parameter will not produce large changes in the quantity of interested variables.

1.3 Summary

Population is a changing entity. The growth rate of a population is the number of organisms added to the population per unit time. Each population has an inherent power to grow. As varying from place-to-place, population density also varies in time. Population may remain constant, they may fluctuate, they may steadily increase or decrease, or may move from one place to other.

After having studied the various characteristics of population, we attempt to follow the change in it owing to several factors as discussed earlier. In the following ten chapters we will formulate and analyze the dynamics of different population interactions in temporal and spatio-temporal domains.

Chapter 2

Discrete-Time Bifurcation Behavior of a Prey-Predator System with Generalized Predator

2.1 Introduction

The prey-predator species, each with non-overlapping generations, which affect each other's population dynamics, have been widely studied by a number of researchers [22–25, 27, 28, 96, 102, 105, 106]. The books by Hassel [157], Peitgen and Richter [158], and Gumowski and Mira [159] presented some interesting results on the dynamic complexity of discrete prey-predator systems.

In this chapter, we investigated the stability and bifurcation of two different discrete-time prey-predator systems with generalized predator (i.e., the predator is partially dependent on prey) using center manifold theorem and bifurcation theory. The chapter is organized as follows. In Section 2.2, the formulation of the model-1 is presented and in Section 2.3, the stability criterion of the model-1 is discussed at the fixed points and obtained the specific conditions for the existence of flip bifurcation and Hopf bifurcation. Again, in Section 2.4 the formulation of the model-2 is presented, followed by the stability analysis of the model-2 at the fixed points and conditions for the existence of flip bifurcation and Hopf bifurcation in the Section 2.5. Numerical simulations are presented to support our analytical findings in Section 2.6, especially for the period doubling bifurcation and chaotic behavior. Finally, a brief conclusion is given in the last section.

2.2 Formulation of Mathematical Model-1

We have proposed a mathematical model for prey-predator dynamics with the following assumptions:

(i) In a particular habitat, there are two populations; one is prey and other is a predator. At any time t, the density of prey population is x and density of predator population is y.

(ii) The prey population grows with logistic rate and the per capita growth rate of the prey in the absence of predator is $a\left(1-\frac{x}{k}\right)$, where a is the intrinsic growth rate of prey and k is carrying capacity of the prey in a particular habitat.

(iii) Predator also depends on alternative resources for growth.

(iv) The parameter b is the predation rate of the prey and l is the half saturation period.

(v) The predator catches the prey and their interactions follow the Leslie-Gower [160, 161] type.

The proposed prey-predator system with generalized predator is of the form:

$$\frac{dx}{dt} = ax\left(1-\frac{x}{k}\right) - \frac{bxy}{x+l}, \tag{2.2.1}$$

$$\frac{dy}{dt} = \left[1 - \frac{my}{nx+q} - d\right] y, \tag{2.2.2}$$

with initial conditions:

$$x(0) = x_0 > 0,\ y(0) = y_0 > 0, \tag{2.2.3}$$

where d denotes the death rate of predator; m is the maximum value which per capita reduction rate of predator can attend; n is a measure of food quality that the prey provides for conversion into predator births; q is the extent to which alternatives are provided for the growth of predator.

Applying forward Euler's scheme to the system of Eqs. (2.2.1)–(2.2.2), we obtain the discrete-time prey-predator system as:

$$x \rightarrow x+\delta\left[ax\left(1-\frac{x}{k}\right)-\frac{bxy}{x+l}\right], \tag{2.2.4}$$

$$y \rightarrow y+\delta\left[1-\frac{my}{nx+q}-d\right]y, \tag{2.2.5}$$

where δ is the step size. Numerical solution to the initial-value problem obtained from Euler's method with step size δ and total number of steps N_0 satisfies $0<\delta\leq\frac{L_0}{N_0}$, where L_0 is the length of the interval.

2.3 Discrete Dynamical Behavior of Model-1

In this section, we discuss the stability criterion of the model-1 at the fixed points and obtain the specific conditions for the existence of flip bifurcation and Hopf bifurcation.

The fixed points of the system (2.2.4)–(2.2.5) are $O_1\,(k,0)$, $A_1\left(0,\frac{(1-d)q}{m}\right)$ and $B_1\,(x^*,y^*)$, where x^*,y^* satisfy

$$\begin{cases} a\left(1-\frac{x^*}{k}\right)-\frac{by^*}{x^*+l}=0, \\ 1-\frac{my^*}{nx^*+q}-d=0. \end{cases} \tag{2.3.1}$$

The Jacobian matrix of (2.2.4)–(2.2.5) at the fixed point (x,y) is written as:

$$J=\begin{bmatrix} 1+\delta\left(a-\frac{2ax}{k}-\frac{bly}{(x+l)^2}\right) & -\frac{b\delta x}{(x+l)} \\ \frac{\delta mny^2}{(nx+q)^2} & 1+\delta\left(1-\frac{2my}{nx+q}-d\right) \end{bmatrix}.$$

The characteristic equation of the Jacobian matrix is given by

$$\lambda^2+p(x,y)\lambda+q(x,y)=0, \tag{2.3.2}$$

where

$$p(x,y) = -trJ = -2-\delta\left(1+a-d-\frac{2ax}{k}-\frac{bly}{(x+l)^2}-\frac{2my}{nx+q}\right),$$

$$q(x,y) = detJ = \left[1+\delta\left(a-\frac{2ax}{k}-\frac{bly}{(x+l)^2}\right)\right]$$

$$\times \left[1+\delta\left(1-\frac{2my}{nx+q}-d\right)\right]+\frac{\delta^2 bmnxy^2}{(x+l)(nx+q)^2}.$$

Now, we state the following lemma as similar as given in Refs. [25, 26]:

Lemma 2.3.1. *Let $F(\lambda) = \lambda^2 + B\lambda + C$. Suppose that $F(1) > 0$; λ_1 and λ_2 are roots of $F(\lambda) = 0$. Then, we have:*

(i) $|\lambda_1| < 1$ *and* $|\lambda_2| < 1$ *if and only if* $F(-1) > 0$ *and* $C < 1$;

(ii) $|\lambda_1| < 1$ *and* $|\lambda_2| > 1$ *(or* $|\lambda_1| > 1$ *and* $|\lambda_2| < 1$*) if and only if* $F(-1) < 0$;

(iii) $|\lambda_1| > 1$ *and* $|\lambda_2| > 1$ *if and only if* $F(-1) > 0$ *and* $C > 1$;

(iv) $\lambda_1 = -1$ *and* $|\lambda_2| \neq 1$ *if and only if* $F(-1) = 0$ *and* $B \neq 0, 2$;

(v) λ_1 *and* λ_2 *are complex and* $|\lambda_1| = |\lambda_2| = 1$ *if and only if* $B^2 - 4C < 0$ *and* $C = 1$.

Let λ_1 and λ_2 be the roots of (2.3.2), which are known as eigen values of the fixed point (x,y). The fixed point (x,y) is a sink or locally asymptotically stable if $|\lambda_1| < 1$ and $|\lambda_2| < 1$. The fixed point (x,y) is a source or locally unstable if $|\lambda_1| > 1$ and $|\lambda_2| > 1$. The fixed point (x,y) is non-hyperbolic if either $|\lambda_1| = 1$ or $|\lambda_2| = 1$. The fixed point (x,y) is a saddle if $|\lambda_1| > 1$ and $|\lambda_2| < 1$ (or $|\lambda_1| < 1$ and $|\lambda_2| > 1$).

Proposition 2.3.2. *The fixed point $O_1(k,0)$ is source if $\delta > \frac{2}{a}$, saddle if $0 < \delta < \frac{2}{a}$, and non-hyperbolic if $\delta = \frac{2}{a}$.*

One can see that when $\delta = \frac{2}{a}$, one of the eigen values of the fixed point $O_1(k,0)$ is –1 and magnitude of other is not equal to 1. Thus the flip bifurcation occurs when the parameter changes in small neighborhood of $\delta = \frac{2}{a}$.

Proposition 2.3.3. *There exist different topological types of* $A_1\left(0, \frac{(1-d)q}{m}\right)$ *for possible parameters.*

(i) $A_1\left(0, \frac{(1-d)q}{m}\right)$ *is sink if* $bq(1-d) > alm$,
and $0 < \delta < min\left\{\frac{2}{1-d}, \frac{2lm}{bq(1-d)-alm}\right\}$.

(ii) $A_1\left(0, \frac{(1-d)q}{m}\right)$ *is source if* $bq(1-d) > alm$,
and $\delta > max\left\{\frac{2}{1-d}, \frac{2lm}{bq(1-d)-alm}\right\}$.

(iii) $A_1\left(0, \frac{(1-d)q}{m}\right)$ *is non-hyperbolic if* $bq(1-d) > alm$ *and either* $\delta = \frac{2}{1-d}$ *or* $\delta = \frac{2lm}{bq(1-d)-alm}$.

(iv) $A_1\left(0, \frac{(1-d)q}{m}\right)$ *is saddle for all values of the parameters, except for that values which lies in (i) to (iii).*

The term *(iii)* of Proposition 2.3.3 implies that the parameters lie in the set

$$\begin{aligned} F_{A_1} = \ & \{(a,b,d,k,l,m,n,q,\delta),\ \delta = \tfrac{2}{1-d},\ \delta \neq \tfrac{2lm}{bq(1-d)-alm} \text{ and} \\ & bq(1-d) > alm,\ a,b,d,k,l,m,n,q,\delta > 0\}. \end{aligned}$$

If the term *(iii)* of Proposition 2.3.3 holds, then one of the eigen values of the fixed point $A_1\left(0, \frac{(1-d)q}{m}\right)$ is –1 and the magnitude of the other is not equal to 1. The point $A_1\left(0, \frac{(1-d)q}{m}\right)$ undergoes flip bifurcation when the parameter changes in small neighborhood of F_{A_1}.

The characteristic equation of the Jacobian matrix J of the system (2.2.4)–(2.2.5) at the fixed point $B_1(x^*, y^*)$ is written as

$$\lambda^2 + p(x^*, y^*)\lambda + q(x^*, y^*) = 0, \tag{2.3.3}$$

where

$$\begin{aligned} p(x^*, y^*) &= -2 - G_1\delta, \\ q(x^*, y^*) &= 1 + G_1\delta + H_1\delta^2, \end{aligned}$$

and

$$G_1 = 1+a-d-\frac{2ax^*}{k}-\frac{bly^*}{(x^*+l)^2}-\frac{2my^*}{nx^*+q},$$

$$H_1 = \left[a-\frac{2ax^*}{k}-\frac{bly^*}{(x^*+l)^2}\right]\left[1-\frac{2my^*}{nx^*+q}-d\right]+\frac{bmnx^*y^{*2}}{(x^*+l)(nx^*+q)^2}.$$

Now

$$F(\lambda) = \lambda^2-(2+G_1\delta)\lambda+(1+G_1\delta+H_1\delta^2).$$

Therefore

$$F(1) = H_1\delta^2,\ F(-1) = 4+2G_1\delta+H_1\delta^2.$$

Using Lemma 2.3.1, we get the following proposition:

Proposition 2.3.4. *There exist different topological types of $B_1(x^*,y^*)$ for all possible parameters.*

(i) $B_1(x^*,y^*)$ is a sink if either condition (i.1) or (i.2) holds:

(i.1) $G_1 < -2\sqrt{H_1}$ and $0 < \delta < \frac{-G_1-\sqrt{G_1^2-4H_1}}{H_1}$,

(i.2) $-2\sqrt{H_1} \leq G_1 < 0$ and $0 < \delta < -\frac{G_1}{H_1}$.

(ii) $B_1(x^*,y^*)$ is source if either condition (ii.1) or (ii.2) holds:

(ii.1) $G_1 < -2\sqrt{H_1}$ and $\delta > \frac{-G_1+\sqrt{G_1^2-4H_1}}{H_1}$,

(ii.2) $-2\sqrt{H_1} \leq G_1 < 0$ and $\delta > -\frac{G_1}{H_1}$.

(iii) $B_1(x^*,y^*)$ is non-hyperbolic if either condition (iii.1) or (iii.2) holds:

(iii.1) $G_1 < -2\sqrt{H_1}$ and $\delta = \frac{-G_1\pm\sqrt{G_1^2-4H_1}}{H_1}$,

(iii.2) $-2\sqrt{H_1} \leq G_1 < 0$ and $\delta = -\frac{G_1}{H_1}$.

(iv) $B_1(x^*,y^*)$ is saddle for all values of the parameters, except for that values which lies in (i) to (iii).

If the term *(iii.1)* of Proposition 2.3.4 holds, then one of the eigen values of the fixed point $B_1(x^*, y^*)$ is –1 and the magnitude of the other is not equal to 1. The term *(iii.1)* of Proposition 2.3.4 may be written as follows:

$$F_{B_{11}} = \{(a,b,d,k,l,m,n,q,\delta): \ \delta = \tfrac{-G_1-\sqrt{G_1^2-4H_1}}{H_1}, \ G_1 < -2\sqrt{H_1} \text{ and } a,b,d,k,l,m,n,q,\delta > 0\}$$

and

$$F_{B_{12}} = \{(a,b,d,k,l,m,n,q,\delta): \ \delta = \tfrac{-G_1+\sqrt{G_1^2-4H_1}}{H_1}, \ G_1 < -2\sqrt{H_1} \text{ and } a,b,d,k,l,m,n,q,\delta > 0\}.$$

If the term *(iii.2)* of Proposition 2.3.4 holds, then the eigen values of the fixed point $B_1(x^*, y^*)$ are a pair of complex conjugate numbers with modulus 1. The term *(iii.2)* of Proposition 2.3.4 may be written as follows:

$$H_{B_1} = \{(a,b,d,k,l,m,n,q,\delta): \ \delta = -\tfrac{G_1}{H_1}, \ -2\sqrt{H_1} \le G_1 < 0 \text{ and } a,b,d,k,l,m,n,q,\delta > 0\}.$$

Now, we will study the flip bifurcation and Hopf bifurcation of the system (2.2.4)–(2.2.5) at the fixed point $B_1(x^*, y^*)$.

2.3.1 Flip Bifurcation

Consider the system (2.2.4)–(2.2.5) with arbitrary parameter $(a,b,d,k,l,m,n,q,\delta_1) \in F_{B_{11}}$, which is described as follows:

$$x \to x + \delta_1 \left[ax\left(1 - \frac{x}{k}\right) - \frac{bxy}{x+l}\right], \tag{2.3.4}$$

$$y \to y + \delta_1 \left[1 - \frac{my}{nx+q} - d\right] y. \tag{2.3.5}$$

$B_1(x^*, y^*)$ is fixed point of the system (2.3.4)–(2.3.5), where x^*, y^* is given by (2.3.1) and

$$\delta_1 = \frac{-G_1 - \sqrt{G_1^2 - 4H_1}}{H_1}.$$

The eigen values of $B_1(x^*, y^*)$ are $\lambda_1 = -1$, $\lambda_2 = 3 + G_1\delta_1$ with $|\lambda_2| \neq 1$ by Proposition 2.3.4.

Consider the perturbation of (2.3.4)–(2.3.5) as below:

$$x \rightarrow x+(\delta_1+\delta_1^*)\left[ax\left(1-\frac{x}{k}\right)-\frac{bxy}{x+l}\right], \tag{2.3.6}$$

$$y \rightarrow y+(\delta_1+\delta_1^*)\left[1-\frac{my}{nx+q}-d\right]y, \tag{2.3.7}$$

where $|\delta_1^*| \ll 1$ is a small perturbation parameter.

Let $u = x-x^*$ and $v = y-y^*$.

After the transformation of the fixed point $B_1(x^*, y^*)$ of the system (2.3.6)–(2.3.7) to the point $(0,0)$, we obtain

$$\begin{pmatrix} u \\ v \end{pmatrix} \rightarrow \begin{pmatrix} a_{11}u+a_{12}v+a_{13}u^2+a_{14}uv+b_{11}\delta_1^*u+b_{12}\delta_1^*v \\ +b_{13}\delta_1^*u^2+b_{14}\delta_1^*uv+O(|u|,|v|,|\delta_1^*|)^3 \\ a_{21}u+a_{22}v+a_{23}u^2+a_{24}uv+a_{25}v^2+b_{21}\delta_1^*u+b_{22}\delta_1^*v \\ +b_{23}\delta_1^*u^2+b_{24}\delta_1^*uv+b_{25}\delta_1^*v^2+O(|u|,|v|,|\delta_1^*|)^3 \end{pmatrix}, \tag{2.3.8}$$

where

$$a_{11} = 1+\delta_1\left[-\frac{a}{k}x^*+\frac{bx^*y^*}{(x^*+l)^2}\right],\ a_{12} = -\frac{b\delta_1 x^*}{x^*+l},$$

$$a_{13} = \delta_1\left[-\frac{a}{k}+\frac{bly^*}{(x^*+l)^3}\right],\ a_{14} = -\frac{\delta_1 bl}{(x^*+l)^2},$$

$$b_{11} = -\frac{a}{k}x^*+\frac{bx^*y^*}{(x^*+l)^2},\ b_{12} = -\frac{bx^*}{x^*+l},$$

$$b_{13} = -\frac{a}{k}+\frac{bly^*}{(x^*+l)^3},\ b_{14} = -\frac{bl}{(x^*+l)^2}, \tag{2.3.9}$$

$$a_{21} = \frac{\delta_1 mny^{*2}}{(nx^*+q)^2},\ a_{22} = 1+\delta_1(1-d)-\frac{2\delta_1 my^*}{nx^*+q},$$

$$a_{23} = -\frac{\delta_1 mn^2y^{*2}}{(nx^*+q)^3},\ a_{24} = \frac{2\delta_1 mny^*}{(nx^*+q)^2},\ a_{25} = -\frac{\delta_1 m}{nx^*+q},$$

$$b_{21} = \frac{mny^*2}{(nx^*+q)^2},\ b_{22} = 1-d-\frac{2my^*}{nx^*+q},\ b_{23} = -\frac{mn^2y^{*2}}{(nx^*+q)^3},$$

$$b_{24} = \frac{2mny^*}{(nx^*+q)^2},\ b_{25} = -\frac{m}{nx^*+q}.$$

Consider the following translation:

$$\begin{pmatrix} u \\ v \end{pmatrix} = T\begin{pmatrix} \tilde{x} \\ \tilde{y} \end{pmatrix},$$

where

$$T = \begin{pmatrix} a_{12} & a_{12} \\ -1-a_{11} & \lambda_2 - a_{11} \end{pmatrix}.$$

Taking T^{-1} on both sides of Eq. (2.3.8), we get

$$\begin{pmatrix} \tilde{x} \\ \tilde{y} \end{pmatrix} \to \begin{pmatrix} -1 & 0 \\ 0 & \lambda_2 \end{pmatrix}\begin{pmatrix} \tilde{x} \\ \tilde{y} \end{pmatrix} + \begin{pmatrix} f(u,v,\delta_1^*) \\ g(u,v,\delta_1^*) \end{pmatrix}, \qquad (2.3.10)$$

where

$$\begin{aligned} f(u,v,\delta_1^*) = {} & \frac{[a_{13}(\lambda_2-a_{11})-a_{12}a_{23}]u^2}{a_{12}(\lambda_2+1)} + \frac{[a_{14}(\lambda_2-a_{11})-a_{12}a_{24}]uv}{a_{12}(\lambda_2+1)} - \frac{a_{12}a_{25}v^2}{a_{12}(\lambda_2+1)} \\ & + \frac{[b_{11}(\lambda_2-a_{11})-a_{12}b_{21}]\delta_1^* u}{a_{12}(\lambda_2+1)} + \frac{[b_{12}(\lambda_2-a_{11})-a_{12}b_{22}]\delta_1^* v}{a_{12}(\lambda_2+1)} \\ & + \frac{[b_{13}(\lambda_2-a_{11})-a_{12}b_{23}]\delta_1^* u^2}{a_{12}(\lambda_2+1)} + \frac{[b_{14}(\lambda_2-a_{11})-a_{12}b_{24}]\delta_1^* uv}{a_{12}(\lambda_2+1)} - \frac{a_{12}b_{25}\delta_1^* v^2}{a_{12}(\lambda_2+1)} \\ & + O(|u|,|v|,|\delta_1^*|)^3, \end{aligned}$$

$$\begin{aligned} g(u,v,\delta_1^*) = {} & \frac{[a_{13}(1+a_{11})+a_{12}a_{23}]u^2}{a_{12}(\lambda_2+1)} + \frac{[a_{14}(1+a_{11})+a_{12}a_{24}]uv}{a_{12}(\lambda_2+1)} + \frac{a_{12}a_{25}v^2}{a_{12}(\lambda_2+1)} \\ & + \frac{[b_{11}(1+a_{11})+a_{12}b_{21}]\delta_1^* u}{a_{12}(\lambda_2+1)} + \frac{[b_{12}(1+a_{11})+a_{12}b_{22}]\delta_1^* v}{a_{12}(\lambda_2+1)} \\ & + \frac{[b_{13}(1+a_{11})+a_{12}b_{23}]\delta_1^* u^2}{a_{12}(\lambda_2+1)} + \frac{[b_{14}(1+a_{11})+a_{12}b_{24}]\delta_1^* uv}{a_{12}(\lambda_2+1)} + \frac{a_{12}b_{25}\delta_1^* v^2}{a_{12}(\lambda_2+1)} \\ & + O(|u|,|v|,|\delta_1^*|)^3, \end{aligned}$$

$$u = a_{12}(\tilde{x}+\tilde{y}),\ \ v = -(1+a_{11})\tilde{x} + (\lambda_2 - a_{11})\tilde{y}.$$

Applying the center manifold theorem to the Eq. (2.3.10) at the origin in the limited neighborhood of $\delta_1^* = 0$. The center manifold $W^c(0,0)$ can be approximately presented as:

$$W^c(0,0) = \left\{ (\tilde{x},\tilde{y}) :\ \tilde{y} = a_0\delta_1^* + a_1\tilde{x}^2 + a_2\tilde{x}\delta_1^* + a_3\delta_1^{*2} + O\left((|\tilde{x}| + |\delta_1^*|)^3 \right) \right\},$$

where $O\left((|\tilde{x}| + |\delta_1^*|)^3 \right)$ is a function with at least third orders in variables $(\tilde{x},\ \delta_1^*)$.

By simple calculations for center manifold, we have

$$a_0 = 0,$$

$$a_1 = \frac{[a_{13}(1+a_{11})+a_{12}a_{23}]a_{12}-[a_{14}(1+a_{11})+a_{12}a_{24}](1+a_{11})+a_{25}(1+a_{11})^2}{1-\lambda_2^2},$$

$$a_2 = \frac{-[b_{11}(1+a_{11})+a_{12}b_{21}]a_{12}+[b_{12}(1+a_{11})+a_{12}b_{22}](1+a_{11})}{a_{12}(\lambda_2+1)^2},$$

$$a_3 = 0.$$

Now, consider the map restricted to the center manifold $W^c(0,0)$ as below:

$$f:\tilde{x} \to -\tilde{x}+h_1\tilde{x}^2+h_2\tilde{x}\delta_1^*+h_3\tilde{x}^2\delta_1^*+h_4\tilde{x}\delta_1^{*2}+h_5\tilde{x}^3+O\left((|\tilde{x}|+|\delta_1^*|)^4\right),$$

where

$$h_1 = \frac{[a_{13}(\lambda_2-a_{11})-a_{12}a_{23}]a_{12}}{(\lambda_2+1)} - \frac{[a_{14}(\lambda_2-a_{11})-a_{12}a_{24}](1+a_{11})}{(\lambda_2+1)} - \frac{a_{12}a_{25}(1+a_{11})^2}{a_{12}(\lambda_2+1)},$$

$$h_2 = \frac{[b_{11}(\lambda_2-a_{11})-a_{12}b_{21}]}{(\lambda_2+1)} - \frac{[b_{12}(\lambda_2-a_{11})-a_{12}b_{22}](1+a_{11})}{a_{12}(\lambda_2+1)},$$

$$\begin{aligned} h_3 = {} & \frac{[a_{13}(\lambda_2-a_{11})-a_{12}a_{23}]2a_2a_{12}}{(\lambda_2+1)} + \frac{[a_{14}(\lambda_2-a_{11})-a_{12}a_{24}](\lambda_2-2a_{11}-1)a_2}{(\lambda_2+1)} \\ & + \frac{2a_{25}(1+a_{11})(\lambda_2-a_{11})a_2}{(\lambda_2+1)} + \frac{[b_{11}(\lambda_2-a_{11})-a_{12}b_{21}]a_1}{(\lambda_2+1)} \\ & + \frac{[b_{12}(\lambda_2-a_{11})-a_{12}b_{22}](\lambda_2-a_{11})a_1}{a_{12}(\lambda_2+1)} + \frac{[b_{13}(\lambda_2-a_{11})-a_{12}b_{23}]a_{12}}{(\lambda_2+1)} \\ & - \frac{[b_{14}(\lambda_2-a_{11})-a_{12}b_{24}](1+a_{11})}{(\lambda_2+1)} - \frac{b_{25}(1+a_{11})^2}{(\lambda_2+1)}, \end{aligned}$$

$$h_4 = \frac{[b_{11}(\lambda_2-a_{11})-a_{12}b_{21}]a_2}{(\lambda_2+1)} + \frac{[b_{12}(\lambda_2-a_{11})-a_{12}b_{22}](\lambda_2-a_{11})a_2}{a_{12}(\lambda_2+1)},$$

$$\begin{aligned} h_5 = {} & \frac{[a_{13}(\lambda_2-a_{11})-a_{12}a_{23}]2a_{12}a_1}{(\lambda_2+1)} + \frac{[a_{14}(\lambda_2-a_{11})-a_{12}a_{24}](\lambda_2-2a_{11}-1)a_1}{(\lambda_2+1)} \\ & + \frac{2a_{25}(1+a_{11})(\lambda_2-a_{11})a_1}{(\lambda_2+1)}. \end{aligned}$$

According to Flip bifurcation, the discriminatory quantities γ_1 and γ_2 are given by:

$$\gamma_1 = \left(\frac{\partial^2 f}{\partial\tilde{x}\partial\delta_1^*} + \frac{1}{2}\frac{\partial f}{\partial\delta_1^*}\frac{\partial^2 f}{\partial\tilde{x}^2}\right)\Bigg|_{(0,0)},$$

$$\gamma_2 = \left(\frac{1}{6}\frac{\partial^3 f}{\partial\tilde{x}^3} + \left(\frac{1}{2}\frac{\partial^2 f}{\partial\tilde{x}^2}\right)^2\right)\Bigg|_{(0,0)}.$$

After simple calculations, we obtain $\gamma_1 = h_2$ and $\gamma_2 = h_5 + h_1^2$.

Analyzing above and the flip bifurcation conditions discussed in [149], we write the following theorem:

Theorem 2.3.5. *If $\gamma_2 \neq 0$, and the parameter δ_1^* alters in the limiting region of the point (0,0), then the system (2.3.6)–(2.3.7) passes through flip bifurcation at the point $B_1(x^*, y^*)$. Also, the period-2 points that bifurcate from fixed point $B_1(x^*, y^*)$ are stable (resp., unstable) if $\gamma_2 > 0$ (resp., $\gamma_2 < 0$).*

2.3.2 Hopf Bifurcation

Consider the system (2.2.4)–(2.2.5) with arbitrary parameter $(a, b, d, k, l, m, n, q, \delta_2) \in H_{B_1}$, which is described as follows:

$$x \rightarrow x + \delta_2 \left[ax\left(1 - \frac{x}{k}\right) - \frac{bxy}{x+l} \right], \quad (2.3.11)$$

$$y \rightarrow y + \delta_2 \left[1 - \frac{my}{nx+q} - d \right] y. \quad (2.3.12)$$

$B_1(x^*, y^*)$ is fixed point of the system (2.3.11)–(2.3.12), where x^*, y^* is given by (2.3.1) and

$$\delta_2 = -\frac{G_1}{H_1}.$$

Consider the perturbation of the system (2.3.11)–(2.3.12) as given below:

$$x \rightarrow x + (\delta_2 + \delta_2^*) \left[ax\left(1 - \frac{x}{k}\right) - \frac{bxy}{x+l} \right], \quad (2.3.13)$$

$$y \rightarrow y + (\delta_2 + \delta_2^*) \left[1 - \frac{my}{nx+q} - d \right] y, \quad (2.3.14)$$

where $|\delta_2^*| \ll 1$ is small perturbation parameter.

The characteristic equation of the system (2.3.13)–(2.3.14) at $B_1(x^*, y^*)$ is given by

$$\lambda^2 + p(\delta_2^*)\lambda + q(\delta_2^*) = 0,$$

where

$$p(\delta_2^*) = -2 - G_1(\delta_2 + \delta_2^*),$$

$$q(\delta_2^*) = 1 + G_1(\delta_2 + \delta_2^*) + H_1(\delta_2 + \delta_2^*)^2.$$

Since the parameter $(a,b,d,k,l,m,n,q,\delta_2) \in H_{B_1}$, the eigen values of $B_1(x^*,y^*)$ are a pair of complex conjugate numbers $\overline{\lambda}$ and λ with modulus 1 by Proposition 2.3.4, where

$$\overline{\lambda},\ \lambda = \frac{-p(\delta_2^*) \mp i\sqrt{4q(\delta_2^*) - p^2(\delta_2^*)}}{2}.$$

Therefore

$$\overline{\lambda},\ \lambda = 1 + \frac{G_1(\delta_2 + \delta_2^*)}{2} \mp \frac{i(\delta_2 + \delta_2^*)\sqrt{4H_1 - G_1^2}}{2}.$$

Now we have

$$|\lambda| = (q(\delta_2^*))^{1/2},\ l = \left.\frac{d|\lambda|}{d\delta_2^*}\right|_{\delta_2^*=0} = -\frac{G_1}{2} > 0.$$

When δ_2^* varies in limited neighborhood of $\delta_2^* = 0$, then $\overline{\lambda}$, $\lambda = \alpha \mp i\beta$, where

$$\alpha = 1 + \frac{\delta_2 G_1}{2},\ \beta = \frac{\delta_2\sqrt{4H_1 - G_1^2}}{2}.$$

Hopf bifurcation requires that when $\delta_2^* = 0$, then $\overline{\lambda}^j, \lambda^j \neq 1$ $(j = 1,\ 2,\ 3,\ 4)$ which is equivalent to $p(0) \neq -2,\ 0,\ 1,\ 2$.

Since the parameter $(a,b,d,k,l,m,n,q,\delta_2) \in H_{B_1}$, therefore $p(0) \neq -2,\ 2$. It is the only requirement that $p(0) \neq 0,\ 1$, which follows that

$$G_1^2 \neq 2H_1,\ 3H_1. \tag{2.3.15}$$

Let $u = x - x^*$ and $v = y - y^*$.

After the transformation of the fixed point $B_1(x^*,y^*)$ of system (2.3.13)–(2.3.14) to the point $(0,0)$, we have

$$\begin{pmatrix} u \\ v \end{pmatrix} \to \begin{pmatrix} a_{11}u + a_{12}v + a_{13}u^2 + a_{14}uv + O(|u|,|v|)^3 \\ a_{21}u + a_{22}v + a_{23}u^2 + a_{24}uv + a_{25}v^2 + O(|u|,|v|)^3 \end{pmatrix}, \tag{2.3.16}$$

where a_{11}, a_{12}, a_{13}, a_{14}, a_{21}, a_{22}, a_{23}, a_{24}, a_{25} are given in (2.3.9) by substituting δ_2 for $\delta_2 + \delta_2^*$.

Now, we discuss the normal form of (2.3.16) when $\delta_2^* = 0$.
Consider the translation as below:

$$\begin{pmatrix} u \\ v \end{pmatrix} = T \begin{pmatrix} \tilde{x} \\ \tilde{y} \end{pmatrix},$$

where

$$T = \begin{pmatrix} a_{12} & 0 \\ \alpha - a_{11} & -\beta \end{pmatrix}.$$

Taking T^{-1} on both sides of (2.3.16), we get

$$\begin{pmatrix} \tilde{x} \\ \tilde{y} \end{pmatrix} \to \begin{pmatrix} \alpha & -\beta \\ \beta & \alpha \end{pmatrix} \begin{pmatrix} \tilde{x} \\ \tilde{y} \end{pmatrix} + \begin{pmatrix} \tilde{f}(\tilde{x},\tilde{y}) \\ \tilde{g}(\tilde{x},\tilde{y}) \end{pmatrix},$$

where

$$\begin{aligned} \tilde{f}(\tilde{x},\tilde{y}) = & \ \tfrac{a_{13}}{a_{12}} u^2 + \tfrac{a_{14}}{a_{12}} uv + O(|u|,|v|)^3, \\ \tilde{g}(\tilde{x},\tilde{y}) = & \ \tfrac{[a_{13}(\alpha - a_{11}) - a_{12}a_{23}]}{a_{12}\beta} u^2 + \tfrac{[a_{14}(\alpha - a_{11}) - a_{12}a_{24}]}{a_{12}\beta} uv \\ & -\tfrac{a_{25}}{\beta} v^2 + O(|u|,|v|)^3, \\ & u = a_{12}\tilde{x}, \ \ v = (\alpha - a_{11})\tilde{x} - \beta\tilde{y}. \end{aligned}$$

Now

$$\tilde{f}_{\tilde{x}\tilde{x}} = 2a_{12}a_{13} + 2a_{14}(\alpha - a_{11}), \ \ \tilde{f}_{\tilde{x}\tilde{y}} = -a_{14}\beta, \ \ \tilde{f}_{\tilde{y}\tilde{y}} = 0,$$

$$\tilde{f}_{\tilde{x}\tilde{x}\tilde{x}} = 0, \ \ \tilde{f}_{\tilde{x}\tilde{x}\tilde{y}} = 0, \ \ \tilde{f}_{\tilde{x}\tilde{y}\tilde{y}} = 0, \ \ \tilde{f}_{\tilde{y}\tilde{y}\tilde{y}} = 0,$$

$$\begin{aligned} \tilde{g}_{\tilde{x}\tilde{x}} = & \ \tfrac{2a_{12}}{\beta} [a_{13}(\alpha - a_{11}) - a_{12}a_{23}] + \tfrac{2(\alpha - a_{11})}{\beta} [a_{14}(\alpha - a_{11}) - a_{12}a_{24}] \\ & -\tfrac{2a_{25}}{\beta} (\alpha - a_{11})^2, \end{aligned}$$

$$\tilde{g}_{\tilde{x}\tilde{y}} = -[a_{14}(\alpha - a_{11}) - a_{12}a_{24}] + 2a_{25}(\alpha - a_{11}), \ \ \tilde{g}_{\tilde{y}\tilde{y}} = -2a_{25}\beta,$$

$$\tilde{g}_{\tilde{x}\tilde{x}\tilde{x}} = 0, \ \ \tilde{g}_{\tilde{x}\tilde{x}\tilde{y}} = 0, \ \ \tilde{g}_{\tilde{x}\tilde{y}\tilde{y}} = 0, \ \ \tilde{g}_{\tilde{y}\tilde{y}\tilde{y}} = 0.$$

According to Hopf bifurcation, the discriminatory quantity s is given by

$$s = -Re\left[\frac{(1-2\overline{\lambda})\overline{\lambda}^2}{1-\lambda}\varphi_{11}\varphi_{20}\right] - \frac{1}{2}\|\varphi_{11}\|^2 - \|\varphi_{02}\|^2 + Re(\overline{\lambda}\varphi_{21}), \tag{2.3.17}$$

where

$$\varphi_{20} = \frac{1}{8}\left[(\tilde{f}_{\tilde{x}\tilde{x}} - \tilde{f}_{\tilde{y}\tilde{y}} + 2\tilde{g}_{\tilde{x}\tilde{y}}) + i\left(\tilde{g}_{\tilde{x}\tilde{x}} - \tilde{g}_{\tilde{y}\tilde{y}} - 2\tilde{f}_{\tilde{x}\tilde{y}}\right)\right],$$

$$\varphi_{11} = \frac{1}{4}\left[(\tilde{f}_{\tilde{x}\tilde{x}} + \tilde{f}_{\tilde{y}\tilde{y}}) + i\left(\tilde{g}_{\tilde{x}\tilde{x}} + \tilde{g}_{\tilde{y}\tilde{y}}\right)\right],$$

$$\varphi_{02} = \frac{1}{8}\left[(\tilde{f}_{\tilde{x}\tilde{x}} - \tilde{f}_{\tilde{y}\tilde{y}} - 2\tilde{g}_{\tilde{x}\tilde{y}}) + i\left(\tilde{g}_{\tilde{x}\tilde{x}} - \tilde{g}_{\tilde{y}\tilde{y}} + 2\tilde{f}_{\tilde{x}\tilde{y}}\right)\right],$$

$$\varphi_{21} = \frac{1}{16}\left[(\tilde{f}_{\tilde{x}\tilde{x}\tilde{x}} + \tilde{f}_{\tilde{x}\tilde{y}\tilde{y}} + \tilde{g}_{\tilde{x}\tilde{x}\tilde{y}} + \tilde{g}_{\tilde{y}\tilde{y}\tilde{y}}) + i\left(\tilde{g}_{\tilde{x}\tilde{x}\tilde{x}} + \tilde{g}_{\tilde{x}\tilde{y}\tilde{y}} - \tilde{f}_{\tilde{x}\tilde{x}\tilde{y}} - \tilde{f}_{\tilde{y}\tilde{y}\tilde{y}}\right)\right],$$

and $\|\varphi_{11}\|$ and $\|\varphi_{02}\|$ are absolute value norms.

Analyzing above and Hopf bifurcation conditions discussed in [149], we write the theorem as below:

Theorem 2.3.6. *If the condition (2.3.15) holds, $s \neq 0$ and the parameter δ_2^* alters in the limited region of the point (0,0), then the system (2.3.13)–(2.3.14) passes through a Hopf bifurcation at the point $B_1(x^*, y^*)$. Moreover, if $s < 0$ (resp., $s > 0$), then an attracting (resp., repelling) invariant closed curve bifurcates from the fixed point $B_1(x^*, y^*)$ for $\delta_2^* > 0$ (resp., $\delta_2^* < 0$).*

2.4 Formulation of Mathematical Model-2

In the model-2, we proposed another prey-predator system with generalized predator and crowding effect with the same assumptions (i)–(iv) of model-1, along with one new assumption that the predator catches the prey and their interactions follow the Holling type-II. The proposed system is of the form:

$$\frac{dx}{dt} = ax\left(1 - \frac{x}{k}\right) - \frac{bxy}{x+l}, \tag{2.4.1}$$

$$\frac{dy}{dt} = cy + \frac{mbxy}{x+l} - dy^2, \tag{2.4.2}$$

with initial conditions:

$$x(0) = x_0 > 0, \; y(0) = y_0 > 0, \tag{2.4.3}$$

where x and y represent the densities of prey and predator populations at any time t, respectively; a denote the intrinsic growth rate of prey and b

is the predation rate of prey; c denotes the growth rate of predator due to alternative resources. Again, d denotes overcrowding rate of predator; l denotes the half saturation constant; m denotes the conversion rate for predator and k denotes carrying capacity of the prey in a particular habitat.

Applying forward Euler's scheme to the system of equations (2.4.1)–(2.4.2), we get the discrete-time system as:

$$x \rightarrow x+\delta\left[ax\left(1-\frac{x}{k}\right)-\frac{bxy}{x+l}\right], \tag{2.4.4}$$

$$y \rightarrow y+\delta\left[cy+\frac{mbxy}{x+l}-dy^2\right], \tag{2.4.5}$$

where δ is the step size.

2.5 Discrete Dynamical Behavior of Model-2

In this section, we discuss the stability criterion of the model-2 at the fixed points and obtain the specific conditions for the existence of flip bifurcation and Hopf bifurcation.

The fixed points of the system (2.4.4)–(2.4.5) are $O_2\left(k,0\right)$, $A_2\left(0,\frac{c}{d}\right)$ and $B_2\left(x^*,y^*\right)$, where x^*,y^* satisfy

$$\begin{cases} a\left(1-\frac{x^*}{k}\right)-\frac{by^*}{x^*+l}=0, \\ c+\frac{mbx^*}{x^*+l}-dy^*=0. \end{cases} \tag{2.5.1}$$

The Jacobian matrix of the system (2.4.4)–(2.4.5) at the fixed point (x,y) is written as:

$$J=\begin{bmatrix} 1+\delta\left(a-\frac{2ax}{k}-\frac{bly}{(x+l)^2}\right) & -\frac{b\delta x}{(x+l)} \\ \frac{\delta mbly}{(x+l)^2} & 1+\delta\left(c+\frac{mbx}{x+l}-2dy\right) \end{bmatrix}.$$

The characteristic equation of the Jacobian matrix is given by

$$\lambda^2+p\left(x,y\right)\lambda+q\left(x,y\right)=0, \tag{2.5.2}$$

where

$$p\left(x,y\right)=-trJ=-2-\delta\left(a-\frac{2ax}{k}-\frac{bly}{(x+l)^2}+c+\frac{mbx}{x+l}-2dy\right),$$

$$q(x,y) = detJ = \left[1+\delta\left(a-\frac{2ax}{k}-\frac{bly}{(x+l)^2}\right)\right] \times \left[1+\delta\left(c+\frac{mbx}{x+l}-2dy\right)\right]+\frac{\delta^2 mb^2 lxy}{(x+l)^3}$$

Proposition 2.5.1. *The fixed point* $O_2(k,0)$ *is source if* $\delta > \frac{2}{a}$*, saddle if* $0 < \delta < \frac{2}{a}$*, and non-hyperbolic if* $\delta = \frac{2}{a}$*, similar to Proposition 2.3.2.*

Proposition 2.5.2. *There exist different topological types of* $A_2\left(0,\frac{c}{d}\right)$ *for possible parameters, similar to Proposition 2.3.3.*

(i) $A_2\left(0,\frac{c}{d}\right)$ *is sink if* $bc-adl>0$ *and* $0<\delta<min\left\{\frac{2}{c},\frac{2dl}{(bc-adl)}\right\}$.

(ii) $A_2\left(0,\frac{c}{d}\right)$ *is source if* $bc-adl>0$ *and* $\delta>max\left\{\frac{2}{c},\frac{2dl}{(bc-adl)}\right\}$.

(iii) $A_2\left(0,\frac{c}{d}\right)$ *is non-hyperbolic if* $\delta=\frac{2}{c}$ *or* $\delta=\frac{2dl}{(bc-adl)}$ *and* $bc-adl>0$.

(iv) $A_2\left(0,\frac{c}{d}\right)$ *is saddle for all values of the parameters, except for that values which lies in (i) to (iii).*

The term *(iii)* of Proposition 2.5.2 implies that the parameters lie in the set

$$F_{A_2} = \{(a,b,c,d,k,l,m,\delta),\quad \delta=\tfrac{2}{c},\ \delta\neq\tfrac{2dl}{(bc-adl)} \text{ and } bc-adl>0,\ a,b,c,d,k,l,m,\delta>0\}.$$

The point $A_2\left(0,\frac{c}{d}\right)$ undergoes flip bifurcation when the parameter changes in small neighborhood of F_{A_2}.

The characteristic equation of the Jacobian matrix J of the system (2.4.4)–(2.4.5) at the fixed point $B_2(x^*,y^*)$ is written as

$$\lambda^2+p(x^*,y^*)\lambda+q(x^*,y^*)=0, \tag{2.5.3}$$

where

$$p(x^*,y^*) = -2-G_2\delta,$$

$$q(x^*,y^*) = 1+G_2\delta+H_2\delta^2,$$

$$G_2 = a - \frac{2ax^*}{k} - \frac{bly^*}{(x^*+l)^2} + c + \frac{mbx^*}{x^*+l} - 2dy^*,$$

$$H_2 = \left[a - \frac{2ax^*}{k} - \frac{bly^*}{(x^*+l)^2}\right]\left[c + \frac{mbx^*}{x^*+l} - 2dy^*\right] + \frac{mb^2lx^*y^*}{(x^*+l)^3}.$$

Now

$$F(\lambda) = \lambda^2 - (2 + G_2\delta)\lambda + (1 + G_2\delta + H_2\delta^2).$$

Therefore

$$F(1) = H_2\delta^2,\ F(-1) = 4 + 2G_2\delta + H_2\delta^2.$$

Using Lemma 2.3.1, we get the following proposition;

Proposition 2.5.3. *There exist different topological types of $B_2\,(x^*, y^*)$ for all possible parameters, similar to Proposition 2.3.4 and the corresponding regions for the flip bifurcation and Hopf bifurcations are given by:*

$$F_{B_{21}} = \{(a,b,c,d,k,l,m,\delta):\ \delta = \tfrac{-G_2-\sqrt{G_2^2-4H_2}}{H_2},\ G_2 < -2\sqrt{H_2} \text{ and } a,b,c,d,k,l,m,\delta > 0\},$$

$$F_{B_{22}} = \{(a,b,c,d,k,l,m,\delta):\ \delta = \tfrac{-G_2+\sqrt{G_2^2-4H_2}}{H_2},\ G_2 < -2\sqrt{H_2} \text{ and } a,b,c,d,k,l,m,\delta > 0\}$$

and

$$H_{B_2} = \{(a,b,c,d,k,l,m,\delta):\ \delta = -\tfrac{G_2}{H_2}, -2\sqrt{H_2} \le G_2 < 0 \text{ and } a,b,c,d,k,l,m,\delta > 0\}.$$

Now, we will study the flip bifurcation and Hopf bifurcation of the system (2.4.4)–(2.4.5) at the fixed point $B_2\,(x^*, y^*)$.

2.5.1 Flip Bifurcation

Consider the system (2.4.4)–(2.4.5) with arbitrary parameter $(a,b,c,d,k,l,m,\delta_1) \in F_{B_{21}}$, which is described as follows:

$$x \rightarrow x+\delta_1\left[ax\left(1-\frac{x}{k}\right)-\frac{bxy}{x+l}\right], \tag{2.5.4}$$

$$y \rightarrow y+\delta_1\left[cy+\frac{mbxy}{x+l}-dy^2\right]. \tag{2.5.5}$$

$B_2(x^*,y^*)$ is fixed point of the system (2.5.4)–(2.5.5), where x^*,y^* is given by (2.5.1) and

$$\delta_1 = \frac{-G_2-\sqrt{G_2^2-4H_2}}{H_2}.$$

The eigen values of $B_2(x^*,y^*)$ are $\lambda_1 = -1$, $\lambda_2 = 3+G_2\delta_1$ with $|\lambda_2| \neq 1$ by Proposition 2.5.3.

Consider the perturbation of (2.5.4)–(2.5.5) as below:

$$x \rightarrow x+(\delta_1+\delta_1^*)\left[ax\left(1-\frac{x}{k}\right)-\frac{bxy}{x+l}\right], \tag{2.5.6}$$

$$y \rightarrow y+(\delta_1+\delta_1^*)\left[cy+\frac{mbxy}{x+l}-dy^2\right], \tag{2.5.7}$$

where $|\delta_1^*| \ll 1$ is a small perturbation parameter.

Analyzing the flip bifurcation conditions for model-2 similar to model-1, we write the following theorem similar to Theorem 2.3.5 as follows:

Theorem 2.5.4. *If $\gamma_2 \neq 0$, and the parameter δ_1^* alters in the limiting region of the point (0,0), then the system (2.5.6)–(2.5.7) passes through flip bifurcation at the point $B_2(x^*,y^*)$. Also, the period-2 points that bifurcate from fixed point $B_2(x^*,y^*)$ are stable (resp., unstable) if $\gamma_2 > 0$ (resp., $\gamma_2 < 0$).*

2.5.2 Hopf Bifurcation

Consider the system (2.4.4)–(2.4.5) with arbitrary parameter $(a,b,c,d,k,l,m,\delta_2) \in H_{B_2}$, which is described as follows:

$$x \to x+\delta_2\left[ax\left(1-\frac{x}{k}\right)-\frac{bxy}{x+l}\right], \tag{2.5.8}$$

$$y \to y+\delta_2\left[cy+\frac{mbxy}{x+l}-dy^2\right]. \tag{2.5.9}$$

$B_2(x^*,y^*)$ is fixed point of the system (2.5.8)–(2.5.9), where x^*,y^* is given by (2.5.1) and

$$\delta_2 = -\frac{G_2}{H_2}.$$

Consider the perturbation of (2.5.8)–(2.5.9) as given below:

$$x \to x+(\delta_2+\delta_2^*)\left[ax\left(1-\frac{x}{k}\right)-\frac{bxy}{x+l}\right], \tag{2.5.10}$$

$$y \to y+(\delta_2+\delta_2^*)\left[cy+\frac{mbxy}{x+l}-dy^2\right]. \tag{2.5.11}$$

where $|\delta_2^*| \ll 1$ is small perturbation parameter.

The characteristic equation of map (2.5.10)–(2.5.11) at $B_2(x^*,y^*)$ is given by

$$\lambda^2+p(\delta_2^*)\lambda+q(\delta_2^*)=0,$$

where

$$p(\delta_2^*) = -2-G_2(\delta_2+\delta_2^*),$$

$$q(\delta_2^*) = 1+G_2(\delta_2+\delta_2^*)+H_2(\delta_2+\delta_2^*)^2.$$

Since the parameter $(a,b,c,d,l,m,\delta_2) \in H_{B_2}$, therefore $p(0) \neq -2,\ 2$. It is the only requirement that $p(0) \neq 0,\ 1$, which follows that

$$G_2{}^2 \neq 2H_2,\ 3H_2. \tag{2.5.12}$$

Analyzing Hopf bifurcation conditions as discussed for model-1, we write the theorem similar to Theorem 2.3.6 as below:

Theorem 2.5.5. *If the condition (2.5.12) holds, $s \neq 0$ and the parameter δ_2^* alters in the limited region of the point (0,0), then the system (2.5.10)–(2.5.11) passes through a Hopf bifurcation at the point $B_2\,(x^*, y^*)$. Moreover, if $s < 0$ (resp., $s > 0$), then an attracting (resp., repelling) invariant closed curve bifurcates from the fixed point $B_2\,(x^*, y^*)$ for $\delta_2^* > 0$ (resp., $\delta_2^* < 0$).*

2.6 Numerical Simulations

To verify the theoretical analysis, bifurcation diagrams, largest Lypunov exponents and phase portraits for the both systems (2.2.4)–(2.2.5) and (2.4.4)–(2.4.5) are presented. These diagrams show the complete dynamical behavior of the both systems at their respective fixed points. For the first system, we discussed flip and Hopf bifurcation respectively in the cases 1 and 2 by keeping the parameters $b = 0.12$, $k = 4$, $l = 3$, $m = 0.1$, $n = 0.2$, $q = 0.5$ as fixed and varying the parameter values of a and d. Similarly for the second system, we presented flip and Hopf bifurcation respectively in the cases 3 and 4 by taking $a = 0.8$, $b = 0.8$, $c = 0.4$, $d = 0.2$, $m = 0.1$ as fixed and varying the values of the parameters k and l.

Case 1: In this case, we take $a = 0.2$, $d = 0.14$ with initial value of $(x, y) = (3.5, 1.6)$ and obtained $\gamma_1 = -3.10$ and $\gamma_2 = 8.59$. From the Figure 2.1(a), it is observed that the fixed point $(0.46, 5.10)$ of the system (2.2.4)–(2.2.5) is stable for $\delta < 2.406$, loses its stability and flip bifurcation appears at $\delta = 2.406$. It shows that the Theorem 2.3.5 is true. The phase portraits show that there are orbits of period-2, 4, 8 at δ = 2.41, 3.0, 3.1 respectively, and chaotic sets at δ = 3.12, 3.15 (see Figure 2.2). Moreover, the Largest Lypunov exponents corresponding to $\delta = 3.12$ and 3.15 are positive that confirm the existence of chaotic sets (see Figure 2.1(b)).

Case 2: In this case, we take $a = 0.8$, $d = 0.44$ with initial value of $(x, y) = (3.5, 1.6)$ and obtained $s = -0.00503$. From the Figure 2.3(a), it is observed that the fixed point $(3.38, 6.59)$ of the system (2.2.4)–(2.2.5) is stable for $\delta < 3.066$, loses its stability and Hopf bifurcation emerges at $\delta = 3.066$. It suggests that the Theorem 2.3.6 is satisfied. The phase portraits in Figure 2.4 show that a smooth invariant circle bifurcates from the fixed point $(3.38, 6.59)$ and its radius increases with

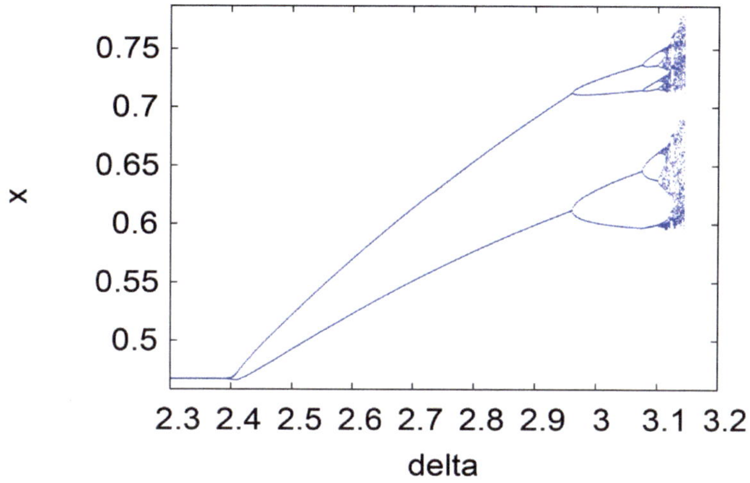

(a)

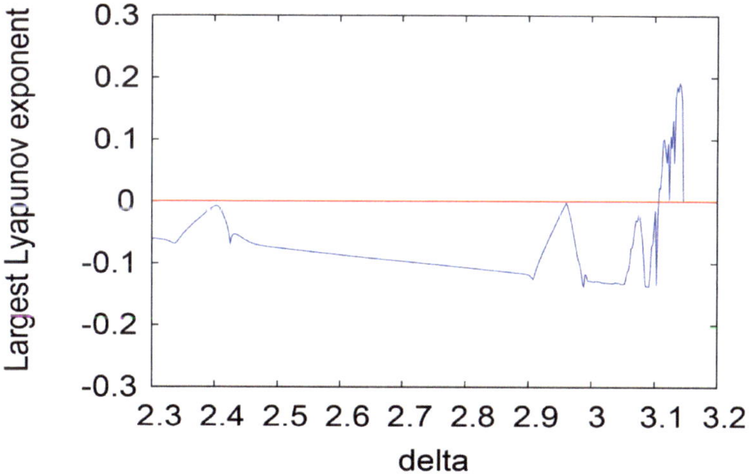

(b)

FIGURE 2.1 (a) Bifurcation diagram of the system (2.2.4)–(2.2.5) for $a = 0.2$, $b = 0.12$, $d = 0.14$, $k = 4$, $l = 3$, $m = 0.1$, $n = 0.2$, $q = 0.5$ and δ covering [2.3, 3.2]. (b) Largest Lyapunov exponents related to (a).

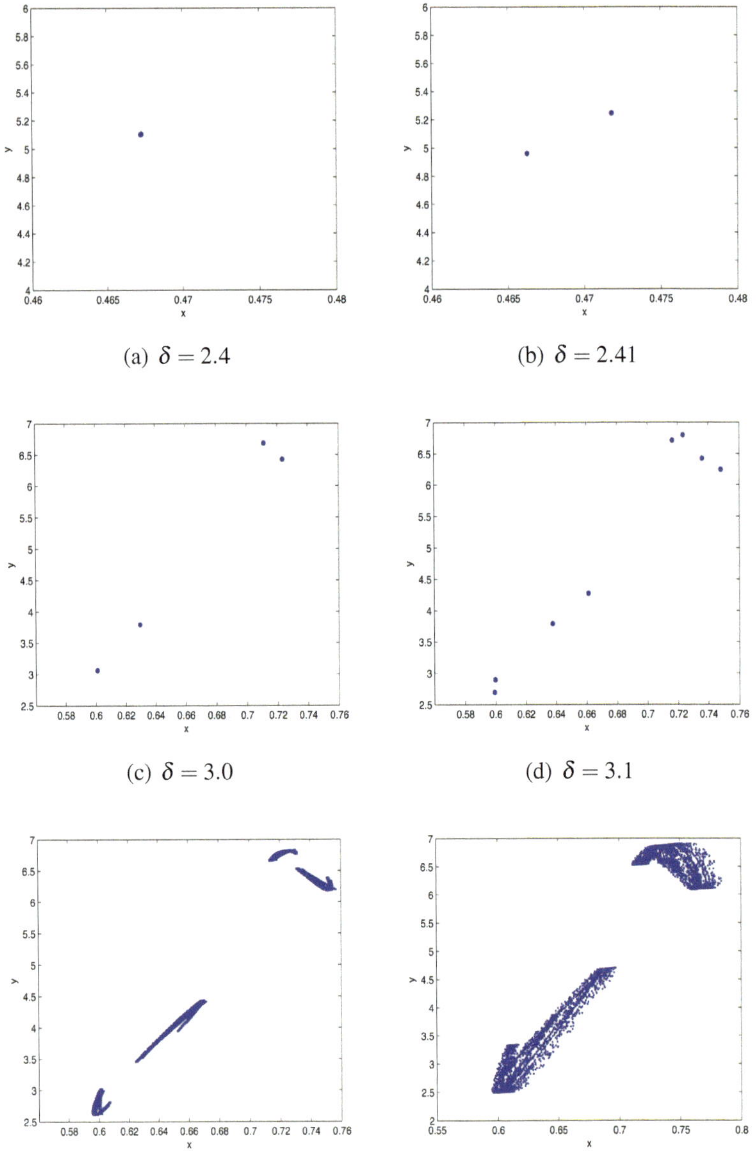

(a) $\delta = 2.4$

(b) $\delta = 2.41$

(c) $\delta = 3.0$

(d) $\delta = 3.1$

(e) $\delta = 3.12$

(f) $\delta = 3.15$

FIGURE 2.2 Phase portraits for several values of δ from 2.4 to 3.15 related to Figure 2.1 (a).

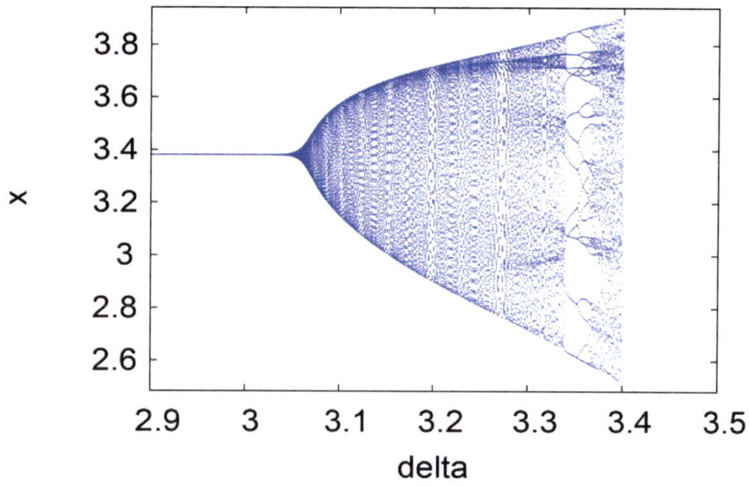

(a)

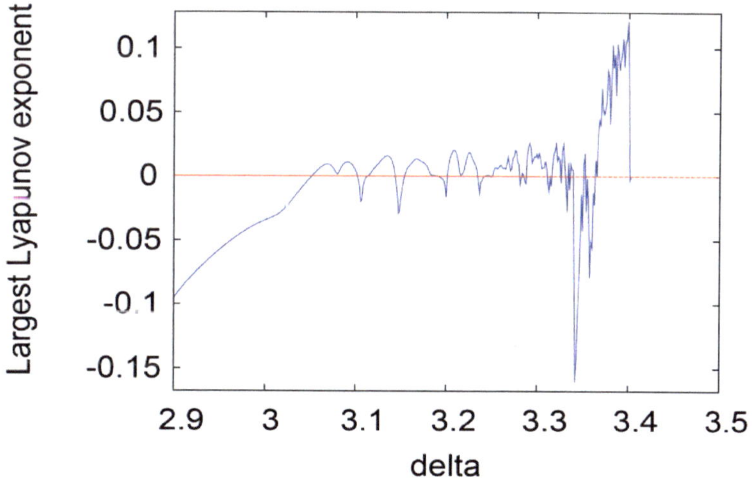

(b)

FIGURE 2.3 (a) Bifurcation diagram of the system (2.2.4)–(2.2.5) for $a = 0.8$, $b = 0.12$, $d = 0.44$, $k = 4$, $l = 3$, $m = 0.1$, $n = 0.2$, $q = 0.5$ and δ covering [2.9, 3.5]. (b) Largest Lyapunov exponents related to (a).

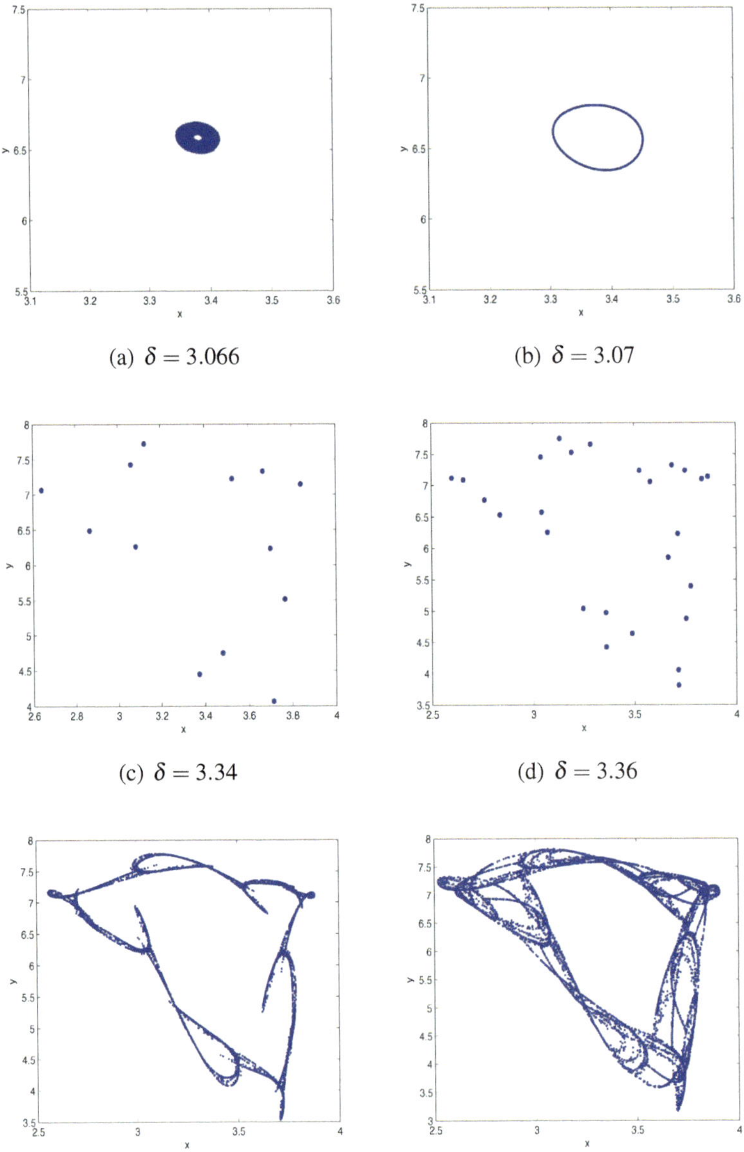

(a) $\delta = 3.066$ (b) $\delta = 3.07$

(c) $\delta = 3.34$ (d) $\delta = 3.36$

(e) $\delta = 3.38$ (f) $\delta = 3.4$

FIGURE 2.4 Phase portraits for various values of δ from 3.066 to 3.4 related to Figure 2.3 (a).

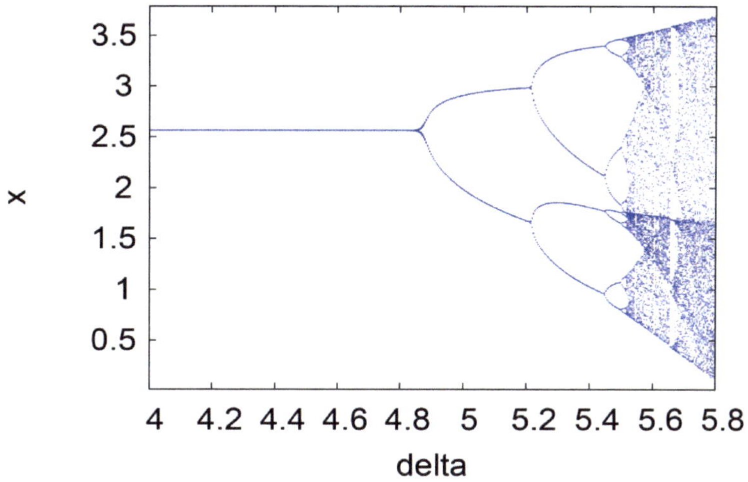

(a)

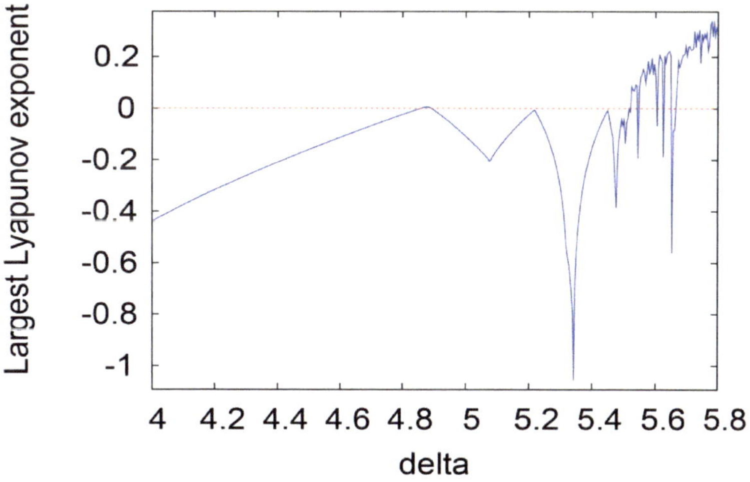

(b)

FIGURE 2.5 (a) Bifurcation diagram of the system (2.4.4)–(2.4.5) for $a = 0.8$, $b = 0.8$, $c = 0.4$, $d = 0.2$, $k = 5$, $l = 2$, $m = 0.1$ with the initial value of $(x, y) = (3, 2)$ and δ covering [4, 5.8]. (b) Largest Lyapunov exponents related to (a).

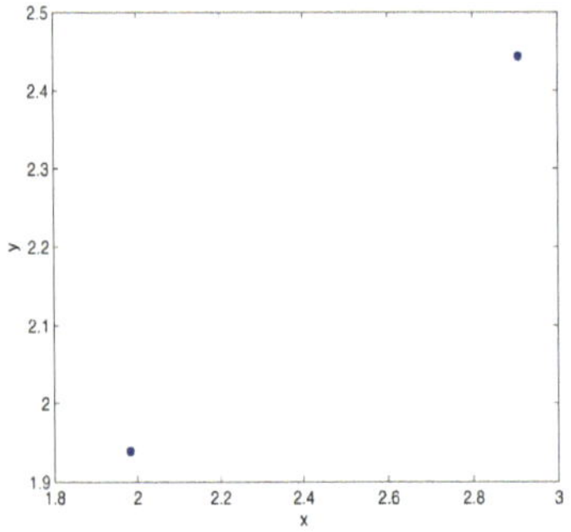

(a) $\delta = 5$

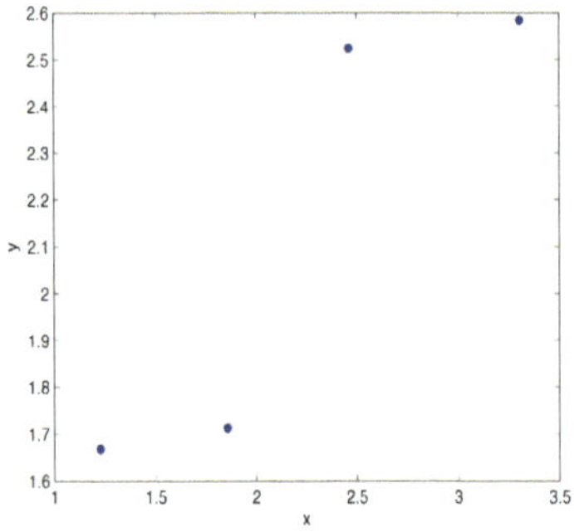

(b) $\delta = 5.3$

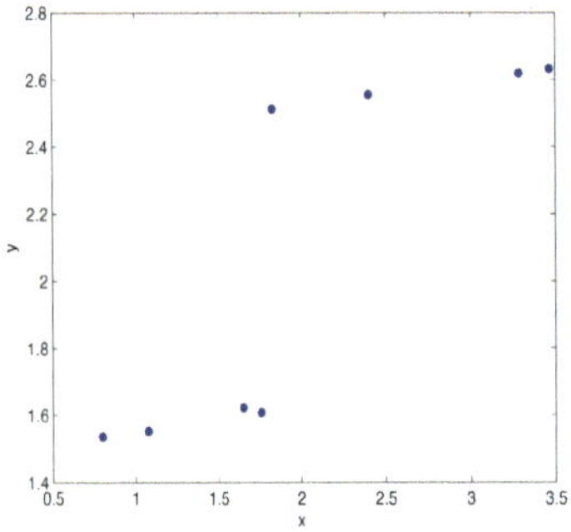

(c) $\delta = 5.5$

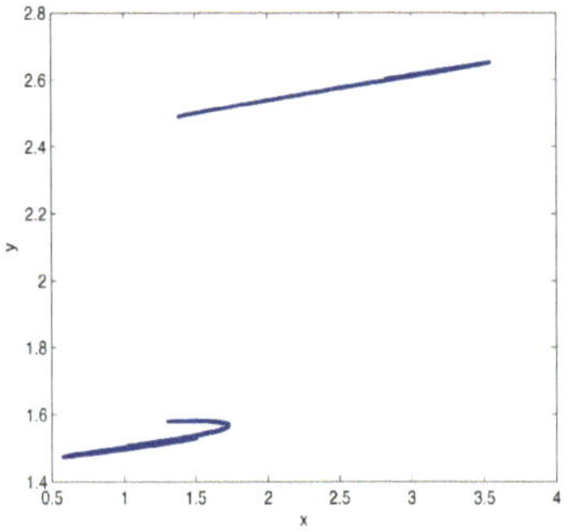

(d) $\delta = 5.6$

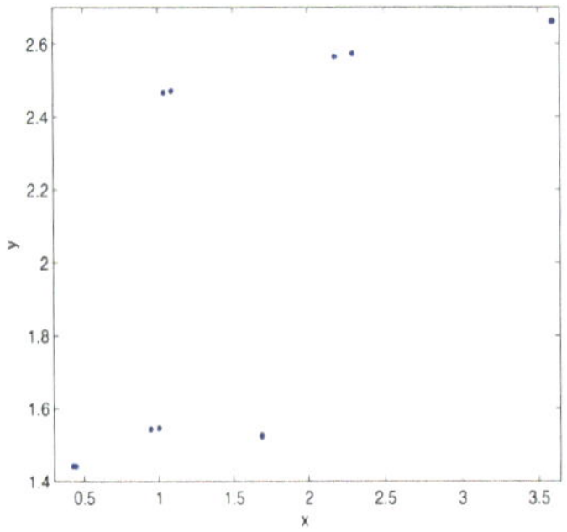

(e) $\delta = 5.662$

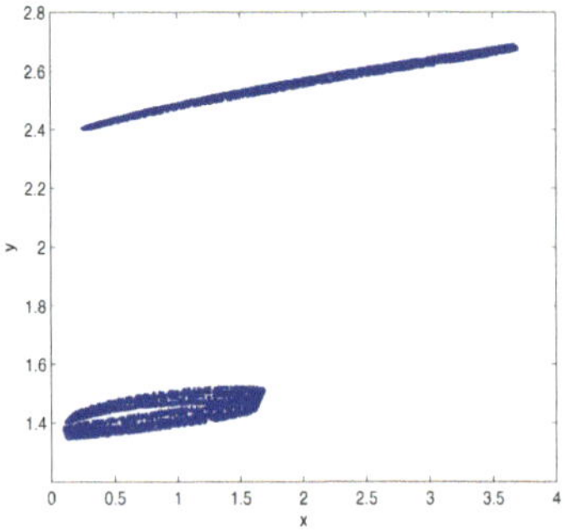

(f) $\delta = 5.8$

FIGURE 2.6 Phase portraits for several values of δ from 5 to 5.8 related to Figure 2.5 (a).

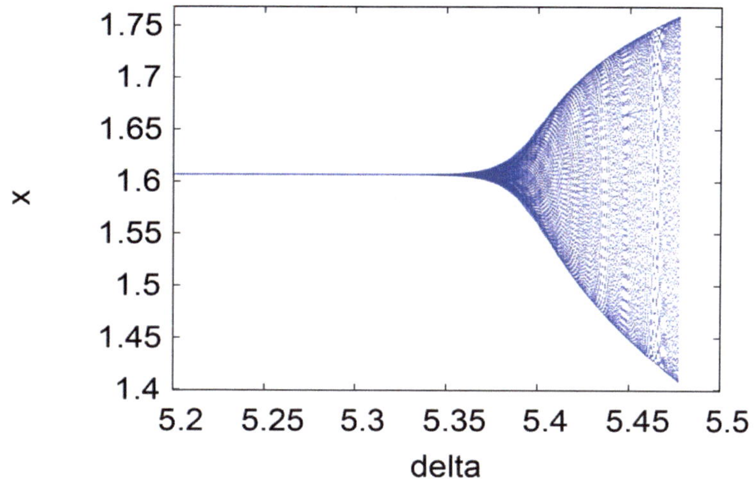

(a)

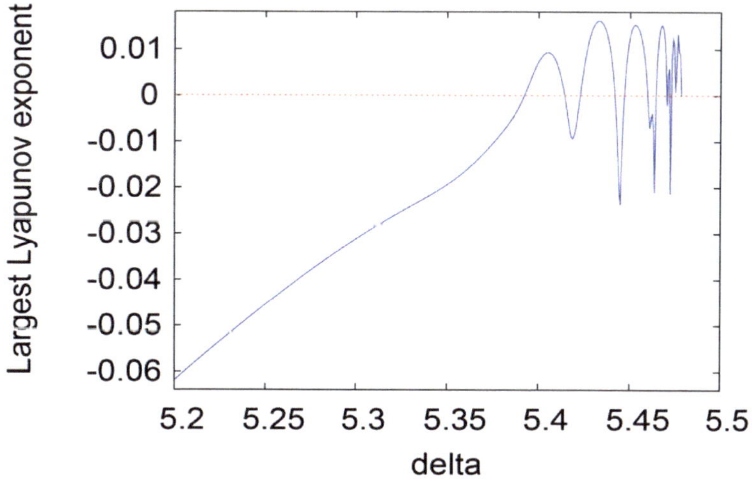

(b)

FIGURE 2.7 (a) Bifurcation diagram of the system (2.4.4)–(2.4.5) for $a = 0.8,\ b = 0.8,\ c = 0.4,\ d = 0.2,\ k = 3,\ l = 3,\ m = 0.1$ with the initial value of $(x,y) = (1.5,\ 2)$ and δ covering [5.2, 5.5]. (b) Largest Lyapunov exponents related to (a).

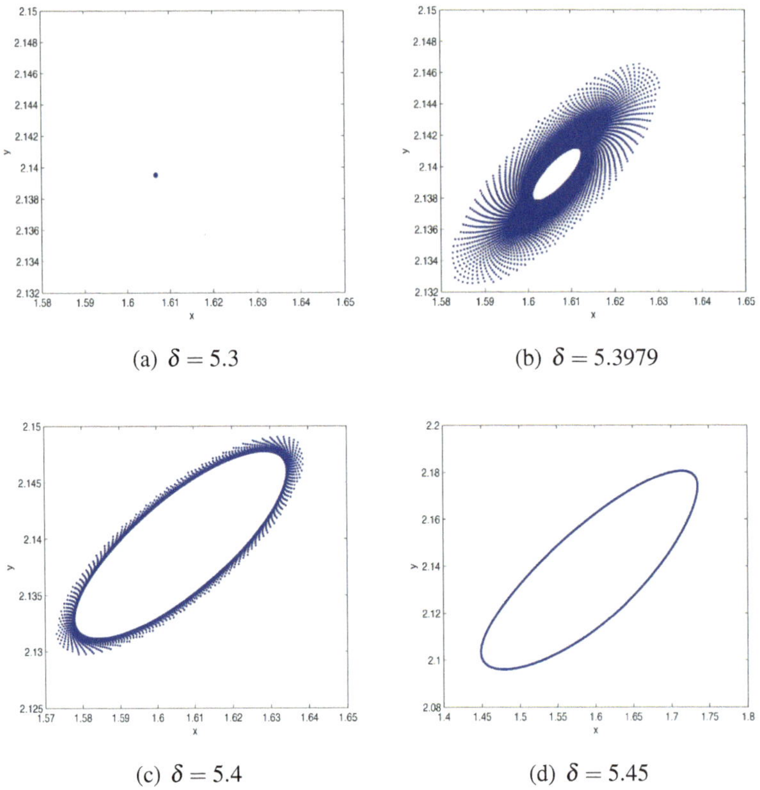

(a) $\delta = 5.3$ (b) $\delta = 5.3979$

(c) $\delta = 5.4$ (d) $\delta = 5.45$

FIGURE 2.8 Phase portraits for several values of δ from 5.3 to 5.45 related to Figure 2.7 (a).

the increase of δ. There are windows of the period-13, 26 at δ = 3.34, 3.36 respectively, and chaotic attractors at δ = 3.38 and 3.4. Moreover, the Largest Lypunov exponents corresponding to $\delta = 3.38$ and 3.4 are positive that confirm the chaotic sets (see Figure 2.3(b)).

Case 3: Taking $k = 5$, $l = 2$ with the initial value of $(x, y) = (3, 2)$, it is observed that from the fixed point $(2.56155, 2.22462)$, a flip bifurcation appears at $\delta = 4.87985$. In this case $\gamma_1 = -0.330478$ and $\gamma_2 = -0.212551$. It established the Theorem 2.5.4. From the Figure 2.5(a), we can see that the fixed point of the system (2.4.4)–(2.4.5) is stable for $\delta < 4.87985$, loses its stability at $\delta = 4.87985$ and there appears period doubling bifurcation for $\delta > 4.87985$. The phase portraits show that there are orbits of period 2, 4, 8 for $\delta \in [5, 5.5]$ and chaotic sets at $\delta = 5.6$ and 5.8 (see Figure 2.6). Moreover, the Largest Lypunov exponents corresponding to $\delta = 5.6$ and 5.8 are positive that confirm the chaotic sets (see Figure 2.5(b)). There is a window of period 9 orbit at $\delta = 5.662$ within the chaotic region $\delta \in [5.6, 5.8]$ (see Figure 2.6).

Case 4: Taking $k = 3$, $l = 3$ with the initial value of $(x, y) = (1.5, 2)$, we see that at the fixed point $(1.6067, 2.1395)$, a Hopf bifurcation emerges at $\delta = 5.3979$. Here $\alpha = -0.9615$, $\beta = 0.2746$ and $s = -259.05$. It shows that the Theorem 2.5.5 holds. From the Figure 2.7(a), we can see that the fixed point of the system (2.4.4)–(2.4.5) is stable for $\delta < 5.3979$, loses its stability at $\delta = 5.3979$ and an invariant circle appears as $\delta > 5.3979$. The phase portraits in Figure 2.8 show that a smooth invariant circle bifurcates from the fixed point and its radius increases with increase of δ.

2.7 Summary

In this chapter, we investigated the stability and bifurcation analysis of two different discrete-time prey-predator systems with predator partially dependent on prey in the closed first quadrant R^2_+. The stability of the both systems at their respective fixed points is discussed. Both the systems undergo flip bifurcation and Hopf bifurcation at the interior fixed points under specific conditions when δ varies in small neighborhood of particular domain(s) of respective system. For a particular set of parameters, numerical simulations of the model-1 display orbits of period-2, 4, 8 and chaotic sets in case of flip bifurcation; and smooth invariant circle, period-13, 26 windows and chaotic attractors in case of Hopf bifurcation. For another particular set of parameters, numerical simulations of the model-2 display cascade of period-doubling bifurcation in orbits of period-2, 4, 8, chaotic sets and stable window of period-9 orbit in case of flip bifurcation; and smooth invariant circles in case of Hopf bifurcation. It means that the predator co-exists with the prey at the period-n orbits and smooth invariant circle. These results show that the discrete system has a rich and complex dynamical behavior.

Chapter 3

A Single Species Harvesting Model with Diffusion in a Two-Patch Habitat

3.1 Introduction

Biotic populations are usually distributed heterogeneously in their habitat, and the distribution itself is often patchy, due to the patchiness of the habitat which arises from a variety of mechanisms and processes under various conditions including deforestation in the case of a forest habitat. It would thus seem natural to study the population dynamics of a single species by including diffusional effects, in a patchy habitat. Many investigators [40, 41, 44, 55] have shown that in a homogeneous habitat, the diffusion, increases the stability of a system. But these may not always be true if the habitat is patchy [47, 54, 57, 162].

It has been found that the opportunities for movement and habitat diversification provided by the spatial aspect of the environment make possible, in a variety of ways, coexistence of species which could not otherwise survive together. If the environment is heterogeneous, different combinations of species are likely to be favored in the various local regions and maintained elsewhere principally by dispersal from more favored regions, and this will act to increase the overall species richness.

A model of a single species population living in two patch habitats with migration between them across a barrier was proposed by Freedman and Waltman [163]. The model was extended by [53, 162] to include the case where species (animals) leaving one habitat does not necessarily reach the other habitat, the existence of a positive equilibrium as a function of barrier strengths was examined.

Also Freedman et al. [54] studied a single species diffusion model by assuming that the habitat consists of two patches and has shown that there exists a positive, monotonic, continuous non-uniform steady state solution that is linearly asymptotically stable under both reservoir and no-flux boundary conditions but it is not globally stable because of patchiness.

Keeping the above [53, 54,163] in view, in this chapter, we consider the dynamics of a diffusing single species population undergoing harvesting in two adjoining patches with a continuous flux matching condition at the interface. The existence of positive, monotonic, continuous nonuniform steady state solution with continuous flux, under both reservoir and no-flux boundary conditions, are studied. Also, the stability of both linear and non-linear systems are discussed. This model is proposed keeping in view the patchiness caused by many man-made projects in the Doon Valley (India) [164]. It is also applicable to the Burwash caribou herd, which lives on both sides of the Shakwak Trench in the Kluane Mountains of the Yukon territories, Canada. The dynamics of this herd has been discussed in [165].

The organization of this chapter is as follows. In Section 3.2, we describe the general mathematical model for two patches. In Section 3.3, we analyzed our model under reservoir and no-flux boundary conditions in Subsection 3.3.1 and 3.3.2, respectively, and the uniform steady state case is discussed in Subsection 3.3.3. Finally in Section 3.4, summary is given.

3.2 Formulation of Mathematical Model

Consider a habitat consisting of two distinct patches labeled by the running variable $i = 1,2$. There are no restrictions on the way the environment is partitioned into these patches. They may be identical or different in size; they may represent identical regimes of climate and soil or nutrient factors, or they may represent distinct such environments, or might simply represent a partitioning of a homogeneous environment. The population dynamics of a single species of logistic type is given by the form of a system of parabolic partial differential equations in the two patches as follows:

$$\frac{\partial N_i(s,t)}{\partial t} = N_i(s,t)\mathbf{g}_i(N_i(s,t)) - N_i\mathbf{p}_i(N_i(s,t)) + D_i\frac{\partial^2 N_i(s,t)}{\partial s^2}, \quad (3.2.1)$$

$$i = 1,2, \qquad 0 \le s \le L_2.$$

Here the growth rate function $\mathbf{g}_i(N_i)$ and the harvesting function $\mathbf{p}_i(N_i)$ are such that

(H.1): $\mathbf{g}_i(N_i),\ \mathbf{p}_i(N_i) \in C^2[0,\infty)$,
$\mathbf{g}_i(0) > 0$, and $\forall N_i \ge 0$, $\mathbf{g}_i'(N_i) \le 0$,
$\mathbf{p}_i(0) = 0$, and $\forall N_i \ge 0$, $\mathbf{p}_i'(N_i) \ge 0$,
and when the habitat has carrying capacity K_i in the i-th patch respectively, then $\mathbf{g}_i(K_i) = 0$.

Further we assume that
(H.2): $\exists\ K_i^* > 0$ such that $\mathbf{g}_i(K_i^*) - \mathbf{p}_i(K_i^*) = 0$.
It follows that $K_i^* \le K_i$ and the equality only holds when $\mathbf{p}_i(N_i) = 0$. Since $\forall N_i \ne K_i^*$, therefore,

$$\frac{\mathbf{g}_i(N_i) - \mathbf{p}_i(N_i)}{N_i - K_i^*} = \frac{\mathbf{g}_i(N_i) - \mathbf{g}_i(K_i^*)}{N_i - K_i^*} - \frac{\mathbf{p}_i(N_i) - \mathbf{p}_i(K_i^*)}{N_i - K_i^*} = \mathbf{g}_i'(\xi_i) - \mathbf{p}_i'(\xi_i) < 0,$$

where $min\{N_i, K_i^*\} \le \xi_i \le max\{N_i, K_i^*\}$. Hence,

$$(N_i - K_i^*)[\mathbf{g}_i(N_i) - \mathbf{p}_i(N_i)] < 0, \ \ \forall N_i \ne K_i^*. \quad (3.2.2)$$

At the interface $s = L_1$ and the continuous flux matching conditions are written as

$$D_1\frac{\partial N_1(L_1,t)}{\partial s} = D_2\frac{\partial N_2(L_1,t)}{\partial s} \text{ and } N_1(L_1,t) = N_2(L_1,t). \quad (3.2.3)$$

The model is studied under two set (namely, reservoir and no-flux) of boundary conditions. In the case of reservoir boundary conditions, we take

$$N_1(0,t) = K_1^* \text{ and } N_2(L_2,t) = K_2^*. \tag{3.2.4}$$

In the case of no-flux boundary conditions, we take

$$\frac{\partial N_1(0,t)}{\partial s} = 0 = \frac{\partial N_2(L_2,t)}{\partial s}. \tag{3.2.5}$$

Finally, the model is completed by assuming some positive initial distribution, that is,

$$N_i(s,0) = \chi_i(s) > 0, \; L_{i-1} \leq s \leq L_i, \; i = 1,2, \tag{3.2.6}$$

such that $N_1(0,0) = K_1^*$, and $N_2(L_2,0) = K_2^*$. An example of $\chi_i(s)$ may be consider as follows:

$$\chi_i(s) = K_1^* + \frac{(K_2^* - K_1^*)}{L_2} s.$$

The existence of non-negative, smooth solutions of the above type of system are shown in Ref. [166]. We also noted that in the case of no diffusion, the behavior of solutions of our model is well known (see Ref. [10]). At each s in the i-th patch, $N_i(s,t) \to K_i^*$ as $t \to \infty$. Clearly, if $K_1^* \neq K_2^*$, then a continuous solution of $N_i(s,t)$ in s is impossible provided the problem must be analyzed by using the techniques of two point boundary value problems [167, 168].

3.3 The Analysis of the Model

3.3.1 Under Reservoir Boundary Conditions

In this section we show the existence of nonuniform steady state solution of our model (3.2.1), (3.2.3), (3.2.4), and (3.2.6). This steady state solution is given by

$$D_i \frac{d^2 u_i}{ds^2} + u_i \mathbf{g}_i(u_i) - u_i \mathbf{p}_i(u_i) = 0, \quad i = 1,2. \tag{3.3.1}$$

The reservoir boundary conditions are given by

$$u_1(0) = K_1^* \text{ and } u_2(L_2) = K_2^*. \tag{3.3.2}$$

At the interface $s = L_1$, we have,

$$D_1 \frac{du_1(L_1)}{ds} = D_2 \frac{du_2(L_1)}{ds}, \quad u_1(L_1) = u_2(L_1). \tag{3.3.3}$$

We use the result of Freedman and Kriszti [47] to show the existence of the positive steady-state solutions in the form of the following theorem.

Theorem 3.3.1. *The steady-state problem (3.3.1), has a unique positive solution* u_i.

Since the functions, $\mathbf{G}_i(u_i) = \mathbf{g}_i(u_i) - \mathbf{p}_i(u_i)$ are such that $\mathbf{G}_i(0) > 0$, $\mathbf{G}_i'(u_i) \le 0$, $\forall u_i \ge 0$ and $\mathbf{G}_i(K_i^*) = 0$. Then $\mathbf{G}_i(u_i) < 0$, if $u_i > max\ \{K_1^*, K_2^*\}$ and $\mathbf{G}_i(u_i) > 0$, if $0 < u_i < min\ \{K_1^*, K_2^*\}$. The positive unique steady-state solution u_i of (3.3.1) is respectively concave or convex on connected subsets if

$\{s \in (0, L_2) : s \neq 0, L_1, L_2;\ u_i(s) > max\ \{K_1^*, K_2^*\}\}$

or $\{s \in (0, L_2) : s \neq 0, L_1, L_2;\ 0 < u_i(s) < min\ \{K_1^*, K_2^*\}\}$.

Hence the unique solution u_i of (3.3.1) satisfies

$$min\ \{K_1^*, K_2^*\} \le u_i(s) \le max\ \{K_1^*, K_2^*\}.$$

We now consider without loss of generality $0 < K_1^* < K_2^*$. Therefore, $K_1^* \le u_i \le K_2^*$.

Let $p_i(s, \alpha_i)$, $L_{i-1} \le s \le L_i$, are the unique solution of the equation (3.3.1), for i = 1, 2, and $p_i(s, \alpha_i)$ are such that

$$\frac{\partial p_1}{\partial s}(0, \alpha_1) = \alpha_1, \quad p_1(0, \alpha_1) = K_1^*,$$

$$\frac{\partial p_2}{\partial s}(L_2, \alpha_2) = \alpha_2, \quad p_2(L_2, \alpha_2) = K_2^*.$$

Multiplying both sides of (3.3.1) by $2du_i/ds$, and integrating from 0 if $i = 1$ and from L_2 if $i = 2$, we get

$$\left[\frac{du_i}{ds}\right]^2 - \alpha_i^2 = -\frac{2}{D_i} \int_{K_i^*}^{u_i(s)} \xi_i(s) \left[\mathbf{g}_i(\xi_i(s)) - \mathbf{p}_i(\xi_i(s))\right] d\xi_i \tag{3.3.4}$$

Hence the following Lemma holds.

Lemma 3.3.2. *If* $\alpha_1 > 0$, *then*

$$\frac{\partial p_1(s,\alpha_1)}{\partial s} > \alpha_1 \text{ on } 0 < s \leq L_1.$$

Proof. From (3.3.4) , we get,

$$\left[\frac{\partial p_1(s,\alpha_1)}{\partial s}\right]^2 = \alpha_1^2 - \frac{2}{D_1}\int_{K_1^*}^{p_1(s,\alpha_1)} \xi_1[\mathbf{g}_1(\xi_1) - \mathbf{p}_1(\xi_1)]d\xi_1. \quad (3.3.5)$$

Since

$$\frac{\partial p_1(0,\alpha_1)}{\partial s} = \alpha_1 > 0\ ,\ p_1(0,\alpha_1) = K_1^*\ ,$$

then there exists $s_1 > 0$ such that $p_1(s,\alpha_1) > K_1^*$ on $0 < s < s_1$. If not, let $s_0, 0 < s_0 \leq L_1$, be the first positive value, if it exists, such that $p_1(s_0,\alpha_1) = K_i^*$. Then by the mean value theorem there exists $\bar{s}$ such that $0 < \bar{s} < s_0$ and $\partial p_1(\bar{s},\alpha_1)/\partial s = 0$; that is,

$$\alpha_1^2 = \frac{2}{D_1}\int_{K_1^*}^{p_1(\bar{s},\alpha_1)} \xi_1[\mathbf{g}_1(\xi_1) - \mathbf{p}_1(\xi_1)]d\xi_1. \quad (3.3.6)$$

Now since $p_1(s,\alpha_1) > K_1^*$ for $0 < s \leq \bar{s}$ and from (3.2.2), we have, $\mathbf{g}_1(\xi_1) - \mathbf{p}_1(\xi_1) < 0$. Hence the right hand side of (3.3.6) is negative, giving a contradiction. Therefore, $p_1(s,\alpha_1) > K_1^*$ and $\partial p_1(s,\alpha_1)/\partial s > 0$. □

Lemma 3.3.3. *If* $0 < p_2 < K_2^*$ *and* $\alpha_2 > 0$, *then*

$$\frac{\partial p_2(s,\alpha_2)}{\partial s} > \alpha_2,\ \ L_1 \leq s < L_2.$$

Proof. From (3.3.4),we have,

$$\left[\frac{\partial p_2(s,\alpha_2)}{\partial s}\right]^2 = \alpha_2^2 - \frac{2}{D_2}\int_{K_2^*}^{p_2(s,\alpha_2)} \xi_2[\mathbf{g}_2(\xi_2) - \mathbf{p}_2(\xi_2)]d\xi_2.$$

Since $0 < p_2 < K_2^*$, hence from (3.2.2), $\xi_2[\mathbf{g}_2(\xi_2) - \mathbf{p}_2(\xi_2)] > 0$. Therefore, $\partial p_2(s,\alpha_2)/\partial s > \alpha_2, L_1 \leq s < L_2$ for $0 < p_2 < K_2^*$. □

Lemma 3.3.4. *Define $F_i(\alpha_i)$ by $F_i(\alpha_i) = p_i(L_1, \alpha_i)$. Then there exists $\hat{\alpha}_i > 0$, such that*

$$F_1 : [0, \hat{\alpha}_1] \to [K_1^*, K_2^*],$$

$$F_2 : [0, \hat{\alpha}_2] \to [K_2^*, K_1^*].$$

Proof. Note that $F_i(\alpha_i)$, if it exists, is continuous. The existence of $\hat{\alpha}_1 > 0$ follows from the following, we note that $F_1(0) = K_1^*$, $F_1(\alpha_1) > K_1^*$ if $\alpha_1 > 0$ (by Lemma 3.3.2), and that $F_1(\infty) = \infty$. Hence, we choose $\hat{\alpha}_i > 0$ to be the least value of α_1 such that $F_1(\hat{\alpha}_1) = K_2^*$.

To show that $\hat{\alpha}_2$ exists, we note that $F_2(0) = K_2^*$. By continuity, $F_2(\alpha_2)$ exists for sufficiently small α_2, $\alpha_2 > 0$. From Lemma 3.3.3, $F_2[(K_2^* - K_1^*)/(L_2 - L_1)]$ is either less than K_1^* or does not exist. Therefore, there exists at least an $\hat{\alpha}_2$, such that $\hat{\alpha}_2 = K_1^*$, hence the lemma. □

Theorem 3.3.5. *There exists a continuous, monotonic solution of system (3.3.1) with continuous flux at L_1.*

Proof. Lemmas 3.3.2 and 3.3.3 follow that any solution, we construct must be monotonic. By Lemma 3.3.4, for each $0 \leq \alpha_2 \leq \hat{\alpha}_2$, we can find an α_1 such that $0 \leq \alpha_1 \leq \hat{\alpha}_1$ for which $p_1(L_1, \alpha_1) = p_2(L_1, \alpha_2)$. Hence, α_1 can be solved as a function of α_2, $\alpha_1 = h(\alpha_2)$, to give a continuous solution of (3.3.1) with (3.3.2) and (3.3.4).

Let

$$\mathscr{G}(\alpha_2) = D_1 \frac{\partial p_1(L_1, h(\alpha_2))}{\partial s} - D_2 \frac{\partial p_2(L_1, \alpha_2)}{\partial s}.$$

Clearly $\mathscr{G}(\alpha_2)$ is continuous on $0 \leq \alpha_2 \leq \hat{\alpha}_2$. Then we have

$$\mathscr{G}(0) = D_1 \frac{\partial p_1(L_1, \hat{\alpha}_1)}{\partial s} > 0,$$

and

$$\mathscr{G}(\hat{\alpha}_2) = -D_2 \frac{\partial p_2(L_1, \hat{\alpha}_2)}{\partial s} < 0.$$

Hence the theorem. □

Now we find the conditions for asymptotic stability in both linear and non-linear case using Lyapunov direct method.

Theorem 3.3.6. *The steady-state, continuous, monotonic solutions of linear system (3.2.1) with continuous flux matching conditions at the interfaces (3.2.3), and under reservoir boundary conditions (3.2.4), is asymptotically stable if*

$$\frac{d}{du_2}\left(u_2[\mathbf{g}_2(u_2)-\mathbf{p}_2(u_2)]\right)<0, \qquad K_1^* \le u_2 \le K_2^*. \tag{3.3.7}$$

Proof. Linearizing (3.2.1) by using

$$N_i(s,t)=u_i(s)+n_i(s,t), \quad i=1,2. \tag{3.3.8}$$

We have

$$\frac{\partial n_i(s,t)}{\partial t}=n_i\left[\mathbf{g}_i(u_i)+u_i\mathbf{g}_i'(u_i)-\mathbf{p}_i(u_i)-u_i\mathbf{p}_i'(u_i)\right]+D_i\frac{\partial^2 n_i}{\partial s^2}. \tag{3.3.9}$$

Using (3.3.8), the corresponding reservoir boundary conditions and the matching conditions at the interface are as follows:

$$\begin{aligned} n_1(0,t) &= n_2(L_2,t)=0, \\ n_1(L_1,t) &= n_2(L_1,t), \\ D_1\frac{\partial n_1}{\partial s}(L_1,t) &= D_2\frac{\partial n_2}{\partial s}(L_2,t). \end{aligned} \tag{3.3.10}$$

Now we consider the following positive definite function ($L_0=0$),

$$V(t)=\sum_{i=1}^{2}\int_{L_{i-1}}^{L_i}\frac{1}{2}n_i^2\,ds. \tag{3.3.11}$$

Differentiating (3.3.11) and using (3.3.9) and (3.3.10), we get

$$\begin{aligned} \dot V(t) &= \int_0^{L_1} n_1^2\left[\mathbf{g}_1(u_1)+u_1\mathbf{g}_1'(u_1)-\mathbf{p}_1(u_1)-u_1\mathbf{p}_1'(u_1)\right]ds \\ &\quad+\int_{L_1}^{L_2} n_2^2\left[\mathbf{g}_2(u_2)+u_2\mathbf{g}_2'(u_2)-\mathbf{p}_2(u_2)-u_2\mathbf{p}_2'(u_2)\right]ds \\ &\quad+D_1\int_0^{L_1} n_1\frac{\partial^2 n_1}{\partial s^2}ds+D_2\int_{L_1}^{L_2} n_2\frac{\partial^2 n_2}{\partial s^2}ds. \end{aligned}$$

Now, taking the following integral, and using (3.3.10), we get

$$
\begin{aligned}
\mathscr{I} &= D_1\int_0^{L_1} n_1\frac{\partial^2 n_1}{\partial s^2}ds + D_2\int_{L_1}^{L_2} n_2\frac{\partial^2 n_2}{\partial s^2}ds\\
&= D_1 n_1(L_1,t)\frac{\partial n_1}{\partial s}(L_1,t) - D_2 n_2(L_1,t)\frac{\partial n_2}{\partial s}(L_1,t)\\
&\quad -D_1\int_0^{L_1}\left(\frac{\partial n_1}{\partial s}\right)^2 ds - D_2\int_{L_1}^{L_2}\left(\frac{\partial n_2}{\partial s}\right)^2 ds\\
&= -D_1\int_0^{L_1}\left(\frac{\partial n_1}{\partial s}\right)^2 ds - D_2\int_{L_1}^{L_2}\left(\frac{\partial n_2}{\partial s}\right)^2 ds. \qquad (3.3.12)
\end{aligned}
$$

Again since for $0 \le s \le L_1$, $u_1 \ge K_1^*$, $\mathbf{G}_1(u_1) = \mathbf{g}_1(u_1) - \mathbf{p}_1(u_1) < 0$, and $\mathbf{G}_1'(u_1) = \mathbf{g}_1'(u_1) - \mathbf{p}_1'(u_1) < 0$, then the expression $\mathbf{g}_1(u_1) + u_1\mathbf{g}_1'(u_1) - \mathbf{p}_1(u_1) - u_1\mathbf{p}_1'(u_1) < 0$ is negative.

Hence $\dot{V}(t)$ is negative definite if the condition (3.3.7) holds true, thus providing the theorem. □

Remark: For $L_1 \le s < L_2$, $u_2 < K_2^*$, $\mathbf{G}_2(u_2) = \mathbf{g}_2(u_2) - \mathbf{p}_2(u_2) > 0$, and $\mathbf{G}_2'(u_2) < 0$. This implies that the expression in the third integral is negative for u_2 very close to K_2^*. Since it is smooth, it remain so $\forall\, u_2,\ K_1^* \le u_2 < K_2^*$ by (3.3.7).

Finally, we discuss the nonlinear stability of the system.

Theorem 3.3.7. *The steady-state, continuous, monotonic solution of nonlinear system (3.2.1) with continuous flux matching condition at the interface (3.2.3), and under the reservoir boundary conditions (3.2.4), is asymptotically stable if,*

$$\frac{(N_i\mathbf{g}_i(N_i) - u_i\mathbf{g}_i(u_i))}{N_i - u_i} - \frac{(N_i\mathbf{p}_i(N_i) - u_i\mathbf{p}_i(u_i))}{N_i - u_i} \le 0, \qquad (3.3.13)$$

in the subregion of $K_1^* \le N_i, u_i \le K_2^*$, for $i = 1, 2$.

Proof. From (3.2.1), (3.3.1) and (3.3.8), we have

$$\frac{\partial n_i}{\partial t} = (N_i\mathbf{g}_i(N_i) - u_i\mathbf{g}_i(u_i)) - (N_i\mathbf{p}_i(N_i) - u_i\mathbf{p}_i(u_i)) + D_i\frac{\partial^2 n_i}{\partial s^2}. \qquad (3.3.14)$$

Now consider the same positive definite function as given in (3.3.11),

$$V(t) = \sum_{i=1}^{2} \int_{L_{i-1}}^{L_i} (N_i - u_i)^2 ds = \sum_{i=1}^{2} \int_{L_{i-1}}^{L_i} n_i^2 ds.$$

Therefore,

$$\begin{aligned} \dot{V}(t) &= \sum_{i=1}^{2} \int_{L_{i-1}}^{L_i} n_i^2 \left[\frac{(N_i)\mathbf{g}_i(N_i) - u_i \mathbf{g}_i(u_i)}{N_i - u_i} - \frac{(N_i)\mathbf{p}_i(N_i) - u_i \mathbf{p}_i(u_i)}{N_i - u_i} \right] ds \\ &+ \sum_{i=1}^{2} D_i \int_{L_{i-1}}^{L_i} n_i \frac{\partial^2 n_i}{\partial s^2} ds, \end{aligned} \quad (3.3.15)$$

and the second integral is always negative by (3.3.12).

Therefore, $\dot{V}(t) \leq 0$ if the conditions (3.3.13) are satisfied. □

Remark: Using the mean value theorem,

$$\begin{aligned} \frac{(N_i)\mathbf{g}_i(N_i) - u_i \mathbf{g}_i(u_i)}{N_i - u_i} - \frac{(N_i)\mathbf{p}_i(N_i) - u_i \mathbf{p}_i(u_i)}{N_i - u_i} &= \mathbf{g}_i(\xi_i) + \xi_i \mathbf{g}_i'(\xi_i) - \mathbf{p}_i(\xi_i) \\ &\quad - \xi_i \mathbf{p}_i'(\xi_i), \end{aligned} \quad (3.3.16)$$

where ξ_i is a fixed point for $i = 1,2$, lies between N_i and u_i. Since $K_1^* \leq N_i, u_i \leq K_2^*$, therefore, $K_1^* \leq \xi_i \leq K_2^*$. Again from **(H.1)**, $\mathbf{p}_i(\xi_i) \geq 0$, $\mathbf{p}_i'(\xi_i) \geq 0$ and $\mathbf{g}_i'(\xi_i) \leq 0, \forall \xi_i \geq 0$. Also $\mathbf{g}_i(\xi_i) \leq 0$, only when $\xi_i \geq K_i$, therefore, the conditions (3.3.13), for $i = 1$ is always true if both $u_1, N_1 \geq K_1 \geq K_1^*$. Further from (3.3.16) for $i = 1,2$,

$$0 \geq -\xi_i \mathbf{g}_i'(\xi_i) + \mathbf{p}_i(\xi_i) + \xi_i \mathbf{p}_i'(\xi_i) \geq \mathbf{g}_i(\xi_i),$$

is the another form of the conditions (3.3.13). Since the functions are continuous, hence it is feasible.

3.3.2 Under No-Flux Boundary Conditions

Similarly, we analyze the steady state solution under no-flux boundary conditions of our model (3.2.1), (3.2.3), (3.2.5), and (3.2.6). The steady state problem takes the form,

$$D_i \frac{d^2 u_i}{ds^2} + u_i \mathbf{g}_i(u_i) - u_i \mathbf{p}_i(u_i) = 0, \quad i = 1,2. \quad (3.3.17)$$

The no-flux boundary conditions are given by

$$\frac{du_1}{ds}(0) = 0 = \frac{du_2}{ds}(L_2), \tag{3.3.18}$$

and at the interface $s = L_1$, we have

$$D_1 \frac{du_1(L_1)}{ds} = D_2 \frac{du_2(L_1)}{ds}, \quad u_1(L_1) = u_2(L_1). \tag{3.3.19}$$

Let $q_i(s, \beta_i)$, $L_{i-1} \leq s \leq L_i$, are the unique solutions of the equation (3.3.17), for i=1,2, and $q_i(s, \beta_i)$ are such that

$$\frac{\partial q_1}{\partial s}(0, \beta_1) = 0, \quad q_1(0, \beta_1) = \beta_1,$$

$$\frac{\partial q_2}{\partial s}(L_2, \beta_2) = \beta_2, \quad q_2(L_2, \beta_2) = \beta_2.$$

It may be noted here that it is possible to show the existence of a positive, monotonic, continuous with continuous flux solution, if we can show that there exist β_1, β_2 such that

$$D_1 \frac{\partial q_1(L_1, \beta_1)}{\partial s} = D_2 \frac{\partial q_2(L_1, \beta_2)}{\partial s}, \quad q_1(L_1, \beta_1) = q_2(L_1, \beta_2).$$

Multiplying both sides of (3.3.17) by $2du_i/ds$ and integrating from 0 if $i = 1$ and from L_2 if $i = 2$, we get

$$\left[\frac{du_i}{ds}\right]^2 = -\frac{2}{D_i} \int_{\beta_i}^{u_i(s)} \xi_{i_i} [\mathbf{g}_i(\xi_i) - \mathbf{p}_i(\xi_i)] \, d\xi_i. \tag{3.3.20}$$

By using (3.3.20), the following lemmas are proved analogous to their counterparts in the previous section.

Lemma 3.3.8. *If $\beta_1 > K_1^*$, then*

$$\frac{\partial p_1(s, \beta_1)}{\partial s} > 0 \, , \; 0 < s \leq L_1.$$

Proof. From (3.3.20), we get,

$$\left[\frac{\partial p_1(s,\beta_1)}{\partial s}\right]^2 = -\frac{2}{D_{11}}\int_{\beta_1}^{p_1(s,\beta_1)} \xi_1\left[\mathbf{g}_1(\xi_1)-\mathbf{p}_1(\xi_1)\right]d\xi_1. \quad (3.3.21)$$

Since $\partial p_1(0,\beta_1)/\partial s = 0$, $p_1(0,\beta_1)=\beta_1$ there exists $s_1>0$ such that $p_1(s,\beta_1)>\beta_1$ on $0<s<s_1$. If not, let s_0, $0<s_0\le L_1$, be the least positive value , if it exists, such that $p_1(s_0,\beta_1)=\beta_1$. Then by the mean value theorem there exists $\bar{s}$ such that $0<\bar{s}<s_0$ and $\partial p_1(\bar{s},\beta_1)/\partial s=0$; that is

$$0 = -\frac{2}{D_{11}}\int_{\beta_1}^{p_1(\bar{s},\beta_1)} \xi_1\left[\mathbf{g}_1(\xi_1)-\mathbf{p}_1(\xi_1)\right]d\xi_1. \quad (3.3.22)$$

But the right hand side of (3.3.22) is non-zero, since $p_1(s,\beta_1)\neq\beta_1$ on $0<s\le\bar{s}$, giving a contradiction. Hence $p_1(s,\beta_1)>\beta_1$, for all value $0<s\le L_1$. Also $\beta_1>K_1^*$, implies, $p(s,\beta_1)>K_1^*$, on $0<s\le L_1$. Hence by (3.2.2) and (3.3.21), the result follows. □

Lemma 3.3.9. *If $0<p_2(s,\beta_2)\le K_2^*$, then $\beta_2<K_2^*$ which implies $p_2(s,\beta_2)<\beta_2$, for $L_1\le s<L_2$.*

Proof. Since $0<p_2(s,\beta_2)\le K_2^*$, then from (3.2.2), we get,

$$p_2\left[\mathbf{g}_2(p_2)-\mathbf{p}_2(p_2)\right]>0.$$

Now, since $\beta_2<K_2^*$, then $p_2\mathbf{g}_2(p_2)-q_2\mathbf{p}_2(p_2)>0$, $\forall\ \beta_2, p_2$. If possible let $p_2>\beta_2$, then the right hand side of (3.3.20) is negative, which is impossible. Therefore $p_2(s,\beta_2)<\beta_2$. □

Lemma 3.3.10. *Define $\mathscr{H}_i(\beta_i)$ by $\mathscr{H}_i(\beta_i)=p_i(L_1,\beta_i)$. Then such that*

$$\mathscr{H}_1 : \left[K_1^*,\hat{\beta}_1\right] \to \left[K_1^*,K_2^*\right],$$

and

$$\mathscr{H}_2 : \left[\hat{\beta}_2,K_2^*\right] \to \left[K_1^*,K_2^*\right].$$

Proof. Since $p_i(L_1, \beta_i)$ is continuous function, therefore if $\mathcal{H}_i(\beta_i)$ exists, then it must be continuous. We choose $\mathcal{H}_1(K_1^*) = K_1^*$, this is possible since $p_1(0, K_1^*) = K_1^*$ and $\partial p_1/\partial s(0, K_1^*) = 0$. Now from Lemma 3.3.8, $\mathcal{H}_1(\beta_1) > K_1^*$ if $\beta_1 > K_1^*$ and since $\mathcal{H}_1(\beta_1)$ is continuous, therefore, $\mathcal{H}_1(\infty) = \infty$. Hence we can find $\hat{\beta}_1 > K_1^*$ to be the first value of β_1 such that $\mathcal{H}_1(\hat{\beta}_1) = K_2^*$.

Again, choose $\mathcal{H}_2(K_2^*) = p_2(L_2, K_2^*) = K_2^*$ and from Lemma 3.3.9, if $\beta_2 < K_2^*$, then $p_2(L_1, \beta_2) < \beta_2$, and hence $\mathcal{H}_1(\beta_2) < \beta_2 < K_2^*$. Then there exists $\hat{\beta}_2$ such that $\mathcal{H}_2(\hat{\beta}_2) = K_1^*$. Hence, the result. □

Theorem 3.3.11. *There exists a continuous, monotonic solution of system (3.3.17) with continuous flux at L_1.*

Proof. By Lemma 3.3.10, for each $\hat{\beta}_2 \le \beta_2 \le K_2^*$, we can choose a β_1 such that $K_1^* \le \beta_1 \le \hat{\beta}_1$ for which $p_1(L_1, \beta_1) = p_2(L_1, \beta_2)$. Hence β_1 can be solved as a function of β_2 in the form $\beta_1 = f(\beta_2)$ to give a continuous solution of (3.3.17). We now define,

$$\mathcal{I}(\beta_2) = D_1 \frac{\partial p_1}{\partial s}(L_1, f(\beta_2)) - D_2 \frac{\partial p_2}{\partial s}(L_1, \beta_2). \tag{3.3.23}$$

Then

$$\mathcal{I}(\hat{\beta}_2) = -D_2 \frac{\partial p_2}{\partial s}(L_1, \hat{\beta}_2) < 0, \quad \mathcal{I}(K_2^*) = D_1 \frac{\partial p_1}{\partial s}(L_1, \hat{\beta}_1) > 0.$$

Now by continuity, there exists β_2, $\hat{\beta}_2 < \beta_2 < K_2^*$, such that $\mathcal{I}(\beta_2) = 0$.

The monotonicity follows from, since $f(\beta_2) = \beta_1 > K_1^*$, Lemma 3.3.8 shows that our solution is monotonic on $0 \le s \le L_1$. By Lemma 3.3.9, we note that on $L_1 \le s < Ł_2$, the solution $p_2(s, \beta_2) < \beta_2$. If $p_2(s, \beta_2)$ is not monotonic over this interval, then there exists $\bar{s}$, $L_1 < \bar{s} < L_2$, such that $\partial p_2(\hat{s}, \beta_2)/\partial s = 0$. But then, by (3.3.20), $u_2'(\bar{s}) > 0$, $u_2(\bar{s}) > \beta_2$, giving a contradiction. This proves the theorem. □

Finally, the stability conditions under no-flux boundary conditions are similar as in the case of reservoir boundary conditions and proofs are exactly same.

Theorem 3.3.12. *The steady-state, continuous, monotonic solutions of the system (3.2.1) with continuous flux matching condition at the* *interfaces (3.2.3) and under the no-flux boundary conditions (3.2.5), is locally asymptotically stable if*

$$\frac{d}{du_2}(u_2[\mathbf{g}_2(u_2) - \mathbf{p}_2(u_2)]) < 0, \qquad K_1^* \leq u_2 \leq K_2^*. \tag{3.3.24}$$

Theorem 3.3.13. *The steady-state, continuous, monotonic solution of nonlinear system (3.2.1) with continuous flux matching condition at the interface (3.2.3), and under the no-flux boundary conditions (3.2.5), is asymptotically stable if,*

$$\frac{(N_i\mathbf{g}_i(N_i) - u_i\mathbf{g}_i(u_i))}{N_i - u_i} - \frac{(N_i\mathbf{p}_i(N_i) - u_i\mathbf{p}_i(u_i))}{N_i - u_i} \leq 0, \tag{3.3.25}$$

in the subregion of $K_1^* \leq N_i, u_i \leq K_2^*$, for $i = 1, 2$.

Remark: The effect of harvesting is to decrease the equilibrium level and modify the conditions for stability (see [54]). It is to be noted further that harvesting enhances stability, see conditions (3.3.24) and (3.3.25).

3.3.3 The Case of Uniform Equilibrium State

We show that uniform steady state of the system (3.2.1)–(3.2.6) is globally asymptotically stable in the homogeneous habitat, under both set of boundary conditions. In our model, there is a uniform steady state $N(s,t) \equiv K, 0 \leq s \leq L_2,\ t \geq 0$, where K is the common carrying capacity in both the patches.

Theorem 3.3.14. *Let $K_1^* = K_2^* = K$. Then the unique steady state solution to (3.3.1) and either (3.3.2) or (3.3.18), $N(s,t) = K$ is globally asymptotically stable.*

Proof. Let $V(N) = V(t)$ be the positive definite function about $N = K$, given by

$$V(N) = V(t) = \sum_{i=1}^{2} \int_{L_{i-1}}^{L_i} \left[N_i - K - K \ln \frac{N_i}{K} \right] ds.$$

Differentiating with respect to t, and using (3.2.1) we get,

$$\dot{V}(t) = \sum_{i=1}^{2} \int_{L_{i-1}}^{L_i} \frac{(N_i - K)}{N_i} \{N_i \mathbf{g}_i(N_i) - N_i \mathbf{p}_i(N_i)\} ds + \sum_{i=1}^{n} D_i \int_{L_{i-1}}^{L_i} \frac{N_i - K}{N_i} \frac{\partial^2 N_i}{\partial^2 s} ds.$$

Using (3.2.2), the first integral on right hand side becomes negative, for all values of $N_i \neq K$.

Since under both set of boundary conditions,

$$\sum_{i=1}^{n} D_i \int_{L_{i-1}}^{L_i} \frac{N_i - K}{N_i} \frac{\partial^2 N_i}{\partial^2 s} ds = -\sum_{i=1}^{n} D_i \int_{L_{i-1}}^{L_i} \frac{K}{N_i^2} \left(\frac{\partial N_i}{\partial s}\right)^2 ds < 0.$$

Hence $V(N) < 0$, and $\dot{v}(t)(K) = 0$. Therefore, $\dot{V}(N)$ is negative definite over $N > 0$ with respect to $N = K$. Hence, the theorem. □

3.4 Summary

A dynamical model of a single species population in two patch habitats with harvesting and migration has been studied in this chapter. From application point of view, one may think of two adjoining forest stands whose carrying capacities are different due to soil and other environmental conditions.

By analyzing the model, it is shown that there exists a uniquely positive, monotonic, continuous steady state solution in both reservoir and no-flux boundary conditions. Moreover, the stability of the system is discussed for both linear and nonlinear cases. It is also shown that the uniform steady state is globally asymptotically stable. Further, the comparison between the uniform and the non-uniform steady state solutions indicate that the patchiness decreases the stability of the system and the effect of harvesting is to decrease the level of equilibrium but to enhances the stability.

Chapter 4

A Single Species Model with Supplementary Forest Resource in a Two-Patch Habitat

4.1 Introduction

Deforestation of a forest habitat caused by industrialization, pollution, and increasing population, is of great concern to all humankind. A typical example in this regard is the depletion of the forest resources in the Doon Valley located in the foothills of Himalayas, Uttarakhand, India. Here the depletion of the forest has been caused mainly by limestone quarrying, paper, and other wood-based industries and associated population migration [169]. Shukla et al. [164] have proposed a mathematical model for forest depletion caused by resource independent industrialization (population) by considering the spatial distribution of both the forest biomass as well as the density of industrialization. By studying the behavior of uniform steady state solution, they have shown that if industrialization increases without control, the forest biomass may not last long. Freedman and Shukla [41] have proposed and analyzed the effect of diffusion and an alternative resource of predator population on predator-prey systems. They, however, did not consider the effect of patchiness in the habitat.

In real ecological situations when the forest is degraded by industrialization distributed spatially, patchiness is caused in the forest habitat. The associated population distributed non-uniformly and dependent upon resource biomass is also found to be causing patchiness. It is noted that little effort has been made to study such systems using mathematical models [47, 54, 164]. Freedman et al. [54] considered a single species diffusion model by assuming that the habitat consists of two adjoining patches and shown that there exists a positive, monotonic, continuous non-uniform steady state solution that is linear asymptotically stable under both reservoir and no-flux boundary conditions. Freedman and Kriszti [47] have also considered the same problem in three patch habitat and shown that the positive steady state solution is piece-wise monotonic.

It may be expected that in presence of supplementary or alternative resources the steady state distributions of species population will be higher and more stable than the previous cases [47, 54, 55]. In this chapter, we therefore, study the effect of supplementary self-renewable resource on a single species population with diffusion in a two patch habitat. The aim here is to show qualitatively that non-uniform steady state distribution of the species population is positive, continuous and monotonic throughout the habitat and the level of distribution is higher than the case of without supplementary resource. We also obtain the conditions for stability of the system in both linear and nonlinear cases.

The organization of this chapter is as follows. In Section 4.2, we describe the general mathematical model for two patches. In Section 4.3, we analyzed our model without diffusion and with diffusion in Subsections 4.3.1 and 4.3.2, respectively. In Section 4.4, we analyzed our model with diffusion in a two patch habitat. In the Section 4.5, we analyze the model under reserve boundary conditions and under no-flux boundary conditions and in the Section 4.6, we discussed the system when the species population is uniform throughout the habitat. Finally in Section 4.7, the summary is provided.

4.2 Formulation of Mathematical Model

We consider a linear forest habitat $0 \leq s \leq L_2$, consisting of two adjoining patches $L_{i-1} \leq s \leq L_i$, for $i = 1, 2$, where $L_0 = 0$ and L_1 is the interface of the two region. Let $R_i(s,t)$ is the density of the non-diffusing self-renewable supplementary resource and $N_i(s,t)$, be the densities of the species population at location s and time t in the above mentioned i-th patch, for $i = 1,2$. It is assumed that $R_i(s,t)$ grows logistically in both these regions with the different intrinsic growth rates (r_i) and the same carrying capacity (C). Further, we assume that the growth rates $\mathbf{g}_i(N_i)$ of $N_i(s,t)$, $i = 1,2$ is general logistic type in absence of the supplementary resource and is different in each patch. Keeping in view of the above, the model governing the system can be written as follows:

$$\frac{\partial R_i}{\partial t} = r_i R_i (1 - \frac{R_i}{C}) - \beta_i R_i N_i, \tag{4.2.1}$$

$$\frac{\partial N_i}{\partial t} = N_i \mathbf{g}_i(N_i) + \theta_i \beta_i R_i N_i + D_i \frac{\partial^2 N_i}{\partial s^2}, \tag{4.2.2}$$

$$\beta_i,\ \theta_i \geq 0, \quad 0 \leq s \leq L_2, \quad i = 1,2,$$

where β_i and θ_i are, respectively, depletion rates of resource and the conversion rates of resource biomass in the corresponding regions; and D_i are the diffusion coefficient of $N_i(s,t)$ in the i-th region, respectively, for $i = 1,2$.

The growth rate $\mathbf{g}_i(N_i)$ functions are such that

(H.1): $\mathbf{g}_i(N_i) \in C^2[0,\infty)$, $\mathbf{g}_i(0) > 0$, and $\forall\ N_i \geq 0$, $\mathbf{g}_i'(N_i) \leq 0$.

We note that when the habitat has carrying capacity K_i in the i-th patch respectively, then $\mathbf{g}_i(K_i) = 0$.

Further we assume that

(H.2): $\exists\ R_i^*, K_i^* > 0$ such that

$$\mathbf{g}_i(K_i^*) + \theta_i \beta_i R_i^* = 0 \ \text{ and } \ r_i(1 - \frac{R_i^*}{C}) - \beta_i K_i^* = 0.$$

It is clear that the equilibrium level of population increases as the level of supplementary resource density increases and $R_i^* \leq C$ and $K_i^* \geq K_i$ both analytically and numerically.

The model (4.2.1) and (4.2.2) is studied under both reservoir and no-flux boundary conditions separately. In reservoir boundary conditions, we assume,

$$N_1(0,t) = K_1^* \text{ and } N_2(L_2,t) = K_2^*, \tag{4.2.3}$$

and in the case of no-flux boundary conditions, we have

$$\frac{\partial N_1(0,t)}{\partial s} = 0 = \frac{\partial N_2(L_2,t)}{\partial s}. \tag{4.2.4}$$

To study the behavior of non-uniform solutions, we also assume the continuity and flux matching conditions for $N_i(s,t)$ at the interface $s = L_1, \forall\, t \geq 0$, as

$$N_1(L_1,t) = N_2(L_1,t), \; D_1\frac{\partial N_1}{\partial s}(L_1,t) = D_2\frac{\partial N_2}{\partial s}(L_1,t). \tag{4.2.5}$$

Since the resource $R_i(s,t)$ is non-diffusing, these types of boundary and matching conditions are not required as there is no diffusion term in (4.2.1). It is further noted that at $s = L_1$, $R_i(s,t)$ will be continuous or discontinuous according as different levels of depletion rates in the two patches.

Finally the model is completed by assuming some positive initial distribution for both forest resource biomass density and population density, that is,

$$R_i(s,0) = \chi_i(s) > 0, \; L_{i-1} < s < L_i, \tag{4.2.6}$$

$$N_i(s,0) = \delta_i(s) > 0, \; L_{i-1} < s < L_i. \tag{4.2.7}$$

Our main aim is to study the behavior of the non-uniform steady state solutions of the above model, in the region $0 \leq s \leq L_2$, as this will through light on the effect of supplementary resource on the species survival in the habitat.

Before we study our original model, in the following, we state some important results for the corresponding model in a single homogeneous habitat $0 \leq s \leq L_2$ without and with diffusion.

4.3 Analysis of the Model in a Homogeneous Habitat

4.3.1 Model without Diffusion

In this case both the supplementary forest resource biomass and species population are uniformly distributed for all $0 \leq s \leq L_2$ without diffusion. Our model reduces to the following form:

$$\frac{dR}{dt} = rR(1-\frac{R}{C}) - \beta RN, \tag{4.3.1}$$

$$\frac{dN}{dt} = aN(1-\frac{N}{K}) + \theta\beta RN. \tag{4.3.2}$$

From Eqs. (4.3.1) and (4.3.2), it follows that there are four equilibria, namely $E_0 = [0,0]$, $E_C = [0,C]$, $E_K = [K,0]$ and $E^* = [R^*, K^*]$, where

$$R^* = \frac{aC(r-\beta K)}{ra+\beta^2\theta CK}, \quad K^* = \frac{rK(a+\beta\theta C)}{ra+\beta^2\theta CK}, \quad \text{provided } r > \beta K. \tag{4.3.3}$$

It is also noted from (4.3.3) that, $R^* \leq C$ and $K^* \geq K$. The nature of R^* and K^* with respect to various parameters is shown in the following table, which can be checked analytically.

TABLE 4.1 Effects of Various Parameters on R^* and K^*, Where $\uparrow$ and $\downarrow$ Means Increase and Decrease, Respectively

(i)	$r\uparrow$	$R^*\uparrow$	$K^*\uparrow$
(ii)	$a\uparrow$	$R^*\uparrow$	$K^*\downarrow$
(iii)	$C\uparrow$	$R^*\uparrow$	$K^*\uparrow$
(iv)	$M\uparrow$	$R^*\downarrow$	$K^*\uparrow$
(v)	$\theta\uparrow$	$R^*\downarrow$	$K^*\uparrow$
(vi)	$\beta\uparrow$ $R^* > C/2$	$R^*\downarrow$	$K^*\uparrow$

The variational matrix of the system is given by

$$[M] = \begin{bmatrix} r(1-2R/C)-\beta N & -\beta R \\ \theta\beta N & a(1-2N/K)-\theta\beta R \end{bmatrix}. \tag{4.3.4}$$

From (4.3.4) and the standard stability theory, we note the following obvious observations. The equilibria E_0 is always unstable. The equilibrium points E_C and E_K are stable or saddle point according as $a+\theta\beta C$ and $r-\beta K$ are negative or positive respectively. It is also observed that the most interesting interior (non-zero) equilibria E^* is locally stable, if it exists (i.e. $r>\beta K$).

Alternatively, if $r>\beta K$, then by using the following positive definite functions,

$$V(R,N) = d(R-R^*)^2 + (N-K^*)^2, \tag{4.3.5}$$

where d is a positive constant,

$$V(N,R) = \left(R - R^* - R^* ln\frac{R}{R^*}\right) + \theta\left(N - K^* - K^* ln\frac{N}{K^*}\right), \tag{4.3.6}$$

and by Lyapunov direct method, we conclude that the equilibria E^* is locally as well as globally asymptotically stable.

4.3.2 Model with Diffusion

Now, we study the behavior of the uniform steady state solution of the system (4.2.1)–(4.2.7) with diffusion in a single homogeneous habitat. In this case we consider that both the populations are not spatially uniformly distributed. Here, $R_i(s,t)$, $N_i(s,t)$, α_i, K_i, D_i, and β_i becomes $R(s,t)$, $N(s,t)$, a, K, D, and β, respectively, $\forall s\in[0,L_2]$. Then the model in this case can be written as,

$$\frac{\partial R}{\partial t} = rR(1-\frac{R}{C}) - \beta RN, \tag{4.3.7}$$

$$\frac{\partial N}{\partial t}(s,t) = aN(1-\frac{N}{K}) + \theta\beta RN + D\frac{\partial^2 N}{\partial s^2}(s,t), \tag{4.3.8}$$

$$0\le\theta\le 1,\;\; \beta\ge 0,\;\; 0\le s\le L_2.$$

The boundary and initial conditions are respectively,

$$N(0,t) = K^* = N(L_2,t) \tag{4.3.9}$$

or

$$\frac{\partial N(0,t)}{\partial s} = 0 = \frac{\partial N(L_2,t)}{\partial s}, \tag{4.3.10}$$

and

$$R(s,0) = \chi(s) > 0,\ 0 < s < L_2, \tag{4.3.11}$$

$$N(s,0) = \delta(s) > 0,\ 0 < s < L_2. \tag{4.3.12}$$

Theorem 4.3.1. *The uniform steady state of the system, i.e.* (R^*, K^*) *is locally as well as globally asymptotically stable if* $r > \beta K$.

Therefore if an equilibrium is stable in non-diffusing case, it is always stable with diffusion. Hence there is no diffusion instability of the system.

Now we go for our original model, and study the behavior of the non-uniform steady state solutions of the system.

4.4 Analysis of the Model with Diffusion in a Two-Patch Habitat

We consider the steady state problem of the system (4.2.1)–(4.2.7). Our aim is to show that there exists a non-uniform positive, continuous and monotonic steady state distribution of the species population $(u_i(s))$ under reservoir boundary conditions and with continuous flux matching at the interface $s = L_1$. We will note later that the steady state distribution of the supplementary forest resource biomass $(w_i(s), i = 1,2)$ in each region of the habitat are positive, continuous and monotonic but there is a continuous or jump discontinuous at the interface $s = L_1$. The steady-state system takes the form,

$$r_i w_i \left(1 - \frac{w_i}{C}\right) - \beta_i w_i u_i = 0, \tag{4.4.1}$$

$$D_i \frac{d^2 u_i}{ds^2} + u_i g_i(u_i) + \theta_i \beta_i w_i u_i = 0. \tag{4.4.2}$$

The reservoir boundary conditions are

$$u_1(0,t) = K_1^*, \;\; u_2(L_2,t) = K_2^*, \tag{4.4.3}$$

and the continuous and the matching conditions at the interface are

$$u_1(L_1) = u_2(L_1), \;\; D_1 \frac{du_1}{ds}(L_1) = D_2 \frac{du_2}{ds}(L_1). \tag{4.4.4}$$

Again from (4.4.1), we can solve w_i as a function of u_i, as follows

$$w_i = C\left(1 - \frac{\beta_i}{r_i}u_i\right), \;\; i = 1,2. \tag{4.4.5}$$

From (4.4.5) it is clear that if u_i are continuously monotonically increasing (decreasing) then w_i are continuously monotonically decreasing (increasing) with continuity or discontinuity at the interface $s = L_1$, according as

$$\frac{\beta_1}{r_1} = \frac{\beta_2}{r_2}, \;\; \text{or} \;\; \frac{\beta_1}{r_1} \neq \frac{\beta_2}{r_2}. \tag{4.4.6}$$

Now by substituting the value of w_i from (4.4.5) in (4.4.2), we get

$$D_i \frac{d^2 u_i}{ds^2} + u_i \mathbf{G}_i(u_i) = 0, \;\; i = 1,2, \tag{4.4.7}$$

where $\mathbf{G}_i(u_i) = \mathbf{g}_i(u_i) + \theta_i\beta_i C(1 - \beta_i u_i/r_i)$, and $\mathbf{G}_i(0) > 0$, $\mathbf{G}_i'(u_i) \leq 0, \; \forall u_i \neq 0$. Therefore $\mathbf{G}_i(u_i)$ is logistic function.

Exactly as same in previous chapter, there exists an unique steady state solution u of (4.4.7) satisfies

$$min\,\{K_1^*, K_2^*\} \leq u(s) \leq max\,\{K_1^*, K_2^*\}.$$

We now consider without loss of generality $0 < K_1^* \leq u_i \leq K_2^*$.

Let $p_i(s,\alpha_i)$, $L_{i-1} \le s \le L_i$, are the unique solution of the equation (4.4.7), for i = 1, 2. Further $p_i(s,\alpha_i)$ are such that

$$\frac{\partial p_1}{\partial s}(0,\alpha_1) = \alpha_1, \quad p_1(0,\alpha_1) = K_1^*,$$

$$\frac{\partial p_2}{\partial s}(L_2,\alpha_2) = \alpha_2, \quad p_2(L_2,\alpha_2) = K_2^*.$$

To show the existence of the monotonic solutions means that there exists α_1 and α_2 such that

$$p_1(L_1,\alpha_1) = p_2(L_1,\alpha_2), \quad D_1\frac{\partial p_1}{\partial s}(L_1,\alpha_1) = D_2\frac{\partial p_1}{\partial s}(L_1,\alpha_2).$$

Multiplying both side of (4.4.7) by $2du_i/ds$ and integrating from 0 if $i = 1$ and from L_2 if $i = 2$, we get

$$\left[\frac{du_i}{ds}\right]^2 = \alpha_i^2 - \frac{2}{D_i}\int_{K_i^*}^{u_i(s)} \xi_i \mathbf{G}_i(\xi_i)d\xi_i(s). \tag{4.4.8}$$

Hence using (4.4.8) and in similar manner as in the previous chapter, the following Lemma and Theorem hold.

Lemma 4.4.1. *If* $\alpha_1 > 0$ *, then*

$$\frac{\partial p_1(s,\alpha_1)}{\partial s} > \alpha_1 \text{ on } 0 < s \le L_1.$$

Lemma 4.4.2. *If* $0 < p_2 < K_2^*$ *and* $\alpha_2 > 0$*, then*

$$\frac{\partial p_2(s,\alpha_2)}{\partial s} > \alpha_2, \quad L_1 \le s < L_2.$$

Lemma 4.4.3. *Define* $F_i(\alpha_i)$ *by* $F_i(\alpha_i) = p_i(L_1,\alpha_i)$*. Then there exists* $\hat{\alpha}_i > 0$ *such that*

$$F_1 : [0,\hat{\alpha}_1] \to [K_1^*,\, K_2^*],$$

$$F_2 : [0,\hat{\alpha}_2] \to [K_2^*,\, K_1^*].$$

Theorem 4.4.4. *There exists a continuous, monotonic solution u_i of species population with the no-flux boundary conditions (4.4.3) and continuous flux at L_1.*

Proof. Lemmas 4.4.1 and 4.4.2 follows that any solution we construct must be monotonic. By Lemma 4.4.3, for each $0 \leq \alpha_2 \leq \hat{\alpha}_2$, we can find α_1 such that $0 \leq \alpha_1 \leq \hat{\alpha}_1$ for which $p_1(L_1, \alpha_1) = p_2(L_1, \alpha_2)$. Hence α_1 can be solved as a function of α_2, $\alpha_1 = h(\alpha_2)$, to give a continuous solution of (4.4.7) with (4.4.3) and (4.4.4).
Let

$$\mathbf{G}(\alpha_2) = D_1 \frac{\partial p_1(L_1, h(\alpha_2))}{\partial s} - D_2 \frac{\partial p_2(L_1, \alpha_2)}{\partial s}.$$

Clearly $\mathbf{G}(\alpha_2)$ is continuous on $0 \leq \alpha_2 \leq \hat{\alpha}_2$. Then we have

$$\mathbf{G}(0) = D_1 \frac{\partial p_1(L_1, \hat{\alpha}_1)}{\partial s} > 0,$$

and

$$\mathbf{G}(\hat{\alpha}_2) = -D_2 \frac{\partial p_2(L_1, \hat{\alpha}_2)}{\partial s} < 0.$$

Hence the theorem. □

Remark: From the Theorem 4.4.4, it is noted that if $K_1^* > K_2^*$ (or $K_1^* < K_2^*$) then the steady state solution u_i is monotonically increasing (or decreasing), for $0 \leq s \leq L_2$ and accordingly from (4.4.5), w_i is also continuously decreases (or increases) in both the regions, $0 \leq s < L_1$ and $L_1 \leq s \leq L_2$. Further the steady state distribution w_i of forest resource continuous and monotonic in each regions but continuous or discontinuous at the interface of the two adjoining regions (4.4.6).

Now, we find the conditions for asymptotic stability in both linear and non-linear case.

Theorem 4.4.5. *The steady-state continuous, monotonic solutions of system (4.4.2) and (4.4.1) with continuous solutions and flux at the interface $s = L_1$ is locally asymptotically stable if*

$$\mathscr{B}_i = \mathbf{g}_i(u_i) + u_i \mathbf{g}_i'(u_i) + \theta_i \beta_i w_i \leq 0, \tag{4.4.9}$$

and

$$\alpha_i^2 [w_i - \theta_i u_i]^2 \leq 4 \mathscr{A}_i \mathscr{B}_i, \tag{4.4.10}$$

where

$$\mathscr{A}_i = r_i\left(1-\frac{2w_i}{C}\right)-\beta_i u_i = -\frac{r_i w_i}{C} \leq 0, \ \ for\ i=1,2.$$

Proof. Let the steady-state solution of system (4.4.1) be

$$w(s) = \begin{cases} w_1(s),\ 0 \leq s \leq L_1 \\ w_2(s),\ L_1 \leq s \leq L_2, \end{cases}$$

and let the steady-state solution of system (4.4.2) be

$$u(s) = \begin{cases} u_1(s),\ 0 \leq s \leq L_1 \\ u_2(s),\ L_1 \leq s \leq L_2. \end{cases}$$

Linearizing (4.2.1) and (4.2.2) by using,

$$R_i(s,t) = w_i(s) + m_i(s,t), \tag{4.4.11}$$

$$N_i(s,t) = u_i(s) + n_i(s,t). \tag{4.4.12}$$

We have,

$$\frac{\partial m_i}{\partial t} = m_i\left[r_i\left(1-\frac{2w_i}{C}\right)-\beta_i u_i\right] - n_i\beta_i w_i, \tag{4.4.13}$$

$$\frac{\partial n_i}{\partial t} = n_i\left[\mathbf{g}_i(u_i) + u_i\mathbf{g}_i'(u_i) + \theta_i\beta_i w_i\right] + m_i\theta_i\beta_i u_i + D_i\frac{\partial^2 n_i}{\partial s^2}. \tag{4.4.14}$$

Using (4.4.11) the corresponding boundary and matching conditions can be obtained as follows

$$n_1(0,t) = K_1^*,\ \ n_2(L_2,t) = K_2^*, \tag{4.4.15}$$

$$n_1(L_1,t) = n_2(L_1,t),\ \ D_1\frac{\partial n_1}{\partial s}(L_1,t) = D_2\frac{\partial n_2}{\partial s}(L_1,t). \tag{4.4.16}$$

Now we consider the following positive definite function,

$$V(t) = \sum_1^2 \int_{L_{i-1}}^{L_i} \frac{1}{2}\left[m_i^2 + n_i^2\right] ds, \tag{4.4.17}$$

from which we get,

$$\dot{V}(t) = \sum_{1}^{2} \int_{L_{i-1}}^{L_i} \left[m_i \frac{\partial m_i}{\partial t} + n_i \frac{\partial n_i}{\partial t} \right] ds. \qquad (4.4.18)$$

By using (4.4.13), (4.4.14), (4.4.15) and (4.4.16), and integration by parts, we get,

$$\begin{aligned} \dot{V}(t) &= \sum_{1}^{2} \int_{L_{i-1}}^{L_i} m_i^2 \mathscr{A}_i ds - \sum_{1}^{2} \int_{L_{i-1}}^{L_i} n_i m_i [\beta_i w_i - \theta_i \beta_i u_i] ds \\ &\quad + \sum_{1}^{2} \int_{L_{i-1}}^{L_i} n_i^2 \mathscr{B}_i ds - \sum_{1}^{2} D_i \int_{L_{i-1}}^{L_i} \left[\frac{\partial n_i}{\partial s} \right]^2 ds, \qquad (4.4.19) \end{aligned}$$

where

$$\mathscr{A}_i = r_i \left(1 - \frac{2w_i}{C} \right) - \beta_i u_i \text{ and } \mathscr{B}_i = \mathbf{g}_i(u_i) + u_i \mathbf{g}_i'(u_i) + \theta_i \beta_i w_i.$$

Again, by using (4.4.5), for $i = 1, 2$, we get

$$\mathscr{A}_i = -\frac{2r_i w_i}{C} + r_i \left(1 - \frac{\beta_i}{r_i} u_i \right) = -\frac{r_i w_i}{C} \leq 0, \qquad (4.4.20)$$

and for $i = 1$,

$$\mathscr{B}_1 = \mathbf{g}_1(u_1) + u_1 \mathbf{g}_1'(u_1) + \theta_i \beta_i C \left(1 - \frac{\beta_1}{r_1} u_1 \right) \leq 0, \qquad (4.4.21)$$

since $u_1 \geq K_1^* \geq K_1$, therefore $\mathbf{g}_1(u_1) \leq 0$ and $\mathbf{g}_1'(u_1) \leq 0$, $\forall\ u_1$. Hence the condition (4.4.21) is a very weak condition, later, we will show in an example that for simple logistic $\mathbf{g}_1(u_1) = a_1(1 - u_1/K_1)$, the condition is automatically satisfied.

From (4.4.19) it is noted that $\dot{V}(t)$ is negative definite, if the conditions (4.4.9) and (4.4.10) are satisfied, for $i = 1, 2$. □

In a similar manner, the following nonlinear stability result can be proved using positive definite function same as Theorem 4.4.5. We consider the case, when $K_1^* \leq K_2^*$, then $R_1^* \geq R_2^*$.

Theorem 4.4.6. *The steady-state continuous, monotonic solutions of nonlinear system (4.4.2) to (4.4.4) with continuous flux at the interface* $s = L_1$ *is asymptotically stable in the subregion of* $\mathbf{R}$*:* $\{R_2^* \leq R_i, w_i \leq R_1^*;\ K_1^* \leq N_i, u_i \leq K_2^*\}$*, provided the following conditions are satisfied:*

(*i*)
$$\mathscr{F}_{1i} = \frac{N_i \mathbf{g}_i(N_i) - u_i \mathbf{g}_i(u_i)}{N_i - u_i} + \theta_i \beta_i R_i \leq 0,$$

(*ii*)
$$\mathscr{F}_{2i} = r_i \left(1 - \frac{R_i + w_i}{C}\right) - \beta_i N_i \leq 0,$$

(*iii*)
$$\beta_i^2 \left[w_i - \theta_i u_i\right]^2 \leq 4 \mathscr{F}_{1i} \mathscr{F}_{2i}.$$

4.5 A Particular Case

For clarity and simplification, we take an example by considering $\mathbf{g}_i(N_i) = a_i(1 - N_i/K_i)$. Then the corresponding system can be written as,

$$\frac{\partial R_i}{\partial t} = r_i R_i (1 - \frac{R_i}{C}) - \beta_i R_i N_i, \tag{4.5.1}$$

$$\frac{\partial N_i}{\partial t} = a_i N_i (1 - N_i/K_i) + \theta_i \beta_i R_i N_i + D_i \frac{\partial^2 N_i}{\partial s^2}. \tag{4.5.2}$$

The existence of non-negative equilibrium (R^*, K^*) is given by,

$$R_i^* = \frac{\alpha_i C(r_i - \beta_i K_i)}{r\alpha_i + \beta_i^2 \theta_i C K_i}, \quad K_i^* = \frac{r_i K_i(\alpha_i + \beta_i \theta_i C)}{r_i \alpha_i + \beta_i^2 \theta_i C K_i}, \quad \text{provided } r_i > \beta_i K_i.$$

From above it is clear that $R_i^* \leq C$ and $K_i^* \geq K_i$. This shows that the effect of supplementary resource is to increase the equilibrium level of the species population. Also, we note that in absence of interaction (i.e. $\beta_i = 0$), $R_1^* = R_2^* = C$ and the biomass is uniformly distributed in the entire habitat.

The model is completed by taking same boundary, matching and initial conditions as in the general case (4.2.3) $\rightarrow$ (4.2.7).

Similar as the general case we study the above system (4.5.1) and (4.5.2) with (4.2.3) $\rightarrow$ (4.2.7) in two patch habitat ($0 \leq s \leq L_2$).

Case 1: Under Reservoir Boundary Conditions

Consider the following steady state system,

$$r_i w_i \left(1 - \frac{w_i}{C}\right) - \beta_i w_i u_i = 0, \tag{4.5.3}$$

$$D_i \frac{d^2 u_i}{ds^2} + \alpha_i u_i \left(1 - \frac{u_i}{K_i}\right) + \theta_i \beta_i w_i u_i = 0, \tag{4.5.4}$$

with (4.4.3) and (4.4.4).

Again from (4.5.3), we can solve w_i as a function of u_i, as follows

$$w_i = C\left(1 - \frac{\beta_i}{r_i} u_i\right), \ i = 1, 2. \tag{4.5.5}$$

From (4.5.5) it is clear that if u_i are continuously monotonically increasing (decreasing) then w_i are continuously monotonically decreasing (increasing) with continuity or discontinuity at the interface $s = L_1$, according as

$$\frac{\beta_1}{r_1} = \frac{\beta_2}{r_2}, \ \text{ or } \ \frac{\beta_1}{r_1} \neq \frac{\beta_2}{r_2}. \tag{4.5.6}$$

Now by substituting the value of w_i from (4.5.5) in (4.5.4), we get

$$D_i \frac{d^2 u_i}{ds^2} + C_i u_i \left(1 - \frac{u_i}{K_i^*}\right) = 0, \ \ i = 1, 2, \tag{4.5.7}$$

where $C_i = \alpha_i + \theta_i \beta_i C$.

Exactly as same in Chapter 3, there exists an unique steady state solution u of (4.5.7) satisfies

$$min\ \{K_1^*, K_2^*\} \leq u(s) \leq max\ \{K_1^*, K_2^*\}.$$

We now consider without loss of generality $0 < K_1^* \leq u_i \leq K_2^*$.

Let $p_i(s,\alpha_i),\ L_{i-1} \leq s \leq L_i$, are the unique solution of the equation (4.5.7), for $i = 1,2$. Also $p_i(s,\alpha_i)$ are such that

$$\frac{\partial p_1}{\partial s}(0,\alpha_1) = \alpha_1, \quad p_1(0,\alpha_1) = K_1^*,$$

$$\frac{\partial p_2}{\partial s}(L_2,\alpha_2) = \alpha_2, \quad p_2(L_2,\alpha_2) = K_2^*.$$

Multiplying both side of (4.5.7) by $2du_i/ds$ and integrating from 0 if $i = 1$ and from L_2 if $i = 2$, we get

$$\left[\frac{du_i}{ds}\right]^2 = \alpha_i^2 - \frac{2}{D_i}\int_{K_i^*}^{u_i(s)} \left[C_i\xi_i\left(1-\frac{\xi_i}{K_i^*}\right)\right] d\xi_i(s). \tag{4.5.8}$$

Hence by using (4.5.8), the following theorem holds.

Theorem 4.5.1. *There exists a continuous, monotonic solution u_i of species population with the no-flux boundary conditions (4.4.3) and continuous flux at L_1.*

Now we find the most interesting results, the conditions for asymptotic stability in both linear and non-linear case.

Theorem 4.5.2. *The steady-state continuous, monotonic solutions of system (4.5.3) and (4.5.4) with continuous solutions and flux at the interface $s = L_1$ is locally asymptotically stable if*

$$K_1^* \leq u_1 \leq min.\left\{K_2^*, \ \frac{F_1 + (F_1^2 - 4E_1G_1)^{1/2}}{2E_1}\right\}, \tag{4.5.9}$$

and

$$max.\left\{K_1^*, \ \frac{r_2K_2(\alpha_2 + \theta_2\beta_2C)}{2\alpha_2r_2 + \theta_2\beta_2^2CK_2}, \ \frac{F_2 - (F_2^2 - 4E_2G_2)^{1/2}}{2E_2}\right\} \leq u_2 \leq K_2^*. \tag{4.5.10}$$

Proof. Let the steady state solution of system (4.5.3) be

$$w(s) = \begin{cases} w_1(s), & 0 \le s \le L_1 \\ w_2(s), & L_1 \le s \le L_2. \end{cases}$$

Also, let the steady-state solution of system (4.5.4) be

$$u(s) = \begin{cases} u_1(s), & 0 \le s \le L_1 \\ u_2(s), & L_1 \le s \le L_2. \end{cases}$$

Linearizing (4.2.1) and (4.2.2) by using,

$$R_i(s,t) = w_i(s) + m_i(s,t), \tag{4.5.11}$$

and

$$N_i(s,t) = u_i(s) + n_i(s,t). \tag{4.5.12}$$

We have,

$$\frac{\partial m_i}{\partial t} = m_i \left[r\left(1 - \frac{2w_i}{C}\right) - \beta_i u_i \right] - n_i \beta_i w_i, \tag{4.5.13}$$

$$\frac{\partial n_i}{\partial t} = n_i \left[\alpha_i \left(1 - \frac{2u_i}{K_i}\right) + \theta_i \beta_i w_i \right] + m_i \theta_i \beta_i u_i + D_i \frac{\partial^2 n_i}{\partial s^2}. \tag{4.5.14}$$

Using (4.5.11) and (4.5.12) the corresponding boundary and matching conditions can be obtained as follows

$$n_1(0,t) = K_1^*, \;\; n_2(L_2,t) = K_2^*, \tag{4.5.15}$$

$$n_1(L_1,t) = n_2(L_1,t), \;\; D_1 \frac{\partial n_1}{\partial s}(L_1,t) = D_2 \frac{\partial n_2}{\partial s}(L_1,t). \tag{4.5.16}$$

Now we consider the following positive definite function,

$$V(t) = \sum_1^2 \int_{L_{i-1}}^{L_i} \frac{1}{2} \left[m_i^2 + n_i^2 \right] ds. \tag{4.5.17}$$

From which we get,

$$\dot{V}(t) = \sum_1^2 \int_{L_{i-1}}^{L_i} \left[m_i \frac{\partial m_i}{\partial t} + n_i \frac{\partial n_i}{\partial t} \right] ds. \tag{4.5.18}$$

By using (4.5.13), (4.5.14), (4.5.15) and (4.5.16), and integration by parts, we get,

$$\begin{aligned}\dot{V}(t) &= \sum_1^2 \int_{L_{i-1}}^{L_i} m_i^2 \mathscr{A}_i ds - \sum_1^2 \int_{L_{i-1}}^{L_i} n_i m_i [\beta_i w_i - \theta_i \beta_i u_i] ds \\ &\quad + \sum_1^2 \int_{L_{i-1}}^{L_i} n_i^2 \mathscr{B}_i ds - \sum_1^2 D_i \int_{L_{i-1}}^{L_i} \left[\frac{\partial n_i}{\partial s}\right]^2 ds, \qquad (4.5.19)\end{aligned}$$

where

$$\mathscr{A}_i = r_i\left(1 - \frac{2w_i}{C}\right) - \beta_i u_i \text{ and } \mathscr{B}_i = \alpha_i\left(1 - \frac{2u_i}{K_i}\right) + \theta_i \beta_i w_i.$$

Again, by using (4.5.5), for $i = 1,2$, we get

$$\mathscr{A}_i = -\frac{r_i w_i}{C} < 0, \qquad (4.5.20)$$

$$\mathscr{B}_i = (\alpha_i + \theta_i \beta_i C) - \left[\frac{\alpha_i + \theta_i \beta_i C}{N_i^*} + \frac{\alpha_i}{K_i}\right] u_i. \qquad (4.5.21)$$

Let

$$M_i = \alpha_i + \theta_i \beta_i C, \quad \mathscr{N}_i = \frac{M_i}{K_i^*} + \frac{\alpha_i}{K_i}.$$

Now from (4.5.21), we note that for $\mathscr{B}_i \leq 0$, we have

$$u_i \geq \frac{M_i}{\mathscr{N}_i} = \frac{r_i K_i (\alpha_i + \theta_i \beta_i C)}{2\alpha_i r_i + \theta_i \beta_i^2 C K_i}, \quad i = 1,2. \qquad (4.5.22)$$

Since $K_1^* \leq u_i \leq K_2^*$, it is clear from (4.5.22) that $u_1 \geq M_1/\mathscr{N}_1$ is automatically satisfied. Therefore this condition is required only for u_2, for $\mathscr{B}_2 \leq 0$.

From (4.5.19) it is noted that $\dot{V}(t)$ is negative definite, if (4.5.22) is satisfied along with the following condition, for $i = 1,2$,

$$\beta_i^2 [w_i - \theta_i u_i]^2 \leq 4 \mathscr{A}_i \mathscr{B}_i. \qquad (4.5.23)$$

Now from (4.5.23), by using (4.5.5) and solving for u_i, $i = 1,2$, we get

$$K_1^* \leq \frac{F_i - (F_i^2 - 4E_i G_i)^{1/2}}{2E_i} \leq u_i \leq \frac{F_i + (F_i^2 - 4E_i G_i)^{1/2}}{2E_i} \leq K_2^*, \qquad (4.5.24)$$

where

$$E_i = \beta_i^2\left(\theta_i + \frac{\beta_i C}{r_i}\right)^2 + 4\beta_i \mathcal{N}_i,$$

$$F_i = 2\beta_i\left(\theta_i + \frac{\beta_i C}{r_i}\right)C + 4(r_i\mathcal{N}_i + \beta_i K_i),$$

$$G_i = \beta_i^2 C^2 + 4r_i K_i.$$

Since $K_1^* \leq u_i \leq K_2^*$, and by using (4.5.22), (4.5.24), we get the conditions (4.5.9) and (4.5.10). Hence the theorem. □

The following numerical example shows the feasibility of the conditions (4.5.9) and (4.5.10).

Numerical Example: Choosing the system parameter values as

$$r = 0.2, \quad \alpha_1 = 0.2, \quad \alpha_2 = 0.25, \quad \beta_1 = 0.002, \quad \beta_2 = 0.0025,$$
$$C = 1000, \quad K_1 = 40, \quad K_2 = 70, \quad \theta_1 = 0.2, \quad \theta_2 = 0.5,$$

we get,

$$\begin{aligned}
&K_1^* = 66.6667,\\
&F_1 - (F_1^2 - 4E_1G_1)^{1/2}/2E_1 = 0.1098,\\
&F_2 - (F_2^2 - 4E_2G_2)^{1/2}/2E_2 = 0.1146,\\
&K_2^* = 78.1395,\\
&F_1 + (F_1^2 - 4E_1G_1)^{1/2}/2E_1 = 77295.45,\\
&F_2 + (F_2^2 - 4E_2G_2)^{1/2}/2E_2 = 50648.8.
\end{aligned}$$

Hence in this case, (4.5.9) and (4.5.10) becomes

$$K_1^* = 66.6667 \leq u_i \leq K_2^* = 78.1395, \quad i = 1, 2.$$

In a similar manner, the following nonlinear stability result can be proved by using positive definite function as in Theorem 4.4.5 for $K_1^* \leq K_2^*$.

Theorem 4.5.3. *The steady state continuous, monotonic solutions of nonlinear system with continuous flux at the interface $s = L_1$ is asymptotically stable in the subregion of* $\mathbf{R}$: $\{R_2^* \leq R_i, w_i \leq R_1^*;\ N_1^* \leq N_i, u_i \leq N_2^*\}$, *provided the following conditions are satisfied:*

(*i*)
$$\mathscr{F}_{1i} = \alpha_i\left(1 - \frac{N_i + u_i}{K_i}\right) + \theta_i\beta_i R_i \leq 0,$$

(*ii*)
$$\mathscr{F}_{2i} = r_i\left(1 - \frac{R_i + w_i}{C}\right) - \beta_i N_i \leq 0,$$

(iii) $$\beta_i^2\left[w_i-\theta_i u_i\right]^2 \leq 4\mathscr{F}_{1i}\mathscr{F}_{2i}.$$

Proof. By using (4.5.11) and (4.5.12) the nonlinear model (4.2.1) and (4.2.2), we get

$$\frac{\partial n_i}{\partial t}=n_i\left[\alpha_i\left(1-\frac{N_i+u_i}{K_i}\right)+\theta_i\beta_i R_i\right]+m_i\theta_i\beta_i u_i+D_i\frac{\partial^2 n_i}{\partial s^2}, \quad (4.5.25)$$

$$\frac{\partial m_i}{\partial t}=m_i\left[r_i\left(1-\frac{R_i+w_i}{C}\right)-\beta_i N_i\right]-n_i\beta_i w_i. \quad (4.5.26)$$

We consider the following positive definite function,

$$V(t)=\sum_1^2\int_{L_{i-1}}^{L_i}\frac{1}{2}\left[n_i^2+m_i^2\right]ds, \quad (4.5.27)$$

from which we get,

$$\begin{aligned}\dot{V}(t) &= \sum_{i=1}^2\int_{L_{i-1}}^{L_i} n_i^2\left[\alpha_i\left(1-\frac{N_i+u_i}{K_i}\right)+\theta_i\beta_i R_i\right]ds\\ &+ \sum_{i=1}^2\int_{L_{i-1}}^{L_i} m_i^2\left[r_i\left(1-\frac{R_i+w_i}{C}\right)-\beta_i N_i\right]ds\\ &+ \sum_{i=1}^2\int_{L_{i-1}}^{L_i}\beta_i\left(w_i-\theta_i u_i\right)ds+\sum_{i=1}^2 D_i\int_{L_{i-1}}^{L_i} n_i\frac{\partial^2 n_i}{\partial s^2}. \quad (4.5.28)\end{aligned}$$

Hence $\dot{V}(t)$ is negative definite if the conditions (i), (ii) and (iii) of the Theorem 4.5.3 holds. □

Note: The conditions (i) and (ii) are always satisfied if,

$$\alpha_i \leq min\left[\alpha_i\frac{N_i+u_i}{K_i}-\theta_i\beta_i R_i\right] \Rightarrow 1 \leq \frac{2K_1^*}{K_i}-\frac{\theta_i\beta_i}{\alpha_i}R_1^*, \quad (4.5.29)$$

$$r_i \leq min\left[r_i\frac{R_i+w_i}{C}+\beta_i N_i\right] \Rightarrow \frac{2R_2^*}{C}+\frac{\beta_i}{r_i}K_1^* \geq 1. \quad (4.5.30)$$

Now using (4.5.29) and (4.5.30), we get the condition (iii) is always satisfied if

$$\beta_i^2\left[R_1^{*2}+\theta_i^2K_2^{*2}-2\theta_iR_2^*K_1^*\right]$$
$$\leq 4\mathscr{G}\mathscr{F}_{1i}\mathscr{G}\mathscr{F}_{2i}\left[1-\frac{2K_1^*}{K_i}+\frac{\theta_i\beta_i}{\alpha_i}R_1^*\right]\left[1-\frac{2R_2^*}{C}-\frac{\beta_i}{r_i}K_1^*\right]. \tag{4.5.31}$$

Hence, the system is nonlinearly asymptotically stable if (4.5.29)–(4.5.31) are satisfied.

The above results imply that the system will settle down to the steady-state distribution in the two patches under certain conditions, the magnitude of the steady state distribution of supplementary resources biomass density being lower than it's original value but the density distribution of species population being correspondingly higher.

Case 2: Under No-Flux Boundary Conditions

The same analysis and results as in Case 1, are valid for no-flux boundary conditions also. Therefore, the non-uniform steady state is positive, monotonic and the system is linearly as well as nonlinearly stable under same set of condition as in Theorems 4.5.1, 4.5.2, and 4.5.3.

In this case, consider the steady state problem of the system (4.5.3) and (4.5.4) with no-flux boundary condition,

$$\frac{du_1}{ds}(0)=0=\frac{du_2}{ds}(L_2), \tag{4.5.32}$$

and continuity and flux matching conditions at the interface (4.4.4).

In this case also, there exists a non-uniform positive, continuous and monotonic steady state distribution of the species population density ($u_i(s)$). Further, the steady state distribution of the supplementary resource biomass ($w_i(s)$, $i=1,2$) in each region of the habitat are positive, continuous and monotonic, but there is a continuity or jump discontinuity at the interface $s=L_1$. Since,

$$w_i=C\left(1-\frac{\beta_i}{r_i}u_i\right),\ i=1,2. \tag{4.5.33}$$

In this case also, it is clear from the above that if u_i are continuously monotonically increasing (decreasing) then w_i are continuously monotonically decreasing (increasing) with continuity or discontinuity at the interface $s = L_1$, according as (4.4.6).

After substituting the value of w_i from (4.5.33) in (4.5.4), we get

$$D_i \frac{d^2 u_i}{ds^2} + C_i u_i \left(1 - \frac{u_i}{K_i^*}\right) = 0, \quad i = 1, 2, \tag{4.5.34}$$

where $C_i = \alpha_i + \theta_i \beta_i C$.

Let $p_i(s, \beta_i)$, $L_{i-1} \leq s \leq L_i$, are the unique solutions of (4.5.34), for $i = 1, 2$, such that

$$\frac{\partial p_1(0, \beta_1)}{\partial s} = 0 \ , \ p_1(0, \beta_1) = \beta_1, \tag{4.5.35}$$

$$\frac{\partial p_2(L_2, \beta_2)}{\partial s} = 0 \ , \ p_2(L_2, \beta_2) = \beta_2. \tag{4.5.36}$$

We will have shown the existence of the monotonic solutions if there exists β_1 and β_2 such that

$$p_1(L_1, \beta_1) = p_2(L_1, \beta_2) \ , \ D_1 \frac{\partial p_1(L_1, \beta_1)}{\partial s} = D_2 \frac{\partial p_2(L_1, \beta_2)}{\partial s}. \tag{4.5.37}$$

From (4.5.34), multiplying both side by $2du_i/ds$ and then integrating with respect to s from 0 if $i = 1$ and from L_2 if $i = 2$, we get

$$\left[\frac{du_i}{ds}\right]^2 = -\frac{2}{D_i} \int_{\beta_i}^{u_i(s)} \left[C_i u_i \left(1 - \frac{u_i}{N_i^*}\right)\right] du_i(s). \tag{4.5.38}$$

Then by exactly in similar manner as in [54], we can state the following theorem, for proof see the previous section.

Theorem 4.5.4. *There exists a continuous, monotonic solution u_i of species population with the no-flux boundary conditions (4.5.32) and continuous flux at L_1.*

We now study the linear and non-linear asymptotic stability of the non-uniform steady state solutions of the system (4.5.3), (4.5.4) with (4.4.4) and (4.5.32) using the Lyapunov direct method.

Theorem 4.5.5. *The steady-state continuous, monotonic solutions of system (4.5.3) and (4.5.4) with continuous solutions and flux at the interface $s = L_1$ is locally asymptotically stable if*

$$N_1^* \leq u_1 \leq min.\left\{N_2^*, \frac{F_1 + (F_1^2 - 4E_1G_1)^{1/2}}{2E_1}\right\}, \tag{4.5.39}$$

and

$$max.\left\{N_1^*, \frac{rK_2(\alpha_2 + \theta_2\beta_2 C)}{2\alpha_2 r + \theta_2\beta_2^2 CK_2}, \frac{F_2 - (F_2^2 - 4E_2G_2)^{1/2}}{2E_2}\right\} \leq u_2 \leq N_2^*. \tag{4.5.40}$$

Proof. Same as Theorem 4.4.5 and only difference is the condition (4.4.15) becomes,

$$\frac{\partial n_1}{\partial s}(0,t) = 0 = \frac{\partial n_2}{\partial s}(L_2,t). \tag{4.5.41}$$

□

In a similar manner, the following nonlinear stability result can be proved by using positive definite function, for $K_1^* \leq K_2^*$.

Theorem 4.5.6. *The steady state continuous, monotonic solutions of nonlinear system with continuous flux at the interface $s = L_1$ is asymptotically stable in the subregion of* $\mathbf{R}$: $\{R_2^* \leq R_i, w_i \leq R_1^*;\ N_1^* \leq N_i, u_i \leq N_2^*\}$, *provided the following conditions are satisfied:*

(*i*) $$\mathscr{F}_{1i} = \alpha_i\left(1 - \frac{N_i + u_i}{K_i}\right) + \theta_i\beta_i R_i \leq 0,$$

(*ii*) $$\mathscr{F}_{2i} = r_i\left(1 - \frac{R_i + w_i}{C}\right) - \beta_i u_i \leq 0,$$

(*iii*) $$\beta_i^2\left[w_i - \theta_i u_i\right]^2 \leq 4\mathscr{F}_{1i}\mathscr{F}_{2i}.$$

The above theorems imply that the system will settle down to the steady-state distribution in the two patches under certain conditions, the magnitude of the steady-state distribution of resources biomass density being lower than it's original value but the density distribution of industrialization being correspondingly higher.

4.6 When the Species Population is Uniform Throughout the Habitat

Now we consider the case when the species population is uniformly distributed between $[0, L_2]$, i.e., when $N_1(s,t) = N_2(s,t) = I^*$, $\forall\ s \in [0, L_2]$ and $\forall\ t \geq 0$. Since the depletion of supplementary resource $(R_i(s,t))$ due to population is different in different region, i.e., $\beta_1 \neq \beta_2$. Let $R_1(s,t) = R_1^*$, $0 \leq s < L_1$, $\forall\ t \geq 0$ and $R_2(s,t) = R_2^*$, $L_1 < s \leq L_2$, $\forall\ t \geq 0$. Without loss of generality, we choose $\beta_2 > \beta_1$, this implies from (4.4.5) that $R_1^* > R_2^*$. Now, we go for the globally stability of the system.

Theorem 4.6.1. *If $u_1 = u_2 = I^*$, $w_1 = R_1^*$ and $w_2 = R_2^*$, then the system is globally asymptotically stable.*

Proof. Let $V(x,y)$ be the positive definite function about $R_i = R_i^*$, $N_i = I^*$, given by

$$\begin{aligned} V(x,y) &= \sum_1^2 \theta_i \int_{L_{i-1}}^{L_i} \left(R_i - R_i^* - R_i^* ln \frac{R_i}{R_i^*} \right) ds \\ &\quad + \sum_1^2 \int_{L_{i-1}}^{L_i} \left(N_i - I^* - I^* ln \frac{N_i}{I^*} \right) ds. \end{aligned} \tag{4.6.1}$$

Differentiating (4.6.1) with respect to t, and using (4.2.1) and (4.2.2) we get,

$$\begin{aligned} \dot{V}(s,t) &= \sum_1^2 \int_{L_{i-1}}^{L_i} (R_i - R_i^*)^2 \left[-\frac{r\theta_i}{C} \right] ds + \sum_1^2 \int_{L_{i-1}}^{L_i} (N_i - I^*)^2 \left[-\frac{\alpha_i}{K_i} \right] ds \\ &+ \sum_1^2 D_i \int_{L_{i-1}}^{L_i} \frac{N_i - I^*}{N_i} \frac{\partial^2 N_i}{\partial s^2} ds. \end{aligned} \tag{4.6.2}$$

Since under both set of boundary conditions,

$$[x_1(0,t)-K^*]\frac{\partial x_1}{\partial s}(0,t)=[x_2(L_2,t)-K^*]\frac{\partial x_2}{\partial s}(L_2,t)=0. \qquad (4.6.3)$$

Then by using (4.6.3), we get

$$\sum_1^2 D_i\int_{L_{i-1}}^{L_i}\frac{N_i-I^*}{N_i}\frac{\partial^2 N_i}{\partial s^2}ds=-\sum_1^2 D_i\int_{L_{i-1}}^{L_i}\frac{I^*}{N_i^2}\left(\frac{\partial N_i}{\partial s}\right)^2 ds. \qquad (4.6.4)$$

Hence from (4.6.2) and (4.6.3), $\dot{V}<0\ \forall R_i\neq R_i^*,\ \forall N_i\neq I^*$, and $\dot{V}(R_i^*,\ I^*)=0$. Therefore $\dot{V}(R_i,N_i)$ is negative definite, proving the theorem. □

4.7 Summary

In this chapter, a mathematical model is proposed to study the role of supplementary renewable resource on a single species population model in a two patch habitat. In the model, it is assumed that the density of resource biomass is governed by the logistic equation with the different intrinsic growth rate but the same carrying capacity in the entire habitat. It is further assumed that the densities of species population are also governed by the logistic equations in both the regions but with different growth rates and carrying capacities. The rate of depletion of resource biomass density due to population is also considered to be different in the two regions.

It is shown that there exists a positive, monotonically increasing, a continuous steady-state solution with continuous flux, in the no-flux boundary conditions, for both forest resource biomass and species population. Moreover, the system is asymptotically stable in the both linear and non-linear cases under some conditions. It has been noted here that forest resources may remain at steady-state but a lower the level then it's carrying capacity.

Chapter 5

A Two Competing Species Model with Diffusion in a Homogeneous and Two-Patch Forest Habitats

5.1 Introduction

The mathematical modeling of competing populations in a habitat has become quite rigorous after the work of Lotka and Volterra. It is only during the last few decades that the environmental and ecological effects have been considered in the evolutionary processes of interacting species. These effects have been taken into account by identifying species migration which might have continuously varying properties due to environmental as well as ecological gradients in the habitat, and may depend upon densities as well as space coordinates of the species [41, 56, 170–177].

The patchiness in the habitat arises due to variety of factors such as geographical, climatic, degradation of the resource biomass, etc. It is known that the opportunities for migration and habitat diversification provided by the spatial changes in the environment make co-existence of species possible which could not otherwise survive. If the environment is heterogeneous, different combinations of species are likely to be favored in some regions and maintained elsewhere. It may be noted here that one of the methods for study the stability of interacting species model with space dependent properties is to divide the habitat in some patches with interaction and diffusion for each species [47, 54, 55, 176]. Freedman et al. [54] studied a single species diffusion model by assuming that the habitat consisted of two patches and shown that the steady-state solution is monotonically increasing and linear asymptotically stable under both reservoir and no-flux boundary conditions. Later, authors of Refs. [47, 55] discussed the single species diffusion model in multi-patch environment and also studied the global stability of the system.

Keeping the above in view in this chapter, we study the co-existence of two competing species with logistic type growth and diffusion in both homogeneous single habitat and the habitat consisting of two patches. In Section 5.2, the complete model of two competing species in a two-patch habitat is written. In Section 5.3, we study the model in a non-patchy homogeneous habitat without and with diffusion and comparing the stability behavior of both the system. In Section 5.4, we study our model in a two-patch habitat for both uniform and non-uniform steady state cases under both reservoir and no-flux boundary conditions. In the Section 5.5, summary is given.

5.2 Formulation of Mathematical Model

Here, we consider a general two species competing model diffusing between two homogeneous patches in a given patchy habitat. Let $x_i(s,t)$ and $y_i(s,t)$ be the populations of two species competing for the same resources, then each species logistically grows in the absence of the other species and the rate of growth of each species decreases due to the presence of the other species in the i-th patch. The system is then governed by the following autonomous partial differential equations:

$$\frac{\partial x_i(s,t)}{\partial t} = x_i(s,t)\mathbf{g}_i\left(x_i(s,t)\right) - y_i(s,t)\mathbf{p}_i\left(x_i(s,t)\right) + D_{1i}\frac{\partial^2 x_i(s,t)}{\partial s^2}, \tag{5.2.1}$$

$$\frac{\partial y_i(s,t)}{\partial t} = y_i(s,t)\mathbf{f}_i\left(y_i(s,t)\right) - x_i(s,t)\mathbf{q}_i\left(y_i(s,t)\right) + D_{2i}\frac{\partial^2 y_i(s,t)}{\partial s^2}, \tag{5.2.2}$$

$$0 \le s \le L_2, \quad i = 1, 2,$$

where the i-th patch is assumed to lie along the spatial length $L_{i-1} \le s \le L_i$ $(L_0 = 0)$, $\mathbf{g}_i(x_i)$ and $\mathbf{f}_i(y_i)$ are the respective specific growth rates, $\mathbf{p}_i(x_i)$, $\mathbf{q}_i(y_i)$ are interaction rates of $x_i(s,t)$ and $y_i(s,t)$, and D_{1i} and D_{2i} are the diffusion coefficient of x_i and y_i in the i-th patch respectively.

We assume the following assumption for $\mathbf{g}_i(x_i)$, $\mathbf{f}_i(y_i)$, $\mathbf{p}_i(x_i)$ and $\mathbf{q}_i(y_i)$

H_1: $\mathbf{g}_i(x_i), \mathbf{f}_i(y_i), \mathbf{p}_i(x_i), \mathbf{q}_i(y_i) \in \mathbf{C}^2[0,\infty)$,

$\mathbf{g}_i(0) > 0, \mathbf{f}_i(0) > 0, \mathbf{p}_i(0) = 0, \mathbf{q}_i(0) = 0$,

For $x_i > 0$, $\mathbf{g}_i'(x_i) \le 0$, $\mathbf{p}_i'(x_i) > 0$,

For $y_i > 0$, $\mathbf{f}_i'(y_i) \le 0$, $\mathbf{q}_i'(y_i) > 0$.

When the first and second species has a carrying capacity K_i, M_i respectively in the i-th patch, then

H_2: $\mathbf{g}_i(K_i) = 0, \mathbf{f}_i(M_i) = 0, \; i = 1, 2.$

We also assume that,

H_3: $\exists\, x_i^* > 0$, $y_i^* > 0$ such that

$$x_i^* \mathbf{g}_i(x_i^*) - y_i^* \mathbf{p}_i(x_i^*) = 0, \tag{5.2.3}$$

$$y_i^* \mathbf{f}_i(y_i^*) - x_i^* \mathbf{q}_i(y_i^*) = 0. \tag{5.2.4}$$

There are only two possibility of existence of positive equilibria (x_i^*, y_i^*), either

$$\text{(i) } K_i > \frac{\mathbf{f}_i(0)}{\mathbf{q}_i'(0)}, \quad M_i > \frac{\mathbf{g}_i(0)}{\mathbf{p}_i'(0)} \quad \text{or (ii) } K_i < \frac{\mathbf{f}_i(0)}{\mathbf{q}_i'(0)}, \quad M_i < \frac{\mathbf{g}_i(0)}{\mathbf{p}_i'(0)}.$$

Since from (5.2.3), we have, $x_i^* \mathbf{g}_i(x_i^*) = y_i^* \mathbf{p}_i(x_i^*)$, this implies that $\mathbf{g}_i(x_i^*) \ge 0 = \mathbf{g}_i(K_i)$ and again since from assumption H_1, $\mathbf{g}_i'(x_i) \le 0$, for all $x_i \ge 0$. Hence $x_i^* \le K_i$. Similarly from (5.2.4) and H_1, we get $y_i^* \le M_i$.

We also assume the continuity and flux matching conditions at the interface $s = L_1$. The continuity conditions at the interface $s = L_1$ for this system are,

$$x_1(L_1,t) = x_2(L_1,t) \text{ and } y_1(L_1,t) = y_2(L_1,t), \tag{5.2.5}$$

and the continuous flux matching conditions at the interface $s = L_1$ for $x_i(s,t)$ and $y_i(s,t)$ are written as:

$$D_{11}\frac{\partial x_1(L_1,t)}{\partial s} = D_{12}\frac{\partial x_2(L_1,t)}{\partial s}, \tag{5.2.6}$$

$$D_{21}\frac{\partial \psi_1(L_1,t)}{\partial s} = D_{22}\frac{\partial \psi_2(L_1,t)}{\partial s}. \tag{5.2.7}$$

The model is studied under two set of boundary conditions, i.e., reservoir and no-flux. In the case of reservoir boundary conditions, we take

$$x_1(0,t) = x_1^*\,,\ x_2(L_2,t) = x_2^*, \text{ and } y_1(0,t) = y_1^*\,,\ y_2(L_2,t) = y_2^*. \tag{5.2.8}$$

In the case of no-flux boundary conditions, we have

$$\frac{\partial x_1(0,t)}{\partial s} = 0 = \frac{\partial x_2(L_2,t)}{\partial s} \text{ and } \frac{\partial y_1(0,t)}{\partial s} = 0 = \frac{\partial y_2(L_2,t)}{\partial s} \tag{5.2.9}$$

Finally the model is completed by assuming some positive initial distributions, that is,

$$x_i(s,0) = \chi_i(s) > 0,\ L_{i-1} < s < L_i, \tag{5.2.10}$$

$$y_i(s,0) = \delta_i(s) > 0,\ L_{i-1} < s < L_i. \tag{5.2.11}$$

We first study the existence and stability behavior of the system (5.2.1) and (5.2.2) in a homogeneous habitat without patchiness, the effect of patchiness will be investigated later.

5.3 Analysis of the Model in a Homogeneous Habitat

5.3.1 Model without Diffusion

In this case $x_i = x$, $y_i = y$, $\mathbf{g}_i(x_i) = \mathbf{g}(x)$, $\mathbf{f}_i(y_i) = \mathbf{f}(y)$, $\mathbf{p}_i(x_i) = \mathbf{p}(x)$, $i = 1,2$. Thus the system (5.2.1) and (5.2.2) reduces to the following form:

$$\frac{dx}{dt} = x\mathbf{g}(x) - y\mathbf{p}(x), \tag{5.3.1}$$

$$\frac{dy}{dt} = y\mathbf{f}(y) - x\mathbf{q}(y). \tag{5.3.2}$$

This is a competition model, in absence of other each species grows logistically. The functions $\mathbf{g}(x)$, $\mathbf{f}(y)$ and $\mathbf{p}(x)$ satisfy the same type of assumption as mentioned in $\mathbf{H_1}$ and $\mathbf{H_2}$. And the assumption $\mathbf{H_3}$ can be written as, $\exists\, x^* > 0$ and $y^* > 0$ such that,

$$x^*\mathbf{g}(x^*) - y^*\mathbf{p}(x^*) = 0, \tag{5.3.3}$$

$$y^*\mathbf{f}(y^*) - x^*\mathbf{q}(y^*) = 0, \tag{5.3.4}$$

$$(x - x^*)[x\mathbf{g}(x) - y^*\mathbf{p}(x)] < 0, \;\; \forall\, x \neq x^*,\; y \neq y^*, \tag{5.3.5}$$

$$(y - y^*)[y\mathbf{f}(y) - x^*\mathbf{q}(y)] < 0, \;\; \forall\, x \neq x^*,\; y \neq y^*. \tag{5.3.6}$$

The assumptions (5.3.5) and (5.3.6) ensure the uniquely existence of positive equilibria of the above system.

From equations (5.3.3) and (5.3.4), it follows that there are four equilibria, namely (i) $E_0 = [0,0]$, (ii) $E_K = [K,0]$, (iii) $E_M = [0,M]$ and (iv) $E^* = [x^*, y^*]$. The existence of E^*, the interior equilibrium can be ensure in both the cases, either

$$\text{Case (i) } K > \frac{\mathbf{f}(0)}{\mathbf{q}'(0)},\;\; M > \frac{\mathbf{g}(0)}{\mathbf{p}'(0)} \;\text{ or Case (ii) } K < \frac{\mathbf{f}(0)}{\mathbf{q}'(0)},\;\; M < \frac{\mathbf{g}(0)}{\mathbf{p}'(0)}.$$

Later we will shown that first one is unstable and second one is stable.

The variational matrix in the general case is given by

$$[M] = \begin{bmatrix} \mathbf{g}(x) + x\mathbf{g}'(x) - y\mathbf{p}'(x) & -\mathbf{p}(x) \\ -\mathbf{q}(y) & \mathbf{f}(y) + y\mathbf{f}'(y) - x\mathbf{q}'(y) \end{bmatrix}. \tag{5.3.7}$$

Now calculating the variational matrix for each equilibria and noting the hypotheses $\mathbf{H_1} \rightarrow \mathbf{H_3}$ and the standard stability theory of ordinary differential equations, we note the following obvious remarks:

The equilibrium point E_0 is always unstable. The equilibrium point E_K is a stable or saddle point according to $\mathbf{f}(0) - K\mathbf{q}'(0)$ is negative or positive. Similarly the E_M is a stable or saddle point according as $\mathbf{g}(0) - M\mathbf{p}'(0)$ is negative or positive. In general, there is no obvious remark to be made about the stability of the most interesting non-zero equilibria E^*, if it exists.

Therefore, our aim of this section is to obtain local stability and as well as global stability conditions for E^*.

We now state main results of this section in Theorem 5.3.1, and 5.3.3 and Lemma 5.3.2.

Theorem 5.3.1. *The equilibrium E^* is locally asymptotically stable, if the following condition*

$$\mathbf{p}(x^*)\mathbf{q}(y^*) < H_1^* H_2^*, \tag{5.3.8}$$

where

$$H_1^* = x^*\mathbf{g}'(x^*) + \mathbf{g}(x^*) - \frac{x^*\mathbf{g}(x^*)}{\mathbf{p}(x^*)}\mathbf{p}'(x^*),$$

and

$$H_2^* = y^*\mathbf{f}'(y^*) + \mathbf{f}(y^*) - \frac{y^*\mathbf{f}(y^*)}{\mathbf{q}(y^*)}\mathbf{q}'(y^*)$$

is satisfied.

From (5.3.5) and (5.3.6), if we linearizing around the equilibrium point E^*, it follows that $H_1^* < 0$ and $H_2^* < 0$. Now from the two curves

$$y = \frac{x\mathbf{g}(x)}{\mathbf{p}(x)} \quad \text{and} \quad x = \frac{y\mathbf{f}(y)}{\mathbf{q}(y)},$$

the gradients at (x^*, y^*) are respectively,

$$\left(\frac{dy}{dx}\right)_{(x^*,y^*)} = \frac{H_1^*}{\mathbf{p}(x^*)} \text{ and } \left(\frac{dy}{dx}\right)_{(x^*,y^*)} = \frac{\mathbf{q}(y^*)}{H_2^*}.$$

Now from Case (i),

$$-\frac{\mathbf{q}(y^*)}{H_2^*} > -\frac{H_1^*}{\mathbf{p}(x^*)}, \text{ i.e. } \frac{\mathbf{q}(y^*)}{-H_2^*} > \frac{-H_1^*}{\mathbf{p}(x^*)}.$$

Multiplying both side by $-H_2^*\mathbf{p}(x^*)$, we get $\mathbf{p}(x^*)\mathbf{q}(y^*) > H_1^*H_2^*$, which contradicts the condition (5.3.8). Hence in this case positive equilibria E^* is unstable. From Case (ii), by similar manner

$$-\frac{\mathbf{q}(y^*)}{H_2^*} < -\frac{H_1^*}{\mathbf{p}(x^*)} \quad \Rightarrow \quad \mathbf{p}(x^*)\mathbf{q}(y^*) < H_1^*H_2^*.$$

Therefore in this case E^* is locally stable.

Lemma 5.3.2. *The region of attraction for all solutions initiating in the positive quadrant is*

$$\mathscr{A} = \{(x,y) : 0 \le x \le K, 0 \le y \le M\}.$$

Proof. From (5.3.1) and (5.3.2) and hypotheses (H_1) to (H_3), we get,

$$\begin{aligned} \dot{x}(t) \le x(t)\mathbf{g}(x(t)) \quad &\le \mathbf{g}(0)x(t)[1 - x(t)/K], \text{ and} \\ \dot{y}(t) \le y(t)\mathbf{f}(y(t)) \quad &\le \mathbf{f}(0)y(t)[1 - y(t)/M], \end{aligned}$$

then, as $t \rightarrow \infty$,

for $x(0) < K$, $\mathit{lim\ sup}\, x(t) \le K$, and for $x(0) > K$, $\mathit{lim\ sup}\, x(t) \rightarrow K$,
for $y(0) < M$, $\mathit{lim\ sup}\, y(t) \le M$, and for $y(0) > M$, $\mathit{lim\ sup}\, y(t) \rightarrow M$.

Therefore, we note that solutions initiating on $\delta\mathscr{A} \cap \mathit{int}\ \mathscr{R}^+$ enter into $\mathit{int}\ \mathscr{A}$. Hence $\mathscr{A}$ is the region of attraction of the given system. □

Theorem 5.3.3. *Let the condition*

$$\left[\frac{\mathbf{p}(x)}{x}+\frac{\mathbf{q}(y)}{y}\right]^2 < \frac{4}{xy}\left[\frac{x\mathbf{g}(x)-y^*\mathbf{p}(x)}{x-x^*}\right]\left[\frac{y\mathbf{f}(y)-x^*\mathbf{q}(y)}{y-y^*}\right]$$

$$\Rightarrow\ \mathbf{p}(x)\mathbf{q}(y) < \left[\frac{x\mathbf{g}(x)-y^*\mathbf{p}(x)}{x-x^*}\right]\left[\frac{y\mathbf{f}(y)-x^*\mathbf{q}(y)}{y-y^*}\right] \tag{5.3.9}$$

holds. Then E^* (in Case (ii) which is locally stable is also globally asymptotically stable in $\mathscr{A}$.

Now in the following example, we show that the existence of E^* and the conditions for the local and the global stability are feasible.
Example: For simplicity we take,

$$\mathbf{g}(x) = r\left(1-\frac{x}{K}\right),\ \ \mathbf{f}(y) = s\left(1-\frac{y}{M}\right),\ \ \mathbf{p}(x) = \alpha_1 x \text{ and } \mathbf{q}(y) = \alpha_2 y.$$

Then the the equilibrium point $E^*(x^*, y^*)$ is given by

$$x^* = \frac{sK(r-\alpha_1 M)}{rs-\alpha_1\alpha_2 KM},\ \ y^* = \frac{rM(s-\alpha_2 K)}{rs-\alpha_1\alpha_2 KM}. \tag{5.3.10}$$

From (5.3.10) it is clear that positive equilibria exists under two set of conditions, namely
Case 1: $r < \alpha_1 M$, $s < \alpha_2 K$ and $rs < \alpha_1\alpha_2 KM$.
Case 2: $r > \alpha_1 M$, $s > \alpha_2 K$ and $rs > \alpha_1\alpha_2 KM$.

Now we note that , $H_1^* = -rx^*/K < 0$, $H_2^* = -sy^*/M < 0$,

$$\frac{[x\mathbf{g}(x)-y^*\mathbf{p}(x)]}{x-x^*} = -\frac{rx}{K} < 0 \text{ and}$$

$$\frac{[y\mathbf{f}(y)-x^*\mathbf{q}(y)]}{y-y^*} = -\frac{sy}{M} < 0,\ \forall x \neq x^*,\ y \neq y^*.$$

Therefore the condition (5.3.5) and (5.3.6) are automatically satisfied. Further both the local and global stability condition (5.3.8) and (5.3.9) becomes,

$$\alpha_1\alpha_2 < \frac{rs}{KM},$$

which is automatically satisfied in Case 2. Hence E^* is locally as well as globally asymptotically stable in Case 2.

TABLE 5.1 Effect of Various Parameters on x^* and y^*

(i)	$r\uparrow$	$x_i^*\downarrow$	$y_i^*\uparrow$	Case 1
		$x_i^*\uparrow$	$y_i^*\downarrow$	Case 2
(ii)	$s\uparrow$	$x_i^*\uparrow$	$y_i^*\downarrow$	Case 1
		$x_i^*\downarrow$	$y_i^*\uparrow$	Case 2
(iii)	$K\uparrow$	$x_i^*\downarrow$	$y_i^*\uparrow$	Case 1
		$x_i^*\uparrow$	$y_i^*\downarrow$	Case 2
(iv)	$M\uparrow$	$x_i^*\uparrow$	$y_i^*\downarrow$	Case 1
		$x_i^*\downarrow$	$y_i^*\uparrow$	Case 2
(v)	$\alpha_1\uparrow$	$x_i^*\uparrow$	$y_i^*\downarrow$	Case 1
		$x_i^*\downarrow$	$y_i^*\uparrow$	Case 2
(vi)	$\alpha_2\uparrow$	$x_i^*\downarrow$	$y_i^*\uparrow$	Case 1
		$x_i^*\uparrow$	$y_i^*\downarrow$	Case 2

5.3.2 Model with Diffusion

Now, we wish to consider the model (5.3.1) and (5.3.2) with diffusion and analyze the uniform equilibrium E^* under both reservoir and no-flux boundary conditions. The model (5.3.1) and (5.3.2) in this case can be written as,

$$\frac{\partial x}{\partial t} = x\mathbf{g}(x) - y\mathbf{p}(x) + D_1\frac{\partial^2 x}{\partial s^2}, \tag{5.3.11}$$

$$\frac{\partial y}{\partial t} = yf(y) - xq(y) + D_2\frac{\partial^2 y}{\partial s^2}, \tag{5.3.12}$$

$$0 \leq s \leq L,$$

where $D_i \geq 0$ are diffusion coefficients. The reservoir and no-flux boundary conditions are respectively,

$$x(0,t) = x^* = x(L,t) \text{ and } y(0,t) = y^* = y(L,t), \tag{5.3.13}$$

$$\frac{\partial x(0,t)}{\partial s} = 0 = \frac{\partial x(L,t)}{\partial s} \text{ and } \frac{\partial y(0,t)}{\partial s} = 0 = \frac{\partial y(L,t)}{\partial s}. \tag{5.3.14}$$

Now if we take the following positive definite function

$$W(x,y) = \int_0^L V(x,y)ds,$$

around the equilibrium point E^*, we can establish the following theorems for local and global stability of the system.

Theorem 5.3.4. *The equilibrium E^* is locally asymptotically stable, if (5.3.8) holds true.*

Moreover by using Poincare's inequality, it is pointed out that even if (5.3.8) does not holds true, this uniform equilibrium may become stable with diffusion under a condition as given in the following theorem.

Theorem 5.3.5. *The equilibrium E^* is locally asymptotically stable, if*

$$\mathbf{p}(x^*)\mathbf{q}(y^*) < \left(H_1^* - D_1\frac{\pi^2}{L^2}\right)\left(H_2^* - D_2\frac{\pi^2}{L^2}\right)$$

is satisfied.

Therefore the unstable equilibrium (Case (i)), in without diffusion model becomes stable with diffusion if the following condition is true,

$$\left(\frac{H_1^*}{D_1} + \frac{H_2^*}{D_2}\right) < \frac{\pi^2}{L^2}.$$

Theorem 5.3.6. *Let the condition*

$$\mathbf{p}(x)\mathbf{q}(y) < \left[\frac{x\mathbf{g}(x) - y^*\mathbf{p}(x)}{x - x^*}\right]\left[\frac{y\mathbf{f}(y) - x^*\mathbf{q}(y)}{y - y^*}\right]$$

holds. Then E^* is globally asymptotically stable in $\mathscr{A}$.

Thus the uniform equilibrium E^* of the system is locally as well as globally asymptotically stable under the same set of conditions, as in the previous case. Further from Theorem 5.3.5, an equilibrium which is unstable without diffusion can become stable with diffusion.

5.4 Analysis of the Model with Diffusion in a Two-Patch Habitat

In the first subsection we study the model (5.2.1)- (5.2.11), in the case of uniform equilibrium state. In the next section we study the non-uniform case.

5.4.1 The Uniform Equilibrium State Under Both Sets of Boundary Conditions

The result of this section to show that uniform steady-state is globally asymptotically stable. In this case, it is clear that, under both sets of boundary conditions, there is a uniform steady-state, $x(s,t) \equiv K^*$, $0 \leq s \leq L_2$, $t \geq 0$, $y(s,t) \equiv M^*$, $0 \leq s \leq L_2$, $t \geq 0, (i = 1,2)$, where K and M are the common uniform equilibrium point of first species and second species respectively in the two patches. Let $x_1^* = x_2^* = K^*$ and $y_1^* = y_2^* = M^*$. By using similar arguments as in Section 5.3.1, the following theorems for stability can be proved for the system (5.2.1)–(5.2.7) with (5.2.8) or (5.2.9).

Theorem 5.4.1. *The unique uniform steady state solutions (K^*, M^*) is locally asymptotically stable, if $H_j^{i*} < 0$, for $i, j = 1,2$, and the following condition*

$$\mathbf{p}_i(K^*)\mathbf{q}_i(M^*) < H_1^{i*}H_2^{i*} \quad i = 1,2,$$

where

$$H_1^{i*} = K^*\mathbf{g}_i'(K^*) + \mathbf{g}_i(K^*) - \frac{K^*\mathbf{g}_i(K^*)}{\mathbf{p}_i(K^*)}\mathbf{p}_i'(K^*),$$

$$H_2^{i*} = M^*\mathbf{f}_i'(M^*) + \mathbf{f}_i(M^*) - \frac{M^*\mathbf{f}_i(M^*)}{\mathbf{q}_i(M^*)}\mathbf{q}_i'(M^*)$$

are satisfied.

Similarly as Theorem 5.3.5, the above uniform steady state is locally asymptotically stable under less stringent conditions as the following theorem:

Theorem 5.4.2. *The unique uniform steady state solutions (K^*, M^*) is locally asymptotically stable, if $H_j^{i*} - D_{ji}\pi^2/(L_i - L_{i-1})^2 < 0$, for $i, j = 1,2$, and the following condition*

$$\mathbf{p}_i(K^*)\mathbf{q}_i(M^*) < \left(H_1^{i*} - D_{1i}\frac{\pi^2}{(L_i - L_{i-1})^2}\right)\left(H_2^{i*} - D_{2i}\frac{\pi^2}{(L_i - L_{i-1})^2}\right),$$

i = 1,2 are satisfied.

We now state the global stability of the uniform steady state.

Theorem 5.4.3. *The uniform steady-state solutions* $(K^*,\ M^*)$ *is globally asymptotically stable, if (5.2.9),* $x(s,t) \equiv K$, $y(s,t) \equiv M$ *is globally asymptotically stable.*

Proof. Let V(x,y) be the positive definite function about $x = K^*, y = M^*$, given by

$$\begin{aligned} V(t) = V(x,y) &= \sum_1^2 \int_{L_{i-1}}^{L_i} \left(x_i - K^* - K^* \ln\{\frac{x_i}{K^*}\}\right) ds \\ &+ \sum_1^2 \int_{L_{i-1}}^{L_i} \left(y_i - M^* - M^* \ln\{\frac{y_i}{M^*}\}\right) ds. \end{aligned}$$

Differentiating with respect to t, and using (5.2.1) and (5.2.2) we get,

$$\begin{aligned} \dot{V}(t) &= \sum_1^2 \int_{L_{i-1}}^{L_i} \left(\frac{x_i - K^*}{x_i}\right) \frac{\partial x_i}{\partial t} ds + \sum_1^2 \int_{L_{i-1}}^{L_i} \left(\frac{y_i - M^*}{y_i}\right) \frac{\partial y_i}{\partial t} ds \\ &= \sum_1^2 \int_{L_{i-1}}^{L_i} \left(\frac{x_i - K^*}{x_i}\right) [x_i \mathbf{g}_i(x_i) - y_i \mathbf{p}_i(x_i)]\, ds \\ &+ \sum_1^2 \int_{L_{i-1}}^{L_i} D_{1i} \left(\frac{x_i - K^*}{x_i}\right) \frac{\partial^2 x_i}{\partial s^2} ds \qquad (5.4.1) \\ &+ \sum_1^2 \int_{L_{i-1}}^{L_i} \left(\frac{y_i - M^*}{y_i}\right) [y_i \mathbf{f}_i(y_i) - x_i \mathbf{q}_i(y_i)]\, ds \\ &+ \sum_1^2 \int_{L_{i-1}}^{L_i} D_{2i} \left(\frac{y_i - M^*}{y_i}\right) \frac{\partial^2 y_i}{\partial s^2} ds. \end{aligned}$$

Now by assumption (5.4.2), first integral of the right hand side is negative, $\forall\, x_i$, other than K, $i = 1,2$. Similarly by (5.4.3) the third integral of right hand side is negative, $\forall\, y_i$, other than M, $i = 1,2$.
Now consider the integral,

$$I_1 = \sum_1^2 \int_{L_{i-1}}^{L_i} D_{1i} \left(\frac{x_i - K^*}{x_i}\right) \frac{\partial^2 x_i}{\partial s^2} ds.$$

Under both set of boundary conditions,

$$[x_1(0,t) - K^*] \frac{\partial x_1(0,t)}{\partial s} = [x_2(L_2,t) - K^*] \frac{\partial x_2(L_2,t)}{\partial s} = 0.$$

We have

$$I_1 = -\sum_{1}^{2}\int_{L_{i-1}}^{L_i} D_{1i}\frac{K^*}{x_i^2}\left(\frac{\partial x_1}{\partial s}\right)^2 ds < 0.$$

Similarly,

$$I_2 = \sum_{1}^{2}\int_{L_{i-1}}^{L_i} D_{2i}\left(\frac{y_i - M^*}{y_i}\right)\frac{\partial^2 y_i}{\partial s^2} ds < 0.$$

Hence $V(x,y) < 0$, and $\dot{V}(K^*,M^*) = 0$. Therefore $\dot{V}(x,y)$ is negative definite over $x > 0$, $y > 0$ with respect to $x = K^*$, $y = M^*$, proving the theorem. □

5.4.2 The Non-Uniform Equilibrium State

We assume the existence of the unsteady state solutions of the system (5.2.1) to (5.2.11) exists [see [174] (Theorem 1, page 111 and Theorem 3, page 123)].

Our aim here is to show that there exists a positive, monotonic, continuous steady state solution for the each species separately, with continuous flux matching at the interface of these patches, in the cases of both reservoir and no-flux boundary conditions and derive the conditions of asymptotic stability for both linear and non-linear models.

There are four possible cases:

(1) $x_2^* > x_1^*$ and $y_2^* > y_1^*$.
(2) $x_2^* > x_1^*$ and $y_2^* < y_1^*$.
(3) $x_2^* < x_1^*$ and $y_2^* < y_1^*$.
(4) $x_2^* < x_1^*$ and $y_2^* > y_1^*$.

Without loss of generality, (3) can be reduced to (1) and (4) can be reduced to (2). Therefore we consider the case (1) and (2) separately under two set of boundary conditions.

To do this we assume the following conditions on x_i and y_i for $i = 1,2$.

$$(x_i - x_i^*)[x_i\mathbf{g}_i(x_i) - y_i\mathbf{p}_i(x_i)] < 0 \ \forall x_i \neq x_i^* \quad \text{and } min.\{y_1^*, y_2^*\} \le y_i \le max.\{y_1^*, y_2^*\}, \tag{5.4.2}$$

$$(y_i - y_i^*)[y_i\mathbf{f}_i(y_i) - x_i\mathbf{q}_i(y_i)] < 0 \ \forall y_i \neq y_i^* \quad \text{and } min.\{y_1^*, y_2^*\} \le y_i \le max.\{y_1^*, y_2^*\}. \tag{5.4.3}$$

5.4.3 The Model Under the Reservoir Boundary Conditions: When $x_2^* > x_1^*$ and $y_2^* > y_1^*$.

We first consider the steady-state problem and show that there exists a non-uniform positive monotonic solutions $u_i(s)$, $v_i(s)$ under reservoir boundary conditions and with continuous flux at the interface.
The steady-state system takes the form

$$D_{1i}\frac{d^2u_i(s)}{ds^2} + u_i\mathbf{g}_i(u_i) - v_i\mathbf{p}_i(u_i) = 0, \tag{5.4.4}$$

$$D_{2i}\frac{d^2v_i(s)}{ds^2} + v_i\mathbf{f}_i(v_i) - u_i\mathbf{q}_i(v_i) = 0. \tag{5.4.5}$$

The reservoir boundary conditions are

$$u_1(0) = x_1^*, u_2(L_2) = x_2^*, \tag{5.4.6}$$

$$v_1(0) = y_1^*, v_2(L_2) = y_2^*. \tag{5.4.7}$$

The continuous solutions and flux matching condition at the interface

$$u_1(L_1) = u_2(L_1); v_1(L_1) = v_2(L_1), \tag{5.4.8}$$

$$D_{11}\frac{du_1(L_1)}{ds} = D_{12}\frac{du_2(L_1)}{ds}, \tag{5.4.9}$$

$$D_{21}\frac{dv_1(L_1)}{ds} = D_{22}\frac{dv_2(L_1)}{ds}. \tag{5.4.10}$$

Let $p_1(s,\alpha_1)$ and $q_1(s,\beta_1), 0 \leq s \leq L_1$ be the unique solutions of (5.4.4) and (5.4.5) respectively, for $i = 1$, such that

$$\frac{\partial p_1(0,\alpha_1)}{\partial s} = \alpha_1, \ \ p_1(0,\alpha_1) = x_1^*, \tag{5.4.11}$$

$$\frac{\partial q_1(0,\beta_1)}{\partial s} = \beta_1, \ \ q_1(0,\beta_1) = y_1^*. \tag{5.4.12}$$

Let $p_2(s,\alpha_2)$ and $q_2(s,\beta_2), L_1 \leq s \leq L_2$ be the unique solutions of (5.4.4) and (5.4.5) respectively, for $i = 2$, such that

$$\frac{\partial p_2(L_2,\alpha_2)}{\partial s} = \alpha_2, \ \ p_2(L_2,\alpha_2) = x_2^*, \tag{5.4.13}$$

$$\frac{\partial q_2(L_2,\beta_2)}{\partial s} = \beta_2,\ \ q_2(L_2,\beta_2) = y_2^*. \tag{5.4.14}$$

We will have shown the existence of the monotonic solutions if we can show that there exists $\alpha_1, \alpha_2, \beta_1$ and β_2 such that

$$p_1(L_1,\alpha_1) = p_2(L_1,\alpha_2)\ ,\ q_1(L_1,\beta_1) = q_2(L_1,\beta_2), \tag{5.4.15}$$

$$D_{11}\frac{\partial p_1(L_1,\alpha_1)}{\partial s} = D_{12}\frac{\partial p_2(L_1,\alpha_2)}{\partial s}\ ,\ D_{21}\frac{\partial q_1(L_1,\beta_1)}{\partial s} = D_{12}\frac{\partial q_2(L_1,\beta_2)}{\partial s}. \tag{5.4.16}$$

From (5.4.4), multiplying both side by $2du_i/ds$ and integrating w.r.to s from 0 if $i=1$ and from L_2 if $i=2$, we get,

$$\left[\frac{du_i}{ds}\right]^2 = \alpha_i^2 - \frac{2}{D_{1i}}\int_{x_i^*}^{u_i(s)} [u_i\mathbf{g}_i(u_i) - v_i\mathbf{p}_i(u_i)]du_i(s). \tag{5.4.17}$$

Similarly from (5.4.5), we have,

$$\left[\frac{dv_i}{ds}\right]^2 = \beta_i^2 - \frac{2}{D_{2i}}\int_{y_i^*}^{v_i(s)} [v_i\mathbf{f}_i(v_i) - u_i\mathbf{q}_i(v_i)]dv_i(s). \tag{5.4.18}$$

In order to construct our required solution we need some preliminary lemmas.

Lemma 5.4.4. *If* $\alpha_1 > 0$, *then*

$$\frac{\partial p_1(s,\alpha_1)}{\partial s} > \alpha_1 \ on\ 0 < s \le L_1.$$

Proof. From (5.4.17), we get,

$$\left[\frac{\partial p_1(s,\alpha_1)}{\partial s}\right]^2 = \alpha_1^2 - \frac{2}{D_{11}}\int_{x_1^*}^{p_1(s,\alpha_1)} [p_1\mathbf{g}_1(p_1) - q_1\mathbf{p}_1(p_1)]dp_1. \tag{5.4.19}$$

Since

$$\frac{\partial p_1(0,\alpha_1)}{\partial s} = \alpha_1 > 0\ ,\ p_1(0,\alpha_1) = x_1^*\ ,$$

then there exists $s_1 > 0$ such that $p_1(s,\alpha_1) > x_1^*$ on $0 < s < s_1$. If not, let $s_0, 0 < s_0 \le L_1$, be the first positive value, if it exists, such that

$p_1(s_0,\alpha_1) = x_1^*$. Then by the mean value theorem there exists $\bar{s}$ such that $0 < \bar{s} < s_0$ and $\partial p_1(\bar{s},\alpha_1)/\partial s = 0$; that is,

$$\alpha_1^2 = \frac{2}{D_{11}} \int_{x_1^*}^{p_1(\bar{s},\alpha_1)} [p_1\mathbf{g}_1(p_1) - q_1\mathbf{p}_1(p_1)]dp_1. \tag{5.4.20}$$

Now since $p_1(s,\alpha_1) > x_1^*$ for $0 < s \leq \bar{s}$, and from (5.4.2), we have, $p_1\mathbf{g}_1(p_1) - q_1\mathbf{p}_1(p_1) < 0$. Hence the right hand side of (5.4.20) is negative , giving a contradiction. Therefore $p_1(s,\alpha_1) > x_1^*$ and $\partial p_1(s,\alpha_1)/\partial s > 0$. □

Lemma 5.4.5. *If* $0 < p_2 < x_2^*$ *and* $\alpha_2 > 0$, *then*

$$\frac{\partial p_2(s,\alpha_2)}{\partial s} > \alpha_2, \ \ L_1 \leq s < L_2.$$

Proof. From (5.4.17), we have,

$$\left[\frac{\partial p_2(s,\alpha_2)}{\partial s}\right]^2 = \alpha_2^2 - \frac{2}{D_{12}} \int_{x_2^*}^{p_2(s,\alpha_2)} [p_2\mathbf{g}_2(p_2) - q_2\mathbf{p}_2(p_2)]dp_2.$$

From (5.4.2), $p_2\mathbf{g}_2(p_2) - q_2\mathbf{p}_2(p_2) > 0$. Hence $\partial p_2(s,\alpha_2)/\partial s > \alpha_2$, $L_1 \leq s < L_2$ for $0 < p_2 < x_2^*$. □

Similarly from (5.4.3) and (5.4.18) we have,

Lemma 5.4.6. *If* $\beta_1 > 0$, *then*

$$\frac{\partial q_1(s,\beta_1)}{\partial s} > \beta_1 \text{ on } 0 < s \leq L_1.$$

Lemma 5.4.7. *If* $0 < q_2 < y_2^*$ *and* $\beta_2 > 0$, *then*

$$\frac{\partial q_2(s,\beta_2)}{\partial s} > \beta_2, \ \ L_1 \leq s < L_2.$$

There exists four continuous functions $F_{ji}(i,j = 1,2)$, for proof see Lemma 3.3.4 in Chapter 3.

Lemma 5.4.8. *Define* $F_{1i}(\alpha_i)$ *by* $F_{1i}(\alpha_i) = p_i(L_1, \alpha_i)$. *Then there exists* $\hat{\alpha}_i > 0$ *such that*

$$F_{11} : [0, \hat{\alpha}_1] \to [x_1^*, x_2^*]$$

$$F_{12} : [0, \hat{\alpha}_2] \to [x_2^*, x_1^*]$$

Lemma 5.4.9. *Define* $F_{1i}(\beta_i)$ *by* $F_{1i}(\beta_i) = p_i(L_1, \beta_i)$. *Then there exists* $\hat{\alpha}_i > 0$ *such that*

$$F_{11} : \left[0, \hat{\beta}_1\right] \to [y_1^*, y_2^*]$$

$$F_{12} : \left[0, \hat{\beta}_2\right] \to [y_2^*, y_1^*]$$

Theorem 5.4.10. *There exists a positive, continuous, monotonic solution of the steady state system (5.4.4) with continuous flux at* L_1.

Proof. Lemmas 5.4.4 and 5.4.5 follows that any solution we construct must be monotonic. By Lemma 5.4.8, for each $0 \le \alpha_2 \le \hat{\alpha}_2$, we can find an α_1 such that $0 \le \alpha_1 \le \hat{\alpha}_1$ for which $p_1(L_1, \alpha_1) = p_2(L_1, \alpha_2)$. Hence α_1 can be solved as a function of α_2, $\alpha_1 = h(\alpha_2)$, to give a continuous solution of (5.4.4) with (5.4.6), (5.4.8) and (5.4.9).

Let

$$\mathbf{G}(\alpha_2) = D_{11} \frac{\partial p_1(L_1, h(\alpha_2))}{\partial s} - D_{12} \frac{\partial p_2(L_1, \alpha_2)}{\partial s}.$$

Clearly $\mathbf{G}(\alpha_2)$ is continuous on $0 \le \alpha_2 \le \hat{\alpha}_2$. Then we have

$$\mathbf{G}(0) = D_{11} \frac{\partial p_1(L_1, \hat{\alpha}_1)}{\partial s} > 0,$$

and

$$\mathbf{G}(\hat{\alpha}_2) = -D_{12} \frac{\partial p_2(L_1, \hat{\alpha}_2)}{\partial s} < 0.$$

Therefore $\exists\ \bar{\alpha}_2$, $0 < \bar{\alpha}_2 < \hat{\alpha}_2$, such that $\mathbf{G}(\bar{\alpha}_2) = 0$. Hence the theorem. □

Similar results are also true for the second species.

Theorem 5.4.11. *There exists a continuous, monotonic solution of the system (5.4.5) with continuous flux at L_1.*

We now study the asymptotic stability of the steady state system (5.4.4) and (5.4.5) to (5.4.10).

Theorem 5.4.12. *The steady state, continuous, monotonic solutions of system (5.4.4) and (5.4.5) with continuous flux at the interface $s = L_1$ is asymptotically stable provided the following conditions are satisfied:*

$$(i) \quad \frac{d}{du_i}[u_i \mathbf{g}_i(u_i)] \leq 0\,,$$

$$(ii) \quad \frac{d}{dv_i}[v_i \mathbf{f}_2(v_i)] \leq 0\,, \text{ and}$$

$$(iii) \quad [\mathbf{p}_i(u_i) + \mathbf{q}_i(v_i)]^2 < 4\left[\frac{d}{du_i}[u_i \mathbf{g}_i(u_i)]\right]\left[\frac{d}{dv_i}[v_i \mathbf{f}_i(v_i)]\right]$$

for $x_1^* \leq u_i \leq x_2^*,\ \ M_1 \leq v_2 \leq M_2$ *and* $i = 1, 2$.

Proof. Let the steady-state solution of system (5.4.4) be

$$u(s) = \begin{cases} u_1(s),\ 0 \leq s \leq L_1 \\ u_2(s),\ L_1 \leq s \leq L_2. \end{cases}$$

Also, let the steady-state solution of system (5.4.5) be

$$v(s) = \begin{cases} v_1(s),\ 0 \leq s \leq L_1 \\ v_2(s),\ L_1 \leq s \leq L_2. \end{cases}$$

Linearizing (5.2.1) and (5.2.2) by using ,

$$x_i(s,t) = u_i(s) + n_i(s,t), \tag{5.4.21}$$

$$y_i(s,t) = v_i(s) + m_i(s,t). \tag{5.4.22}$$

We have,

$$\frac{\partial n_i(s,t)}{\partial t} = n_i\left[\mathbf{g}_i(u_i) + u_i \mathbf{g}_i'(u_i)\right] - n_i v_i \mathbf{p}_i'(u_i) - m_i \mathbf{p}_i(u_i) + D_{1i}\frac{\partial^2 n_i}{\partial s^2}, \tag{5.4.23}$$

$$\frac{\partial m_i(s,t)}{\partial t} = m_i\left[\mathbf{f}_i(v_i)+v_i\mathbf{f}_i'(v_i)\right] - m_iu_i\mathbf{q}_i'(v_i) - n_i\mathbf{q}_i(v_i) + D_{2i}\frac{\partial^2 m_i}{\partial s^2}. \tag{5.4.24}$$

Using (5.4.21) and (5.4.22) the corresponding initial, boundary and matching conditions can be obtained as follows

$$\begin{aligned}
n_i(s,0) &= \chi_i(s) - u_i(s),\ m_i(s,0) = \delta_i(s) - v_i(s),\\
n_1(0,t) &= 0 = n_2(L_2,t)\ ,\ m_1(0,t) = 0 = m_2(L_2,t),\\
n_1(L_1,t) &= n_2(L_1,t)\ ,\ m_1(L_1,t) = m_2(L_1,t).
\end{aligned} \tag{5.4.25}$$

$$D_{11}\frac{\partial n_1}{\partial s}(L_1,t) = D_{12}\frac{\partial n_2}{\partial s}(L_1,t),$$

$$D_{21}\frac{\partial m_1}{\partial s}(L_1,t) = D_{22}\frac{\partial m_2}{\partial s}(L_1,t).$$

Now we consider the following positive definite function,

$$V(t) = \sum_1^2 \int_{L_{i-1}}^{L_i} \frac{1}{2}\left[n_i^2 + m_i^2\right] ds.$$

From which we get,

$$\dot{V}(t) = \sum_1^2 \int_{L_{i-1}}^{L_i} \left[n_i\frac{\partial n_i}{\partial t} + m_i\frac{\partial m_i}{\partial t}\right] ds.$$

By using (5.4.23) and (5.4.24) , we get,

$$\begin{aligned}
\dot{V}(t) \;=\; & \sum_1^2 \int_{L_{i-1}}^{L_i} n_i^2\left[\mathbf{g}_i(u_i)+u_i\mathbf{g}_i'(u_i)\right] ds - \sum_1^2 \int_{L_{i-1}}^{L_i} n_i^2 v_i \mathbf{p}_i'(u_i) ds\\
& -\sum_1^2 \int_{L_{i-1}}^{L_i} n_i m_i \mathbf{p}_i(u_i) ds - \sum_1^2 D_{2i} \int_{L_{i-1}}^{L_i} \left[\frac{\partial m_i}{\partial s}\right]^2 ds\\
& +\sum_1^2 \int_{L_{i-1}}^{L_i} m_i^2\left[\mathbf{f}_i(v_i)+v_i\mathbf{f}_i'(v_i)\right] ds - \sum_1^2 \int_{L_{i-1}}^{L_i} m_i^2 u_i \mathbf{q}_i'(v_i) ds\\
& -\sum_1^2 \int_{L_{i-1}}^{L_i} n_i m_i \mathbf{q}_i(v_i) ds - \sum_1^2 D_{1i} \int_{L_{i-1}}^{L_i} \left[\frac{\partial n_i}{\partial s}\right]^2 ds.
\end{aligned}$$

Since $\mathbf{p}_i'(u_i) > 0,\ \forall x_i \geq 0$. Therefore second integral of the right hand side of above equation is negative. Similarly sixth integral is also negative. Hence $V(t)$ is negative definite if conditions (i), (ii) and (iii) are satisfies, and the theorem is proved. □

Theorem 5.4.13. *The steady-state, continuous, monotonic solutions of non-linear system (5.4.4) to (5.4.10) with continuous flux at the interface $s = L_1$ is asymptotically stable in the subregion of*

$$\mathbf{R} : \{x_1^* \leq x_i,\ u_i \leq x_2^*,\ y_1^* \leq y_i,\ v_i \leq y_2^*,\ \textit{for } i = 1,2\},$$

provided the following conditions are satisfied:

$$(1)\, \frac{x_i \mathbf{g}_i(x_i) - u_i \mathbf{g}_i(u_i)}{x_i - u_i} \leq 0,$$

$$(2)\, \frac{y_i \mathbf{f}_i(y_i) - v_i \mathbf{f}_i(v_i)}{y_i - v_i} \leq 0,$$

$$(3)\, x_i y_i \left[\frac{u_i \mathbf{p}_i(x_i)}{x_i} + \frac{v_i \mathbf{q}_i(y_i)}{y_i}\right]^2 < 4 u_i v_i \left[\frac{x_i \mathbf{g}_i(x_i) - u_i \mathbf{g}_i(u_i)}{x_i - u_i}\right] \left[\frac{y_i \mathbf{f}_i(y_i) - v_i \mathbf{f}_i(v_i)}{y_i - v_i}\right].$$

Proof. From (5.2.1), (5.2.2), (5.4.21) and (5.4.22), we have

$$\frac{\partial n_i}{\partial t} = (u_i + n_i)\mathbf{g}_i(u_i + n_i) - u_i \mathbf{g}_i(u_i) - (v_i + m_i)\mathbf{p}_i(u_i + n_i) + v_i p_i(u_i) + D_{1i} \frac{\partial^2 n_i}{\partial s^2}, \tag{5.4.26}$$

$$\frac{\partial m_i}{\partial t} = (v_i + m_i)\mathbf{f}_i(v_i + m_i) - v_i \mathbf{f}_i(v_i) - (u_i + n_i)\mathbf{q}_i(v_i + m_i) + u_i q_i(v_i) + D_{2i} \frac{\partial^2 m_i}{\partial s^2}. \tag{5.4.27}$$

Now consider the positive definite function,

$$V(t) = \sum_1^2 \int_{L_{i-1}}^{L_i} u_i \left(n_i - u_i \ln \frac{u_i + n_i}{u_i}\right) ds + \sum_1^2 \int_{L_{i-1}}^{L_i} v_i \left(m_i - v_i \ln \frac{v_i + m_i}{v_i}\right) ds.$$

From which we get,

$$\dot{V}(t) = \sum_1^2 \int_{L_{i-1}}^{L_i} \frac{u_i n_i}{u_i + n_i} \frac{\partial n_i}{\partial t} ds + \sum_1^2 \int_{L_{i-1}}^{L_i} \frac{v_i m_i}{v_i + m_i} \frac{\partial m_i}{\partial t} ds.$$

After using equations (5.4.26) and (5.4.27), we get

$$
\begin{aligned}
\dot{V}(t) &= \sum_1^2 \int_{L_{i-1}}^{L_i} \frac{u_i n_i^2}{u_i+n_i}\left[\frac{(u_i+n_i)\mathbf{g}_i(u_i+n_i)-u_i\mathbf{g}_i(u_i)}{n_i}\right] ds \\
&- \sum_1^2 \int_{L_{i-1}}^{L_i} \frac{u_i n_i^2}{u_i+n_i}\left[v_i\left(\frac{\mathbf{p}_i(u_i+n_i)-\mathbf{p}_i(u_i)}{n_i}\right)\right] ds \\
&- \sum_1^2 \int_{L_{i-1}}^{L_i} \frac{u_i n_i m_i}{u_i+n_i}\mathbf{p}_i(u_i+n_i)ds + \sum_1^2 D_{1i}\int_{L_{i-1}}^{L_i} \frac{u_i n_i}{u_i+n_i}\frac{\partial^2 n_i}{\partial s^2} ds \\
&+ \sum_1^2 \int_{L_{i-1}}^{L_i} \frac{v_i m_i^2}{v_i+m_i}\left[\frac{(v_i+m_i)\mathbf{f}_i(v_i+m_i)-v_i\mathbf{f}_i(v_i)}{m_i}\right] ds \\
&- \sum_1^2 \int_{L_{i-1}}^{L_i} \frac{v_i m_i^2}{v_i+m_i}\left[u_i\left(\frac{\mathbf{q}_i(v_i+m_i)-\mathbf{q}_i(v_i)}{m_i}\right)\right] ds \\
&- \sum_1^2 \int_{L_{i-1}}^{L_i} \frac{v_i n_i m_i}{v_i+m_i}\mathbf{q}_i(v_i+m_i)ds + \sum_1^2 D_{2i}\int_{L_{i-1}}^{L_i} \frac{v_i m_i}{v_i+m_i}\frac{\partial^2 m_i}{\partial s^2} ds.
\end{aligned}
$$

Now,

$$\frac{\mathbf{p}_i(u_i+n_i)-\mathbf{p}_i(u_i)}{n_i} \geq 0, \ \forall\, n_i,$$

$$\frac{\mathbf{q}_i(v_i+m_i)-\mathbf{q}_i(v_i)}{m_i} \geq 0, \ \forall\, m_i.$$

Also by using (5.4.25) and $\partial u_i/\partial s > 0$,

$$\sum_1^2 D_{1i}\int_{L_{i-1}}^{L_i} \frac{u_i n_i}{u_i+n_i}\frac{\partial^2 n_i}{\partial s^2} ds = -\sum_1^2 D_{1i}\int_{L_{i-1}}^{L_i} \frac{\partial}{\partial s}\left(\frac{u_i n_i}{u_i+n_i}\right)\frac{\partial n_i}{\partial s} ds < 0.$$

Similarly

$$\sum_1^2 D_{2i}\int_{L_{i-1}}^{L_i} \frac{v_i m_i}{v_i+m_i}\frac{\partial^2 m_i}{\partial s^2} ds < 0.$$

Therefore $\dot{V}(t) \leq 0$ if the conditions (1),(2),(3) holds true. Hence the theorem is proved. □

Example: Let us consider an example by choosing the following function in our model (5.2.1) and (5.2.2),

$$\mathbf{g}_i(x_i) = r_{1i}\left(1 - \frac{x_i}{K_i}\right),\ \mathbf{f}_i(y_i) = r_{2i}\left(1 - \frac{y_i}{M_i}\right),\ \mathbf{p}_i(x_i) = c_{1i}x_i,\ \mathbf{q}_i(y_i) = c_{2i}y_i,$$

$$0 \leq c_{1i},\ c_{2i} < 1,\ i = 1,2,$$

then

$$K_i^* = \frac{r_{2i}K_i[r_{1i} - c_{1i}M_i]}{r_{1i}r_{2i} - c_{1i}c_{2i}K_iM_i},\ \text{and}\ M_i^* = \frac{r_{1i}M_i[r_{2i} - c_{2i}K_i]}{r_{1i}r_{2i} - c_{1i}c_{2i}K_iM_i}.$$

From the above it is clear that $K_i^* \leq K_i$ and $M_i^* \leq M_i$.

Here the conditions (1) and (2) (see Theorem 5.4.13) of non-linear stability becomes,

$$r_{1i}\left(1 - \frac{x_i + u_i}{K_i}\right) \leq 0,\ r_{2i}\left(1 - \frac{y_i + v_i}{M_i}\right) \leq 0.$$

Now the function $G_i(x_i) = x_i\mathbf{g}_i(x_i)$ is decreasing from the point $x_{0i} = K_i/2$. Similarly the function $F_i(y_i) = y_i\mathbf{f}_i(y_i)$ starts decreasing from $y_{0i} = M_i/2$.

Now if we choose r_{1i}, r_{2i}, c_{1i}, c_{2i} are such that $x_i^* \geq K_i/2$ and $y_i^* \geq M_i/2$. Then (1) and (2) (see Theorem 5.4.13) are satisfied in the following region:

$$\{x_1^* \leq x_i,\ u_i \leq x_2^*,\ y_1^* \leq y_i,\ v_i \leq y_2^*,\ \text{for}\ i = 1,2\}.$$

It is pointed out here that the condition (3) (see Theorem 5.4.13) of non-linear stability can also satisfied in above region for a suitable choice of $\mathbf{g}_i$, $\mathbf{f}_i$ and $\mathbf{p}_i$ satisfying $\mathbf{H}_1 \to \mathbf{H}_3$. In this particular case the condition (3), becomes

$$x_iy_i\left[c_{1i}u_i - c_{2i}v_i\right]^2 \leq 4r_{1i}r_{2i}u_iv_i\left[1 - \frac{x_i + u_i}{K_i}\right]\left[1 - \frac{y_i + v_i}{M_i}\right]. \quad (5.4.28)$$

This condition is automatically satisfied if for a particular choice of r_{1i}, r_{2i}, c_{1i} and c_{2i}, the maximum of the left hand side is $\leq$ minimum of right hand side. That is,

$$xx_2^*y_2^*\left[c_{1i}x_2^* - c_{2i}y_1^*\right]^2 \leq 4x_1^*y_1^*r_{1i}r_{2i}\left(\frac{2x_1^*}{K_i} - 1\right)\left(\frac{2y_1^*}{M_i} - 1\right). \quad (5.4.29)$$

It is clear from (5.4.29) that for suitable choice of r_{1i} and r_{2i} the above condition can be satisfied. For particular case taking the parameter values,

$$\begin{array}{llll} r_{11} = 0.34, & r_{12} = 0.35, & r_{21} = 0.574, & r_{22} = 0.49, \\ K_1 = 340, & K_2 = 175, & M_1 = 287, & M_2 = 490, \\ c_{11} = 0.0003, & c_{12} = 0.0003, & c_{21} = 0.0001 & c_{22} = 0.0001, \end{array}$$

Then, we get $x_1^* = 250.15,\ \ x_2^* = 100,\ \ y_1^* = 299.5,\ \ y_2^* = 500.$
In this numerical example the condition (5.4.29) is automatically satisfied.

Now we consider the case when $x_2^* > x_1^*$ and $y_1^* > y_2^*$:

For $x_2^* > x_1^*$ the monotonicity of steady state solution is similar as the above case and for $M_1 > M_2$, the monotonicity just reverse of the above case. Hence the steady state solution is monotonic under both set of boundary conditions.

In this case the linear asymptotic stability conditions for the steady state system under reservoir boundary conditions are similar as the above case.

5.4.4 The Model Under No-Flux Boundary Conditions

In this section we study the steady state model with no-flux boundary conditions, i.e.,

$$\frac{du_1(0)}{ds} = 0 = \frac{du_2(L_2)}{ds};\ \frac{dv_1(0)}{ds} = 0 = \frac{dv_2(L_2)}{ds} \tag{5.4.30}$$

As before, we assume $x_2^* > x_1^*$ and $y_2^* > y_1^*$.
Let $p_1(s, \alpha_1)$ and $q_1(s, \beta_1), 0 \leq s \leq L_1$ are the unique solutions of (5.4.4) and (5.4.5) respectively, for $i = 1$, such that

$$\frac{\partial p_1(0, \alpha_1)}{\partial s} = 0\ ,\ \ p_1(0, \alpha_1) = \alpha_1, \tag{5.4.31}$$

$$\frac{\partial q_1(0, \beta_1)}{\partial s} = 0\ ,\ \ q_1(0, \beta_1) = \beta_1. \tag{5.4.32}$$

Let $p_2(s, \alpha_2)$ and $q_2(s, \beta), L_1 \leq s \leq L_2$ are the unique solutions of (5.4.4) and (5.4.5) respectively, for $i = 2$, such that

$$\frac{\partial p_2(L_2, \alpha_2)}{\partial s} = 0\ ,\ \ p_2(L_2, \alpha_2) = \alpha_2. \tag{5.4.33}$$

$$\frac{\partial q_2(L_2,\beta_2)}{\partial s}=0\ ,\ q_1(L_2,\beta_2)=\beta_2. \tag{5.4.34}$$

We will have shown the existence of the monotonic solutions if we can show that there exists α_1, α_2, β_1 and β_2 such that

$$p_1(L_1,\alpha_1)=p_2(L_1,\alpha_2)\ ,\ q_1(L_1,\beta_1)=q_2(L_1,\beta_2), \tag{5.4.35}$$

$$D_{11}\frac{\partial p_1(L_1,\alpha_1)}{\partial s}=D_{12}\frac{\partial p_2(L_1,\alpha_2)}{\partial s}, \tag{5.4.36}$$

$$D_{21}\frac{\partial q_1(L_1,\beta_1)}{\partial s}=D_{12}\frac{\partial q_2(L_1,\beta_2)}{\partial s}. \tag{5.4.37}$$

From (5.4.4), multiplying both side by $2du_i/ds$ and integrating w.r.to s from 0 if $i=1$ and from L_2 if $i=2$, we get

$$\left[\frac{du_i}{ds}\right]^2=-\frac{2}{D_{1i}}\int_{\alpha_i}^{u_i(s)}[u_i\mathbf{g}_i(u_i)-v_i\mathbf{p}_i(u_i)]du_i(s). \tag{5.4.38}$$

Similarly from (5.4.5), we have

$$\left[\frac{dv_i}{ds}\right]^2=-\frac{2}{D_{2i}}\int_{\beta_i}^{u_i(s)}[v_i\mathbf{f}_i(v_i)-u_i\mathbf{q}_i(v_i)]du_i(s). \tag{5.4.39}$$

Similar type of lemmas as in the case of reservoir boundary conditions as follows:

Lemma 5.4.14. *If $\alpha_1>x_1^*$, then*

$$\frac{\partial p_1(s,\alpha_1)}{\partial s}>0\ ,\ 0<s\leq L_1.$$

Proof. From (5.4.38), we get,

$$\left[\frac{\partial p_1(s,\alpha_1)}{\partial s}\right]^2=-\frac{2}{D_{11}}\int_{\alpha_1}^{p_1(s,\alpha_1)}[p_1\mathbf{g}_1(p_1)-q_1\mathbf{p}_1(p_1)]dp_1. \tag{5.4.40}$$

Since $\partial p_1(0,\alpha_1)/\partial s=0$, $p_1(0,\alpha_1)=\alpha_1$ there exists $s_1>0$ such that $p_1(s,\alpha_1)>\alpha_1$ on $0<s<s_1$. If not, let s_0, $0<s_0\leq L_1$, be the first positive value , if it exists, such that $p_1(s_0,\alpha_1)=\alpha_1$. Then by the mean

value theorem there exists $\bar{s}$ such that $0 < \bar{s} < s_0$ and $\partial p_1(\bar{s}, \alpha_1)/\partial s = 0$; that is,

$$0 = -\frac{2}{D_{11}} \int_{\alpha_1}^{p_1(\bar{s},\alpha_1)} [p_1 \mathbf{g}_1(p_1) - q_1 \mathbf{p}_1(p_1)]\, dp_1. \qquad (5.4.41)$$

But the right-hand side of (5.4.41) is non-zero, since $p_1 > \alpha_1$ on $0 < s \leq \bar{s}$. Also $\alpha_1 > x_1^*$, therefore, $p_1 > x_1^*$. This implies that, $p_1 \mathbf{g}_1(p_1) - q_1 \mathbf{p}_1(p_1) < 0$. Giving a contradiction. Hence $p_1(s, \alpha_1) > \alpha_1$, for all value $0 < s \leq L_1$. Implies, $p(s, \alpha_1) > x_1^*$, on $0 < s \leq L_1$. Hence by (5.4.2) and (5.4.40), the result follows. □

Similarly by using (5.4.39) and (5.4.3) the following lemma follows:

Lemma 5.4.15. *If $\beta_1 > y_1^*$, then*

$$\frac{\partial q_1(s, \beta_1)}{\partial s} > 0\ ,\ 0 < s \leq L_1.$$

Lemma 5.4.16. *If $0 < p_2(s, \alpha_2) \leq x_2^*$, then $\alpha_2 < x_2^*$ implies $p_2(s, \alpha_2) < \alpha_2$, for $L_1 \leq s < L_2$.*

Proof. Since $0 < p_2(s, \alpha_2) \leq x_2^*$, then from (5.4.2), we get, $p_2 \mathbf{g}_2(p_2) - q_2 \mathbf{p}_2(p_2) > 0$. Now Since $\alpha_2 < x_2^*$, then $p_2 \mathbf{g}_2(p_2) - q_2 \mathbf{p}_2(p_2) > 0$, for all α_2, p_2. Hence, from (5.4.38), $p_2 < \alpha_2$. □

Again by using (5.4.3) and (5.4.39) the following lemma follows:

Lemma 5.4.17. *If $0 < q_2(s, \beta_2) \leq y_2^*$, then $\beta_2 < y_2^*$ implies $q_2(s, \beta_2) < \beta_2$, for $L_1 \leq s < L_2$.*

Lemma 5.4.18. *Define $G_{1i}(\alpha_i)$ by $G_{1i}(\alpha_i) = p_i(L_1, \alpha_i)$. Then such that*

$$\mathbf{G}_{11} : [x_1^*, \hat{\alpha}_1] \rightarrow [x_1^*, x_2^*],$$

$$\mathbf{G}_{12} : [\hat{\alpha}_2, x_2^*] \rightarrow [x_1^*, x_2^*].$$

Proof. Similar as Lemma 3.3.4 in Chapter 3 . □

Lemma 5.4.19. *Define $G_{2i}(\beta_i)$ by $G_{2i}(\beta_i) = q_i(L_1, \beta_i)$. Then such that*

$$\mathbf{G}_{21} : \left[y_1^*, \hat{\beta}_1\right] \to [y_1^*, y_2^*],$$

$$\mathbf{G}_{22} : \left[\hat{\beta}_2, y_2^*\right] \to [y_1^*, y_2^*].$$

Proof. Similar as Lemma 3.3.4 in Chapter 3 . □

Theorem 5.4.20. *(i) There exists a continuous, monotonic solution of system (5.4.4) with continuous flux at L_1.*
(ii) There exists a continuous, monotonic solution of system (5.4.5) with continuous flux at L_1.

Proof. Analogous to the Theorem 4.4.4 in Chapter 4 . □

Finally, in a similar manner to the case of reservoir boundary conditions, the following linear and nonlinear stability conditions are as follows:

Theorem 5.4.21. *The steady-state, continuous, monotonic solutions of system (5.4.4) and (5.4.5) with continuous flux at the interface $s = L_1$ is asymptotically stable provided the following conditions are satisfied:*

$$(i) \quad \frac{d}{du_i}\left[u_i \mathbf{g}_i(u_i)\right] \le 0\,,$$

$$(ii) \quad \frac{d}{dv_i}\left[v_i \mathbf{f}_i(v_i)\right] \le 0\,, and$$

$$(iii) \quad \left[\mathbf{p}_i(u_i) + \mathbf{q}_i(v_i)\right]^2 < 4\left[\frac{d}{du_i}\left[u_i \mathbf{g}_i(u_i)\right]\right]\left[\frac{d}{dv_i}\left[v_i \mathbf{f}_i(v_i)\right]\right]$$

for $x_1^* \le u_i \le x_2^*,\ \ y_1^* \le v_i \le y_2^*$ *and* $i = 1, 2$.

Theorem 5.4.22. *The steady-state, continuous ,monotonic solutions of non-linear system (5.4.4), (5.4.5), (5.4.20) and (5.4.30), with continuous flux at the interface $s = L_1$ is asymptotically stable in the subregion of*

$$\mathbf{R} : \{x_1^* \leq x_i,\ u_i \leq x_2^*,\ y_1^* \leq y_i\ v_i \leq y_2^*,\ for\ i = 1,2\},$$

provided the following conditions are satisfied:

$$(1)\frac{x_i\mathbf{g}_i(x_i) - u_i\mathbf{g}_i(u_i)}{x_i - u_i} \leq 0,$$

$$(2)\frac{y_i\mathbf{f}_i(y_i) - v_i\mathbf{f}_i(v_i)}{y_i - v_i} \leq 0,$$

$$(3)x_iy_i\left[\frac{u_i\mathbf{p}_i(x_i)}{x_i} + \frac{v_i\mathbf{q}_i(y_i)}{y_i}\right]^2 < 4u_iv_i\left[\frac{x_i\mathbf{g}_i(x_i) - u_i\mathbf{g}_i(u_i)}{x_i - u_i}\right]\left[\frac{y_i\mathbf{f}_i(y_i) - v_i\mathbf{f}_i(v_i)}{y_i - v_i}\right].$$

Remark: This above theorems imply that the system will settle down to a steady state distribution for each species, in the two patches under certain conditions, the magnitude of the steady state distributions of both the species being lower than it's initial density. Further, the above analysis also suggest that patchiness destabilizes the system.

5.4.5 Both the Spccies have Uniform Steady State in the Second Patch

In this case, the steady-state solutions of both the species are variable in the first patch and constant in second patch, i.e. $u_2 = x_2^*$ and $v_2 = M_2$, $L_1 \leq s \leq L_2, t \geq 0$. As shown in the general case we note that here also the steady state solution is positive, continuous and monotonic in the first patch. For stability analysis we use the positive definite function,

$$\begin{aligned} V(t) &= \int_0^{L_1} u_1\left(x_1 - u_1 - u_1\ln\frac{x_1}{x_1^*}\right)ds + \int_{L_1}^{L_2}\left(x_2 - x_2^* - x_2^*\ln\frac{x_2}{x_2^*}\right)ds \\ &+ \int_0^{L_1} v_1\left(y_1 - v_1 - v_1\ln\frac{y_1}{M_1}\right)ds + \int_{L_1}^{L_2}\left(y_2 - M_2 - M_2\ln\frac{y_2}{M_2}\right)ds. \end{aligned}$$

Theorem 5.4.23. *Let $u_2 = x_2^*$ and $v_2 = y_2^*$. Then the steady-state, continuous, monotonic solutions of non-linear system (5.2.1) to (5.2.7) and* *with either (5.2.8) or (5.2.9) and with continuous flux at the interface* $s = L_1$ *is asymptotically stable in a subregion of* $\mathscr{R}$: $\{K_1 \le x_1 \le K_2, x_1^* \le u_1 \le x_2^*, M_1 \le y_1, v_1 \le M_2\}$, *provided the following conditions are satisfied:*

(1) $$\frac{x_1\mathbf{g}_1(x_1) - u_1\mathbf{g}_1(u_1)}{x_1 - u_1} \le 0,$$

(2) $$\frac{y_1\mathbf{f}_1(y_1) - v_1\mathbf{f}_1(v_1)}{y_1 - v_1} \le 0,$$

(3) $$\frac{u_1[\mathbf{p}_1(x_1)]^2}{x_1} \le 4\frac{v_1}{y_1}\left[\frac{x_1\mathbf{g}_1(x_1) - u_1\mathbf{g}_1(u_1)}{x_1 - u_1}\right]\left[\frac{y_1\mathbf{f}_1(y_1) - v_1\mathbf{f}_1(v_1)}{y_1 - v_1}\right].$$

5.5 Summary

In this chapter, we have considered a general competition model of two species with diffusion in a two patch environment. The model has been given by a system of two autonomous partial differential equations. We have obtained the existence of the positive, monotonic, continuous steady-state solution for each species, with continuous flux at the interface. We obtained the the criteria for asymptotic stability of the system in both linear and nonlinear cases under both reservoir or no-flux boundary conditions. It has been shown that in both cases the non-uniform steady-state is asymptotically stable under appropriate conditions. It is also shown that the uniform steady-state system of uniform equilibrium state is globally asymptotically stable.

Chapter 6

A Competing Species Model with Diffusion in Two-Patch Habitat with a Common Supplementary Resource

6.1 Introduction

The study of resource-based competition model is an important area of research in population biology. Some experimental investigations on micro-organisms using the chemostat [178, 179] have been conducted in the fifties and perhaps the best laboratory idealization of nature for population studies has been described in Ref. [180]. Also some other mathematical investigations related to two competing populations which are wholly dependent on a self-renewable resource in a habitat without diffusion have been presented [181–183].

It may be noted that, the effect of diffusion on the growth and co-existence of interacting species have been discussed by several investigators [41, 44, 173–176], but little attention has been paid to study such problems with alternative resource and diffusion. Freedman and Shukla [41] have studied the effect of an alternative resource for predator on a prey-predator system with diffusion in a homogeneous habitat.

Keeping in view the above, in this chapter, we study the effect of a common supplementary resource on the coexistence of two competing species with diffusion, in a two patch habitat. This chapter is organized as follows. In the next section, we proposed a two competing species system with a common supplementary resource in a two-patch habitat. In Section 6.3, we study our main model in a two-patch habitat for both non-uniform and uniform steady state cases under both reservoir and no-flux boundary conditions. In the Section 6.4, a summary is given.

6.2 Formulation of Mathematical Model

We consider a general two-species competing model diffusing between two homogeneous patches in a given patchy habitat as discussed in the Chapter 5. Let $x_i(s,t)$ and $y_i(s,t)$ be the population densities of two species competing for the same resources, such that each species logistically grows in the absence of the other species, and the rate of growth of each species decreases due to the presence of the other species in the i-th patch. Further we consider that there is a common non-diffusing self-renewable supplementary resource for both the species in the habitat, whose biomass density is $R_i(s,t)$, $i = 1,2$. We assume that the density of each of the competing populations which are logistically growing increase with the increase in the density of the supplementary resource biomass. The system is then governed by the following autonomous partial differential equations:

$$\frac{\partial R_i}{\partial t} = a_i R_i \left(1 - \frac{R_i}{C_i}\right) - \alpha_i R_i x_i - \beta_i R_i y_i, \tag{6.2.1}$$

$$\frac{\partial x_i}{\partial t} = x_i \mathbf{g}_i(x_i) - y_i \mathbf{p}_i(x_i) + \theta \alpha_i R_i x_i + D_{1i} \frac{\partial^2 x_i}{\partial s^2}, \tag{6.2.2}$$

$$\frac{\partial y_i}{\partial t} = y_i \mathbf{f}_i(y_i) - x_i \mathbf{q}_i(y_i) + \phi \beta_i R_i y_i + D_{2i} \frac{\partial^2 y_i}{\partial s^2}, \tag{6.2.3}$$

$$0 \leq s \leq L_2, \quad \text{and } i = 1,2.$$

where the i-th patch is assumed to lie along the spatial length $L_{i-1} \leq s \leq L_i$ $(L_0 = 0)$, C_i, $i = 1,2$ are the carrying capacity of the supplementary resource in the i-th patch and the constants α_i and β_i, $i = 1,2$, are positive interaction rates of the alternative resource with the first and second species respectively in the i-th patch. The functions $\mathbf{g}_i(x_i)$ and $\mathbf{f}_i(y_i)$ are the respective specific growth rates, $\mathbf{p}_i(x_i)$, $\mathbf{q}_i(y_i)$ are interaction rates of $x_i(s,t)$ and $y_i(s,t)$, and D_{1i}, D_{2i} are the diffusion coefficient of x_i and y_i in the i-th patch respectively. The constants θ and ϕ are the conversion rates for the first and second species respectively.

We assume the following assumption for $\mathbf{g}_i(x_i)$, $\mathbf{f}_i(y_i)$, $\mathbf{p}_i(x_i)$ and $\mathbf{q}_i(y_i)$:

AH_1: $\mathbf{g}_i(x_i), \mathbf{f}_i(y_i), \mathbf{p}_i(x_i), \mathbf{q}_i(y_i) \in \mathbf{C}^2[0,\infty)$,

$\mathbf{g}_i(0) > 0, \mathbf{f}_i(0) > 0, \mathbf{p}_i(0) = 0, \mathbf{q}_i(0) = 0$,

For $x_i > 0$, $\mathbf{g}_i'(x_i) \leq 0$, $\mathbf{p}_i'(x_i) > 0$,

For $y_i > 0$, $\mathbf{f}_i'(y_i) \leq 0$, $\mathbf{q}_i'(y_i) > 0$.

When the first and second species has a carrying capacity K_i, M_i respectively in the i-th patch, then

AH_2: $\mathbf{g}_i(K_i) = 0, \mathbf{f}_i(M_i) = 0, \ i = 1,2.$

The model is studied under two set of boundary conditions i.e. reservoir and no-flux. In the case of reservoir boundary conditions, we take

$$x_1(0,t) = x_1^* \ , \ x_2(L_2,t) = x_2^*, \tag{6.2.4}$$

$$y_1(0,t) = y_1^* \ , \ y_2(L_2,t) = y_2^*, \tag{6.2.5}$$

and in the case of no-flux boundary conditions, we have

$$\frac{\partial x_1(0,t)}{\partial s} = 0 = \frac{\partial x_2(L_2,t)}{\partial s}, \tag{6.2.6}$$

$$\frac{\partial y_1(0,t)}{\partial s} = 0 = \frac{\partial y_2(L_2,t)}{\partial s}. \tag{6.2.7}$$

We also assume the continuity and flux matching conditions at the interface $s = L_1$. The continuity conditions at the interface $s = L_1$ for this system are,

$$x_1(L_1,t) = x_2(L_1,t), \ \ y_1(L_1,t) = y_2(L_1,t) \ \text{and} \ R_1(L_1,t) = R_2(L_1,t). \tag{6.2.8}$$

In the continuous flux matching conditions at the interface $s = L_1$ for $x_i(s,t)$ and $y_i(s,t)$ are written as,

$$D_{11}\frac{\partial x_1(L_1,t)}{\partial s} = D_{12}\frac{\partial x_2(L_1,t)}{\partial s}, \tag{6.2.9}$$

$$D_{21}\frac{\partial v_1(L_1,t)}{\partial s} = D_{22}\frac{\partial v_2(L_1,t)}{\partial s}. \tag{6.2.10}$$

Finally the model is completed by assuming some positive initial distribution of each species, for $i = 1,2$, that is,

$$x_i(s,0) = \chi_i(s) > 0,\ L_{i-1} < s < L_i, \tag{6.2.11}$$

$$y_i(s,0) = \delta_i(s) > 0,\ L_{i-1} < s < L_i, \tag{6.2.12}$$

$$R_i(s,0) = R_{0i}(s) > 0,\ L_{i-1} < s < L_i. \tag{6.2.13}$$

Our most important aim is to study the long time behavior of the uniform and non-uniform steady state solution of the above model under both type of boundary conditions (namely, reservoir and no flux) and the continuous flux matching conditions at the interface of the two patches.

6.3 Analysis of the Model in a Two Patch Habitat

6.3.1 The Case of Nonuniform Steady State: Under Both Sets of Boundary Conditions

Let $u_i(s)$, $v_i(s)$ and $w_i(s)$ are the steady state solutions of the first species (x_i), second species (y_i) and the supplementary resource (R_i). Then the steady state system of the above proposed model become

$$w_i = \frac{C_i}{a_i}\left[a_i - \alpha_i u_i - \beta_i v_i\right], \tag{6.3.1}$$

$$D_{1i}\frac{d^2 u_i}{ds^2} + u_i \mathbf{g}_i(u_i) - v_i \mathbf{p}_i(u_i) + \theta \alpha_i w_i u_i = 0, \tag{6.3.2}$$

$$D_{2i}\frac{d^2 v_i}{ds^2} + v_i \mathbf{f}_i(v_i) - u_i \mathbf{q}_i(v_i) + \phi \beta_i w_i v_i = 0. \tag{6.3.3}$$

Now substituting the value of w_i from (6.3.1) into (6.3.2) and (6.3.3), we get,

$$D_{1i}\frac{d^2u_i}{ds^2}+u_i\mathscr{G}_i(u_i)-v_i\mathscr{P}_i(u_i)=0, \tag{6.3.4}$$

$$D_{2i}\frac{d^2v_i}{ds^2}+v_i\mathscr{F}_i(v_i)-u_i\mathscr{Q}_i(v_i)=0, \tag{6.3.5}$$

where

$$\begin{aligned}
\mathscr{G}_i(u_i) &= \mathbf{g}_i(u_i)+\theta\alpha_i\frac{C_i}{a_i}(a_i-\alpha_i u_i),\\
\mathscr{P}_i(u_i) &= \mathbf{p}_i(u_i)+\theta\alpha_i\beta_i\frac{C_i}{a_i}u_i,\\
\mathscr{F}_i(v_i) &= \mathbf{f}_i(v_i)+\phi\beta_i\frac{C_i}{a_i}(a_i-\beta_i v_i),\\
\mathscr{Q}_i(v_i) &= \mathbf{q}_i(v_i)+\phi\alpha_i\beta_i\frac{C_i}{a_i}v_i.
\end{aligned}$$

Again the functions $\mathscr{G}_i(u_i)$ and $\mathscr{F}_i(v_i)$ are logistic type, since

$$\begin{aligned}
&\mathscr{G}_i(0)=\mathbf{g}_i(0)+\theta\alpha_iC_i>0,\quad \mathscr{G}_i'(u_i)=\mathbf{g}_i'(u_i)-\theta\alpha_i^2C_i/a_i\le 0,\ \forall u_i\ne 0,\\
&\mathscr{F}_i(0)=\mathbf{f}_i(0)+\phi\beta_iC_i>0,\quad \mathscr{F}_i'(v_i)=\mathbf{f}_i'(v_i)-\phi\beta_i^2C_i/a_i\le 0,\ \forall v_i\ne 0.
\end{aligned}$$

and since,

$\mathscr{P}_i(0)=0,\ \mathscr{P}_i'(u_i)\le 0\ \forall u_i\ne 0$ and
$\mathscr{Q}_i(0)=0,\ \mathscr{Q}_i'(v_i)\le 0\ \forall v_i\ne 0,$

therefore, the functions $\mathscr{P}_i(u_i)$ and $\mathscr{Q}_i(v_i)$ are interaction type functions. Then the system (6.3.4) and (6.3.5) with boundary and conditions,

$$u_1(0,t)=x_1^*,\ u_2(L_2,t)=x_2^* \text{ and } v_1(0,t)=y_1^*,\ v_2(L_2,t)=y_2^* \tag{6.3.6}$$

or

$$\frac{\partial u_1(0,t)}{\partial s}=0=\frac{\partial u_2(L_2,t)}{\partial s},\ \text{and}\ \frac{\partial v_1(0,t)}{\partial s}=0=\frac{\partial v_2(L_2,t)}{\partial s}, \tag{6.3.7}$$

and the continuity and flux matching conditions at the interface $s=L_1$,

$$u_1(L_1,t)=u_2(L_1,t),\ \ v_1(L_1,t)=v_2(L_1,t), \tag{6.3.8}$$

$$D_{11}\frac{du_1}{ds}(L_1) = D_{12}\frac{du_2}{ds}(L_1), \text{ and } D_{21}\frac{dv_1}{ds}(L_1) = D_{22}\frac{dv_2}{ds}(L_1), \quad (6.3.9)$$

become the exactly same type of steady state system described in the previous chapter, the case of two competing species without supplementary resource. In the presence of the non-diffusing supplementary resource, the steady state problem becomes the same type of steady state system as in the previous chapter with the modified growth rates $\mathscr{G}_i(u_i)$ and $\mathscr{F}_i(v_i)$ and the modified interaction rates $\mathscr{P}_i(u_i)$ and $\mathscr{Q}_i(v_i)$. Therefore the behavior of the steady state solutions will be same, which gives the following theorem:

Theorem 6.3.1. *There exists an unique positive, continuous, monotonic steady state solution for each of the species with continuous flux at* L_1.

Now we go for the linear and nonlinear stability of the system.

Theorem 6.3.2. *The positive continuous steady state solutions of the system is locally asymptotically stable if*

$$\begin{array}{lll} (i) & \mathscr{X}_i \leq 0,\ \mathscr{Y}_i \leq 0,\ \mathscr{Z}_i \leq 0, & (6.3.10) \\ (ii) & \mathscr{U}_i^2 \leq 4\mathscr{X}_i\mathscr{Y}_i, & (6.3.11) \\ (iii) & \mathscr{X}_i\mathscr{Y}_i\mathscr{Z}_i + 2\mathscr{U}_i\mathscr{V}_i\mathscr{W}_i \leq \mathscr{X}_i\mathscr{V}_i^2 + \mathscr{Y}_i\mathscr{W}_i^2 + \mathscr{Z}_i\mathscr{U}_i^2, & (6.3.12) \end{array}$$

where

$$\begin{aligned} \mathscr{X}_i &= \mathbf{g}_i(u_i) + u_i\mathbf{g}_i'(u_i) - v_i\mathbf{p}_i'(u_i) + \theta\alpha_i w_i, \\ \mathscr{Y}_i &= \mathbf{f}_i(v_i) + v_i\mathbf{f}_i'(v_i) - u_i\mathbf{q}_i'(v_i) + \phi\beta_i w_i, \\ \mathscr{Z}_i &= a_i\left(1 - \frac{2w_i}{C_i}\right) - \alpha_i u_i - \beta_i v_i, \\ \mathscr{U}_i &= -\frac{1}{2}[\mathbf{p}_i(u_i) + \mathbf{q}_i(v_i)], \\ \mathscr{V}_i &= \frac{\beta_i}{2}[\phi v_i - w_i], \\ \text{and } \mathscr{W}_i &= \frac{\alpha_i}{2}[\theta u_i - w_i]. \end{aligned} \quad (6.3.13)$$

Proof. Linearizing (6.2.1), (6.2.2) and (6.2.3) by using,

$$R_i(s,t) = w_i(s) + r_i(s,t), \tag{6.3.14}$$

$$x_i(s,t) = u_i(s) + n_i(s,t), \tag{6.3.15}$$

$$y_i(s,t) = v_i(s) + m_i(s,t), \tag{6.3.16}$$

we have,

$$\frac{\partial r_i}{\partial t} = r_i\left[a_i\left(1 - \frac{2w_i}{C_i}\right) - \alpha_i u_i - \beta_i v_i\right] - n_i\alpha_i w_i - m_i\beta_i w_i, \tag{6.3.17}$$

$$\begin{aligned}\frac{\partial n_i}{\partial t} &= n_i[\mathbf{g}_i(u_i) + u_i\mathbf{g}_i'(u_i) - v_i\mathbf{p}_i'(u_i) + \theta\alpha_i w_i] \\ &\quad - m_i\mathbf{p}_i(u_i) + r_i\theta\alpha_i u_i + D_{1i}\frac{\partial^2 n_i}{\partial s^2},\end{aligned} \tag{6.3.18}$$

$$\begin{aligned}\frac{\partial m_i}{\partial t} &= m_i[\mathbf{f}_i(v_i) + v_i\mathbf{f}_i'(v_i) - u_i\mathbf{q}_i'(v_i) + \phi\beta_i w_i] \\ &\quad - n_i\mathbf{q}_i(v_i) + r_i\phi\beta_i v_i + D_{2i}\frac{\partial^2 m_i}{\partial s^2}.\end{aligned} \tag{6.3.19}$$

Using (6.3.14), (6.3.15) and (6.3.16) the corresponding boundary and matching conditions can be obtained as follows:

$$\begin{aligned}
n_1(0,t) &= 0 = n_2(L_2,t),\ m_1(0,t) = 0 = m_2(L_2,t), \\
&\quad \text{(Reservoir case)} \\
\frac{\partial n_1}{\partial s}(0,t) &= \frac{\partial n_2}{\partial s}(L_2,t),\ \frac{\partial m_1}{\partial s}(0,t) = \frac{\partial m_2}{\partial s}(L_2,t), \\
&\quad \text{(No-flux case)} \\
n_1(L_1,t) &= 0 = n_2(L_1,t),\ m_1(L_1,t) = 0 = m_2(L_1,t), \\
D_{11}\frac{\partial n_1}{\partial s}(L_1,t) &= D_{12}\frac{\partial n_2}{\partial s}(L_1,t),\ D_{21}\frac{\partial m_1}{\partial s}(L_1,t) = D_{22}\frac{\partial m_2}{\partial s}(L_1,t).
\end{aligned}$$

Now we consider the following positive definite function,

$$V(t) = \sum_1^2 \int_{L_{i-1}}^{L_i} \frac{1}{2}[r_i^2 + n_i^2 + m_i^2]ds. \tag{6.3.20}$$

From which we get,

$$\dot{V}(t) = \sum_{1}^{2} \int_{L_{i-1}}^{L_i} \left[r_i \frac{\partial r_i}{\partial t} + n_i \frac{\partial n_i}{\partial t} + m_i \frac{\partial m_i}{\partial t} \right] ds.$$

By using (6.3.18), (6.3.19) and (6.3.17), we get,

$$\begin{aligned}
\dot{V}(t) = & \sum_{1}^{2} \int_{L_{i-1}}^{L_i} r_i^2 \left[a_i \left(1 - \frac{2w_i}{C_i}\right) - \alpha_i u_i - \beta_i v_i \right] ds \\
+ & \sum_{1}^{2} \int_{L_{i-1}}^{L_i} n_i^2 [\mathbf{g}_i(u_i) + u_i \mathbf{g}_i'(u_i) - v_i \mathbf{p}_i'(u_i) + \theta \alpha_i w_i] ds \\
+ & \sum_{1}^{2} \int_{L_{i-1}}^{L_i} m_i^2 [\mathbf{f}_i(v_i) + v_i \mathbf{f}_i'(v_i) - u_i \mathbf{q}_i'(v_i) + \phi \beta_i w_i] ds \\
+ & \sum_{1}^{2} \int_{L_{i-1}}^{L_i} n_i m_i [-\mathbf{p}_i(u_i) - \mathbf{q}_i(v_i)] ds + \sum_{1}^{2} \int_{L_{i-1}}^{L_i} n_i r_i \alpha_i [\theta u_i - w_i] ds \\
+ & \sum_{1}^{2} \int_{L_{i-1}}^{L_i} m_i r_i \beta_i [\phi v_i - w_i] ds \\
+ & \sum_{1}^{2} D_{1i} \int_{L_{i-1}}^{L_i} n_i \frac{\partial^2 n_i}{\partial s^2} ds + \sum_{1}^{2} D_{2i} \int_{L_{i-1}}^{L_i} m_i \frac{\partial^2 m_i}{\partial s^2} ds.
\end{aligned}$$

Therefore,

$$\begin{aligned}
\dot{V}(t) = & \sum_{1}^{2} \int_{L_{i-1}}^{L_i} [\mathscr{Z}_i r_i^2 + \mathscr{X}_i n_i^2 + \mathscr{Y}_i m_i^2 + 2\mathscr{W}_i r_i n_i + 2\mathscr{U}_i n_i m_i + 2\mathscr{V}_i m_i r_i] ds \\
- & \sum_{1}^{2} D_{1i} \int_{L_{i-1}}^{L_i} \left(\frac{\partial n_i}{\partial s}\right)^2 ds - \sum_{1}^{2} D_{2i} \int_{L_{i-1}}^{L_i} \left(\frac{\partial m_i}{\partial s}\right)^2 ds.
\end{aligned}$$

where the functions $\mathscr{X}_i$, $\mathscr{Y}_i$, $\mathscr{Z}_i$, $\mathscr{U}_i$, $\mathscr{V}_i$ and $\mathscr{W}_i$ are given in (6.3.13). Hence $\dot{V}$ is negative definite if the conditions (6.3.10)–(6.3.12) holds. □

We now show that there exist a small subregion of $\mathscr{R} : \{min(x_1^*, x_2^*) \leq x_i, u_i \leq max(x_1^*, x_2^*),\ min(y_1^*, y_2^*) \leq y_i, v_i \leq max(y_1^*, y_2^*)\}$, where the system is non-linearly stable. For this let

$$\mathscr{A}_i = \frac{x_i \mathbf{g}_i(x_i) - u_i \mathbf{g}_i(u_i)}{x_i - u_i} - y_i \frac{\mathbf{p}_i(x_i) - \mathbf{p}_i(u_i)}{x_i - u_i} + \theta \alpha_i R_i, \qquad (6.3.21)$$

$$\mathscr{B}_i = \frac{y_i\mathbf{f}_i(y_i) - v_i\mathbf{f}_i(v_i)}{y_i - v_i} - x_i\frac{\mathbf{q}_i(y_i) - \mathbf{q}_i(v_i)}{y_i - v_i} + \phi\beta_i R_i, \tag{6.3.22}$$

$$\mathscr{C}_i = a_i\left(1 - \frac{R_i + w_i}{C_i}\right) - \alpha_i u_i - \beta_i v_i, \tag{6.3.23}$$

$$\mathscr{D}_i = -\frac{1}{2}[\mathbf{p}_i(u_i) + \mathbf{q}_i(v_i)], \tag{6.3.24}$$

$$\mathscr{E}_i = \frac{\beta_i}{2}[\phi v_i - R_i], \tag{6.3.25}$$

$$\mathscr{F}_i = \frac{\alpha_i}{2}[\theta u_i - R_i]. \tag{6.3.26}$$

then the following nonlinear stability theorem is proved.

Theorem 6.3.3. *The positive continuous steady state solutions of the system is nonlinearly asymptotically stable if,*

$$(i) \quad \mathscr{A}_i \le 0,\ \mathscr{B}_i \le 0,\ \mathscr{C}_i \le 0, \tag{6.3.27}$$

$$(ii) \quad \mathscr{D}_i^2 \le 4\mathscr{A}_i\mathscr{B}_i, \tag{6.3.28}$$

$$(iii) \quad \mathscr{A}_i\mathscr{B}_i\mathscr{C}_i + 2\mathscr{D}_i\mathscr{E}_i\mathscr{F}_i \le \mathscr{A}_i\mathscr{E}_i^2 + \mathscr{B}_i\mathscr{F}_i^2 + \mathscr{C}_i\mathscr{D}_i^2. \tag{6.3.29}$$

Proof. By using (6.3.15), (6.3.16) and (6.3.14), we get from (6.2.1), (6.2.2) and (6.2.3),

$$\frac{\partial r_i}{\partial t} = r_i\left[a_i\left(1 - \frac{R_i + w_i}{C_i}\right) - \alpha_i u_i - \beta_i v_i\right] - n_i\alpha_i R_i - m_i\beta_i R_i, \tag{6.3.30}$$

$$\begin{aligned}\frac{\partial n_i}{\partial t} &= n_i\left[\frac{x_i\mathbf{g}_i(x_i) - u_i\mathbf{g}_i(u_i)}{x_i - u_i} - y_i\frac{\mathbf{p}_i(x_i) - \mathbf{p}_i(u_i)}{x_i - u_i} + \theta\alpha_i R_i\right] \\ &\quad - m_i\mathbf{p}_i(u_i) + r_i\theta\alpha_i u_i + D_{1i}\frac{\partial^2 n_i}{\partial s^2},\end{aligned} \tag{6.3.31}$$

$$\begin{aligned}\frac{\partial m_i}{\partial t} &= m_i\left[\frac{y_i\mathbf{f}_i(y_i) - v_i\mathbf{f}_i(v_i)}{y_i - v_i} - x_i\frac{\mathbf{q}_i(y_i) - \mathbf{q}_i(v_i)}{y_i - v_i} + \phi\beta_i R_i\right] \\ &\quad - n_i\mathbf{q}_i(v_i) + r_i\phi\beta_i v_i + D_{2i}\frac{\partial^2 m_i}{\partial s^2}.\end{aligned} \tag{6.3.32}$$

Here also we consider the same positive definite function as in the case of linear stability.

$$V(t)=\sum_1^2\int_{L_{i-1}}^{L_i}\frac{1}{2}[r_i^2+n_i^2+m_i^2]ds.$$

From which we get,

$$\dot{V}(t)=\sum_1^2\int_{L_{i-1}}^{L_i}\left[r_i\frac{\partial r_i}{\partial t}+n_i\frac{\partial n_i}{\partial t}+m_i\frac{\partial m_i}{\partial t}\right]ds.$$

By using (6.3.30), (6.3.31) and (6.3.32), we get,

$$\begin{aligned}\dot{V}(t)= & \sum_1^2\int_{L_{i-1}}^{L_i}n_i^2\left[\frac{x_i\mathbf{g}_i(x_i)-u_i\mathbf{g}_i(u_i)}{x_i-u_i}-y_i\frac{\mathbf{p}_i(x_i)-\mathbf{p}_i(u_i)}{x_i-u_i}+\theta\alpha_iR_i\right]ds\\
+ & \sum_1^2\int_{L_{i-1}}^{L_i}m_i^2\left[\frac{y_i\mathbf{f}_i(y_i)-v_i\mathbf{f}_i(v_i)}{y_i-v_i}-x_i\frac{\mathbf{q}_i(y_i)-\mathbf{q}_i(v_i)}{y_i-v_i}+\phi\beta_iR_i\right]ds\\
+ & \sum_1^2\int_{L_{i-1}}^{L_i}r_i^2\left[a_i\left(1-\frac{R_i+w_i}{C_i}\right)-\alpha_iu_i-\beta_iv_i\right]ds\\
+ & \sum_1^2\int_{L_{i-1}}^{L_i}n_im_i[-\mathbf{p}_i(u_i)-\mathbf{q}_i(v_i)]ds+\sum_1^2\int_{L_{i-1}}^{L_i}m_ir_i\beta_i[\phi v_i-R_i]ds\\
+ & \sum_1^2\int_{L_{i-1}}^{L_i}r_in_i\alpha_i[\theta u_i-R_i]ds\\
+ & \sum_1^2D_{1i}\int_{L_{i-1}}^{L_i}n_i\frac{\partial^2n_i}{\partial s^2}ds+\sum_1^2D_{2i}\int_{L_{i-1}}^{L_i}m_i\frac{\partial^2m_i}{\partial s^2}ds.\end{aligned}$$

Therefore,

$$\begin{aligned}\dot{V}(t)= & \sum_1^2\int_{L_{i-1}}^{L_i}[\mathscr{A}_in_i^2+\mathscr{B}_im_i^2+\mathscr{C}_ir_i^2+2\mathscr{D}_in_im_i+2\mathscr{E}_im_ir_i+2\mathscr{F}_ir_in_i]ds\\
- & \sum_1^2D_{1i}\int_{L_{i-1}}^{L_i}\left(\frac{\partial n_i}{\partial s}\right)^2ds-\sum_1^2D_{2i}\int_{L_{i-1}}^{L_i}\left(\frac{\partial m_i}{\partial s}\right)^2ds.\end{aligned}$$

where the functions $\mathscr{A}_i$, $\mathscr{B}_i$, $\mathscr{C}_i$, $\mathscr{D}_i$, $\mathscr{E}_i$ and $\mathscr{F}_i$ are given by (6.3.21)–(6.3.26). Hence $\dot{V}$ is negative definite if the conditions (6.3.27)–(6.3.29) holds true, for both $i=1,2$. □

Now, we consider the uniform steady state case.

6.3.2 The Case of Uniform Steady State: Under Both Sets of Boundary Conditions

Our purpose of this section to find the conditions for local and global stability of the uniform steady state, i.e. $R_i(s,t) \equiv C^*$, $x_i(s,t) \equiv K^*$ and $y_i(s,t) \equiv M^*$, for $0 \leq s \leq L_2$, $t \geq 0$, of the system, under both sets of boundary conditions.

Theorem 6.3.4. *The equilibrium (C^*, K^*, M^*) is locally asymptotically stable, for $i = 1,2$, if the following conditions are satisfied,*

$$(i) \quad H_i^* + \theta\alpha_i C^* \leq 0, \tag{6.3.33}$$

$$(ii) \quad F_i^* + \phi\beta_i C^* \leq 0, \tag{6.3.34}$$

$$(iii) \quad [\mathbf{p}_i(K^*) + \mathbf{q}_i(M^*)]^2 \leq 4[H_i^* + \theta\alpha_i C^*][F_i^* + \phi\beta_i C^*], \; i = 1,2, \tag{6.3.35}$$

$$(iv) \quad [H_i^* + \theta\alpha_i C^*][F_i^* + \phi\beta_i C^*]\left[\frac{a_i\phi M^*}{C_i}\right] \leq [F_i^* + \phi\beta_i C^*][\theta K^* - \phi M^*]^2 + \left[\frac{a_i\phi M^*}{C_i}\right][\mathbf{p}_i(K^*) + \mathbf{q}_i(M^*)]^2, \tag{6.3.36}$$

where

$$H_i^* = \mathbf{g}_i(K^*) + K^*\mathbf{g}_i'(K^*) - M^*\mathbf{p}_i'(K^*) \; and F_i^* = \mathbf{f}_i(M^*) + M^*\mathbf{f}_i'(M^*) - K^*\mathbf{q}_i'(M^*). \tag{6.3.37}$$

Proof. Linearizing the system (6.2.1)–(6.2.3), by using

$$R_i(s,t) = C^* + r_i(s,t), \tag{6.3.38}$$

$$x_i(s,t) = K^* + n_i(s,t), \tag{6.3.39}$$

$$y_i(s,t) = M^* + m_i(s,t), \tag{6.3.40}$$

we get,

$$\frac{\partial r_i}{\partial t} = r_i\left[-\frac{a_i C^*}{C_i}\right] - n_i\alpha_i C^* - m_i\beta_i C^*, \tag{6.3.41}$$

$$\frac{\partial n_i}{\partial t} = n_i[\mathbf{g}_i(K^*) + K^*\mathbf{g}_i'(K^*) - M^*\mathbf{p}_i'(K^*) + \theta\alpha_i C^*] - m_i\mathbf{p}_i(K^*) + r_i\theta\alpha_i K^* + D_{1i}\frac{\partial^2 n_i}{\partial s^2}, \tag{6.3.42}$$

$$\begin{aligned}\frac{\partial m_i}{\partial t} &= m_i[\mathbf{f}_i(M^*)+M^*\mathbf{f}_i'(M^*)-K^*\mathbf{q}_i'(M^*)+\phi\beta_iC^*] \\ &\quad -n_i\mathbf{q}_i(M^*)+r_i\phi\beta_iM^*+D_{2i}\frac{\partial^2 m_i}{\partial s^2}. \qquad (6.3.43)\end{aligned}$$

We considering the following positive definite function,

$$\mathbf{V}=\frac{1}{2}\sum_1^2\int_{L_{i-1}}^{L_i}\left[(x_i-K^*)^2+(y_i-M^*)^2+d_i(R_i-C^*)^2\right], \qquad (6.3.44)$$

where d_i, $i=1,2$ are positive constants.
Differentiating (6.3.44) and using (6.3.41)–(6.3.43), we get

$$\begin{aligned}\dot{V} = &\sum_1^2\int_{L_{i-1}}^{L_i} n_i^2[H_i^*+\theta\alpha_iC^*]ds+\sum_1^2\int_{L_{i-1}}^{L_i} m_i^2[G_i^*+\phi\beta_iC^*]ds \\ - &\sum_1^2\int_{L_{i-1}}^{L_i} r_i^2\left[\frac{d_ia_iC^*}{C_i}\right]ds-\sum_1^2\int_{L_{i-1}}^{L_i} n_im_i[\mathbf{p}_i(K^*)+\mathbf{q}_i(M^*)]ds \\ + &\sum_1^2\int_{L_{i-1}}^{L_i} n_ir_i\alpha_i[\theta K^*-d_iC^*]ds+\sum_1^2\int_{L_{i-1}}^{L_i} m_ir_i\beta_i[\phi M^*-d_iC^*]ds \\ + &\sum_1^2 D_{1i}\int_{L_{i-1}}^{L_i} n_i\frac{\partial^2 n_i}{\partial s^2}ds+\sum_1^2 D_{2i}\int_{L_{i-1}}^{L_i} m_i\frac{\partial^2 m_i}{\partial s^2}ds. \qquad (6.3.45)\end{aligned}$$

Integrating by parts and using the matching conditions at the interface and for both set of boundary conditions,

$$\sum_1^2\int_{L_{i-1}}^{L_i} D_{1i}n_i\frac{\partial^2 n_i}{\partial s^2}ds = -\sum_1^2 D_{1i}\int_{L_{i-1}}^{L_i}\left(\frac{\partial n_i}{\partial s}\right)^2 ds, \qquad (6.3.46)$$

$$\sum_1^2\int_{L_{i-1}}^{L_i} D_{2i}m_i\frac{\partial^2 m_i}{\partial s^2}ds = -\sum_1^2 D_{2i}\int_{L_{i-1}}^{L_i}\left(\frac{\partial m_i}{\partial s}\right)^2 ds. \qquad (6.3.47)$$

We choose d_i, for $i=1,2$, such that, the coefficients of m_ir_i become zero, i.e. $d_1=d_2=\phi M^*/C^*$. Therefore, from (6.3.45), $\dot{V}$ is negative definite, if the conditions (6.3.33)–(6.3.35) and (6.3.36) are satisfies. □

Using Poincare's Inequality, we can reduce the local stability conditions as follows:

Theorem 6.3.5. *Let $H_i^* + \theta\alpha_i C^* > 0$ and/or $F_i^* + \phi\beta_i C^* > 0$. Then the equilibrium (K^*, M^*, C^*) is locally asymptotically stable, if the conditions (6.3.35) and (6.3.36) along with*

$$H_i^* + \theta\alpha_i C^* \leq D_{1i}\frac{\pi^2}{(L_i - L_{i-1})^2}, \text{ and } F_i^* + \phi\beta_i C^* \leq D_{2i}\frac{\pi^2}{(L_i - L_{i-1})^2}$$

for $i = 1, 2$, holds.

Proof. By using Poincare's Inequality, we get

$$D_{1i}\int_{L_{i-1}}^{L_i}\left[\frac{\partial n_i}{\partial s}\right]^2 ds \leq D_{1i}\frac{\pi^2}{(L_i - L_{i-1})^2}\int_{L_{i-1}}^{L_i} n_i^2 ds,$$

and

$$D_{2i}\int_{L_{i-1}}^{L_i}\left[\frac{\partial m_i}{\partial s}\right]^2 ds \leq D_{2i}\frac{\pi^2}{(L_i - L_{i-1})^2}\int_{L_{i-1}}^{L_i} m_i^2 ds.$$

Therefore from (6.3.45), using (6.3.46) and (6.3.47) and choosing $d_i = \phi M^*/C^*$, for $i = 1, 2$, we get,

$$\begin{aligned}
\dot{V} = \quad & \sum_1^2 \int_{L_{i-1}}^{L_i} n_i^2 [H_i^* + \theta\alpha_i C^* - D_{1i}\frac{\pi^2}{(L_i - L_{i-1})^2}] ds \\
+ \quad & \sum_1^2 \int_{L_{i-1}}^{L_i} m_i^2 [G_i^* + \phi\beta_i C^* - D_{2i}\frac{\pi^2}{(L_i - L_{i-1})^2}] ds \\
- \quad & \sum_1^2 \int_{L_{i-1}}^{L_i} r_i^2 \left[\frac{a_i\phi M^*}{C_i}\right] ds - \sum_1^2 \int_{L_{i-1}}^{L_i} n_i m_i [\mathbf{p}_i(K^*) + \mathbf{q}_i(M^*)] ds \\
+ \quad & \sum_1^2 \int_{L_{i-1}}^{L_i} n_i r_i \alpha_i [\theta K^* - \phi M^*] ds.
\end{aligned}$$

Hence the theorem. □

We now state the global stability of the uniform steady state.

Theorem 6.3.6. *The uniform steady-state (K^*,M^*,c^*) is globally asymptotically stable if*

$$\mathscr{A}_i = \frac{x_i\mathbf{g}_i(x_i) - M^*\mathbf{p}_i(x_i)}{x_i - K^*} + \theta\alpha_i C^* \leq 0, \tag{6.3.48}$$

$$\mathscr{B}_i = \frac{y_i\mathbf{f}_i(y_i) - K^*\mathbf{q}_i(y_i)}{y_i - M^*} + \phi\beta_i C^* \leq 0, \tag{6.3.49}$$

$$\left[\frac{\mathbf{p}_i(x_i)}{x_i} + \frac{\mathbf{q}_i(y_i)}{y_i}\right]^2 \leq 4\frac{\mathscr{A}_i\mathscr{B}_i}{x_i y_i}, \tag{6.3.50}$$

and

$$\frac{\mathscr{A}_i\mathscr{B}_i a_i}{x_i y_i C_i} \leq \beta_i^2\mathscr{A}_i[\phi-1]^2 + \alpha_i^2\mathscr{B}_i[\theta-1]^2 + \frac{a_i}{C_i}\left[\frac{\mathbf{p}_i(x_i)}{x_i} + \frac{\mathbf{q}_i(y_i)}{y_i}\right]^2. \tag{6.3.51}$$

Proof. Let us consider the following positive definite function,

$$\begin{aligned} V(x,y) = \quad & \sum_1^2 \int_{L_{i-1}}^{L_i} \left(x_i - K^* - K^* ln\frac{x_i}{K^*}\right) ds \\ & + \sum_1^2 \int_{L_{i-1}}^{L_i} \left(y_i - M^* - M^* ln\frac{y_i}{M^*}\right) ds \\ & + \sum_1^2 \int_{L_{i-1}}^{L_i} \left(R_i - C^* - C^* ln\frac{R_i}{C^*}\right). \end{aligned} \tag{6.3.52}$$

Differentiating (6.3.52) with respect to t, and using (6.2.1)–(6.2.2), we get

$$\begin{aligned} \dot{V}(s,t) \quad = \quad & \sum_{i=1}^2 \int_{L_{i-1}}^{L_i} \left[\left(\frac{x_i - K^*}{x_i}\right)\frac{\partial x_i}{\partial t} + \left(\frac{y_i - M^*}{y_i}\right)\frac{\partial y_i}{\partial t}\right. \\ & \left. + \left(\frac{R_i - C^*}{R_i}\right)\frac{\partial R_i}{\partial t}\right] ds \end{aligned}$$

$$
\begin{aligned}
\dot{V}(s,t) &= \sum_{i=1}^{2}\int_{L_{i-1}}^{L_i}\frac{(x_i-K^*)^2}{x_i}\left[\frac{x_i\mathbf{g}_i(x_i)-M^*\mathbf{p}_i(x_i)}{x_i-K^*}+\theta\alpha_i C^*\right]ds\\
&+ \sum_{i=1}^{2}\int_{L_{i-1}}^{L_i}\frac{(y_i-M^*)^2}{y_i}\left[\frac{y_i\mathbf{f}_i(y_i)-K^*\mathbf{q}_i(y_i)}{y_i-M^*}+\phi\beta_i C^*\right]ds\\
&- \sum_{1}^{2}\int_{L_{i-1}}^{L_i}(R_i-C^*)^2\left[\frac{a_i}{C_i}\right]ds\\
&- \sum_{1}^{2}\int_{L_{i-1}}^{L_i}(x_i-K^*)(y_i-M^*)\left[\frac{\mathbf{p}_i(x_i)}{x_i}+\frac{\mathbf{q}_i(y_i)}{y_i}\right]ds\\
&+ \sum_{1}^{2}\int_{L_{i-1}}^{L_i}(y_i-M^*)(R_i-C^*)\left[\beta_i(\phi-1)\right]ds\\
&+ \sum_{1}^{2}\int_{L_{i-1}}^{L_i}(R_i-C^*)(x_i-K^*)\left[\alpha_i(\theta-1)\right]ds\\
&+ \sum_{1}^{2}D_{1i}\int_{L_{i-1}}^{L_i}\frac{x_i-K^*}{x_i}\frac{\partial^2 x_i}{\partial s^2}ds+\sum_{1}^{2}D_{2i}\int_{L_{i-1}}^{L_i}\frac{y_i-M^*}{y_i}\frac{\partial^2 y_i}{\partial s^2}ds.
\end{aligned}
$$

Now since under both sets of boundary conditions,

$$[x_1(0,t)-K^*]\frac{\partial x_1}{\partial s}(0,t)=[x_2(L_2,t)-K^*]\frac{\partial x_2}{\partial s}(L_2,t)=0, \quad (6.3.53)$$

$$[y_1(0,t)-M^*]\frac{\partial y_1}{\partial s}(0,t)=[y_2(L_2,t)-M^*]\frac{\partial y_2}{\partial s}(L_2,t)=0. \quad (6.3.54)$$

Then the integrals,

$$I_1=\sum_{1}^{2}D_{1i}\int_{L_{i-1}}^{L_i}\frac{x_i-K^*}{x_i}\frac{\partial^2 x_i}{\partial s^2}ds=-\sum_{1}^{2}D_{1i}\int_{L_{i-1}}^{L_i}\left(\frac{\partial x_i}{\partial s}\right)^2 ds, \quad (6.3.55)$$

and

$$I_2=\sum_{1}^{2}D_{2i}\int_{L_{i-1}}^{L_i}\frac{y_i-M^*}{y_i}\frac{\partial^2 y_i}{\partial s^2}ds=-\sum_{1}^{2}D_{2i}\int_{L_{i-1}}^{L_i}\left(\frac{\partial y_i}{\partial s}\right)^2 ds. \quad (6.3.56)$$

Hence $\dot{V}(K^*,M^*,C^*)=0$ and $\dot{V}(x,y)<0$ if the conditions (6.3.48)–(6.3.51) are satisfied. Therefore $\dot{V}(x,y)$ is negative definite over $x>0$, $y>0$, $R>0$ with respect to $x_i^*=K^*$, $y_i^*=M^*$, $R_i^*=C^*$, proving the theorem. □

Remark: On comparing the analysis of this chapter with earlier chapter we may be concluded that the role of the supplementary resource is to increase the level of non-uniform steady state at each point of the habitat.

6.4 Summary

In this chapter, we have discussed the existence and stability of the non-uniform steady state corresponding to two competing species system in a two patch habitat with diffusion. In this chapter, the same ecological problem modeled and analyzed when there is a non-diffusing renewable common resource for each of the competing population in both the patches. It has been assumed that both the competing population follow a general type of logistic growth in each of the patches as in the previous chapter. Also, the self-renewable supplementary resource is simple logistically growing.

It has been shown; there exists a positive, monotonic, continuous steady state solution with continuous matching at the interface for both the species separately and we also obtained the criteria for asymptotic stability for both linear and nonlinear cases under both sets of boundary conditions. It has been further shown that in the presence of supplementary resource the level of steady state distribution may increase and the effect of patchiness is destabilizing even in the presence of a common self-renewable supplementary resource for both the species.

Chapter 7

Dynamics of a Prey and Generalized-Predator System with Disease in Prey and Gestation Delay for Predator in Single Patch Habitat

7.1 Introduction

The correlation between the disease and the prey-predator system is a topic of significant interest, and the joint study of ecology and epidemiology is a relatively new branch of study, known as eco-epidemiology. It is a well-known fact that the predator is more likely to attack the infected prey because the latter gets weaker and less active due to infection, and hence became more vulnerable to the predator. This concept was modeled by various researchers [87, 88, 184, 185]. But, there is also a possibility that the predator gets infected due to consumption of the infected prey and dies out more rapidly. In this case, the growth of the predator will depend on the healthy prey. Further, there will be a lack of the healthy prey due to disease in the prey population and therefore, the predator starts depending on the alternative foods for their survival. Also, in population dynamics, growth is not instantaneous and the predator populations take some time to give birth to a new offspring after mating is known as gestation delay. The simplest prey-predator models cannot capture the rich variety of dynamics and the inclusion of the gestation delay in these models makes them more realistic [83, 99–101].

In the present chapter, we proposed and analyzed prey-predator system with disease in prey, and predator depending on alternative resources for survival. We have also considered gestation delay for predator. This chapter is organized as follows. In Section 7.2, formulation of model is presented. In Section 7.3, positivity and boundedness of the system has been obtained. In Section 7.4, the system is analyzed for the asymptotic stability at all the feasible equilibrium states and obtained the conditions for the existence of Hopf bifurcation at the disease-free equilibrium and endemic equilibrium states. In Section 7.5, the sensitivity analysis of the state variables at endemic equilibrium state with respect to model parameters is performed. In Section 7.6, we presented some numerical simulations to support our analytical findings. Finally, a brief conclusion is given in the last section.

7.2 Formulation of Mathematical Model

In this chapter, we extend the prey-predator dynamics of model-2 (Chapter 2) by taking into consideration the disease in the prey and gestation delay for predator growth. The assumptions of the proposed system are:

(i) In a particular habitat, there are two populations; prey and predator. There is a disease among the prey population, and the prey population at any time t is divided into two mutually exclusive classes, susceptible S and infective I. The density of predator population at any time t is P. The incidence rate is the classic bilinear βSI and β is the contact rate for every infective prey with susceptible prey.

(ii) The prey population grows with logistic rate, a is the intrinsic growth rate, k is the carrying capacity. We suppose that the infective preys cannot produce offsprings due to the disease. Thus, the

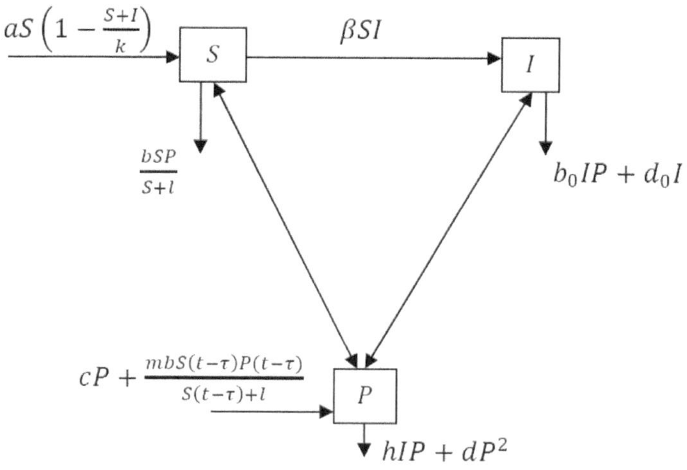

FIGURE 7.1 The schematic diagram of the model.

per capita growth rate of the prey is $a\left(1-\frac{S+I}{k}\right)$ in the absence of the predator.

(iii) The predator catches the susceptible prey, and the predation functional response is Holling type II.

(iv) The predator might get infected due to consumption of infected prey and dies out with a fixed rate h.

(v) τ is a gestation delay for predator growth.

(vi) Due to lack of healthy prey, predator depends on alternative resources.

The proposed system is of the form:

$$\frac{dS}{dt} = aS\left(1-\frac{S+I}{k}\right) - \frac{bSP}{S+l} - \beta SI, \tag{7.2.1}$$

$$\frac{dI}{dt} = \beta SI - b_0IP - d_0I, \tag{7.2.2}$$

$$\frac{dP}{dt} = cP - hIP + \frac{mbS(t-\tau)P(t-\tau)}{S(t-\tau)+l} - dP^2, \tag{7.2.3}$$

with initial conditions:

$$S(\theta)=\phi_1(\theta),\ I(\theta)=\phi_2(\theta),\ P(\theta)=\phi_3(\theta),\quad \phi_1(0)>0,\ \phi_2(0)>0,\ \phi_3(0)>0,$$

where $\theta \in [-\tau,0]$ and $\phi_1(\theta), \phi_2(\theta), \phi_3(\theta) \in \mathscr{C}([-\tau,0],R_+^3)$, the Banach space of continuous functions mapping the interval $[-\tau,0]$ into R_+^3, where $R_+^3 = \{(x_1,x_2,x_3) : x_i \geq 0, i = 1,2,3\}$. The detail description of the parameters is stated in Table 7.1.

TABLE 7.1 Description of Parameters for the System (7.2.1)–(7.2.3)

Parameter	Description	Unit
a	Intrinsic growth rate of prey	days^{-1}
k	Carrying capacity of prey in a particular habitat	–
b	Predation rate of susceptible prey	days^{-1}
l	Half saturation constant	–
β	Contact rate of infective prey with susceptible prey	days^{-1}
b_0	Predation rate of infected prey	days^{-1}
d_0	Death rate for the infective prey	days^{-1}
c	Growth rate of predator due to alternative resources	days^{-1}
h	Death rate of predator due to infected prey	days^{-1}
m	Conversion rate for predator	days^{-1}
d	Overcrowding of predator species	days^{-1}
τ	Gestation delay for predator growth	days

7.3 Positivity and Boundedness of the System

We state and prove the following lemmas for the positivity and boundedness of the solution of the system (7.2.1)–(7.2.3):

Lemma 7.3.1. *The solution of the system (7.2.1)–(7.2.3) with initial conditions are positive, for all $t \geq 0$.*

Proof. Let $(S(t), I(t), P(t))$ be a solution of the system (7.2.1)–(7.2.3) with initial condition. Let us consider $S(t)$ for $t \in [0, \tau]$. We obtain from the equation (7.2.1) that

$$\frac{dS}{dt} \geq -aS\left(\frac{S+I}{k}\right) - \frac{bSP}{S+l} - \beta SI,$$

it follows that

$$S(t) \geq \frac{\exp\left\{-\int_0^t\left(\frac{aI}{k} + \frac{bPS}{S(S+l)} + \beta I\right)du\right\}}{S(0) + \int_0^t a\exp\left\{-\int_0^t\left(\frac{aI}{k} + \frac{bPS}{S(S+l)} + \beta I\right)du\right\}dv} > 0.$$

For $t \in [0, \tau]$, the equation (7.2.2) can be rewritten as

$$\frac{dI}{dt} \geq -b_0 IP - d_0 I,$$

which evidences that

$$I(t) \geq I(0)\exp\left\{-\int_0^t (d_0 + b_0 P)du\right\} > 0.$$

The equation (7.2.3) for $t \in [0, \tau]$ can be rewritten as

$$\frac{dP}{dt} \geq -hIP - dP^2,$$

which implies that

$$P(t) \geq \frac{\exp\{-\int_0^t hIdu\}}{P(0) + \int_0^t d\exp\{-\int_0^t hIdu\}} > 0.$$

In the similar way, we can treat the intervals $[\tau, 2\tau], ..., [n\tau, (n+1)\tau], n \in N$. Thus by induction, we establish that $S(t) > 0$, $I(t) > 0$ and $P(t) > 0$ for all $t \geq 0$. □

Lemma 7.3.2. *The solution of the system of equations (7.2.1)–(7.2.3) with initial conditions is uniformly bounded in* Ω, *where*

$$\Omega = \{(S, I, P) : 0 \leq S(t) + I(t) + P(t) \leq \frac{k_2}{k_1}\},$$

$k_1 = min\{d_1, d_2, d_3\}$ *and* $k_2 = ak + \frac{c^2}{d}$.

Proof. Let $V(t) = S(t) + I(t) + P(t)$. Calculating the derivative of $V(t)$ with respect to t, we have

$$\begin{aligned}\frac{dV(t)}{dt} = &\ aS\left(1 - \frac{S+I}{k}\right) - \frac{bSP}{S+l} - b_0 IP - d_0 I + cP - hIP \\ &+ \frac{mbS(t-\tau)P(t-\tau)}{S(t-\tau)+l} - dP^2.\end{aligned}$$

Now $m < 1$, therefore we have

$$\frac{dV(t)}{dt} \leq aS\left(1 - \frac{S+I}{k}\right) - b_0 IP - d_0 I + cP - hIP - dP^2.$$

Taking $k_1 = min\{a, d_0, c\}$, we obtain that

$$\begin{aligned}\frac{dV(t)}{dt} + k_1 V &\leq 2aS - aS\left(\frac{S+I}{k}\right) - b_0 IP + 2cP - hIP - dP^2. \\ &\leq 2aS - \frac{aS^2}{k} + 2cP - dP^2.\end{aligned}$$

Assume $f(S,P) = 2aS - \frac{aS^2}{k} + 2cP - dP^2$. Solving $\frac{\partial f}{\partial S} = 0$ and $\frac{\partial f}{\partial P} = 0$ simultaneously, we obtain the stationary point $\left(k, \frac{c}{d}\right)$. We can see that function $f(S,P)$ has maximum value at the stationary point $\left(k, \frac{c}{d}\right)$ and maximum value of $f(S,P)$ is $ak + \frac{c^2}{d}$. Therefore, we can assume a positive constant $k_2 = ak + \frac{c^2}{d}$, such that

$$\frac{dV(t)}{dt} + k_1 V \leq k_2.$$

Thus we get

$$0 < V(t) \leq V(0)e^{-k_1 t} + \frac{k_2}{k_1}.$$

As $t \to \infty$, we have

$$0 \leq V(t) \leq \frac{k_2}{k_1}.$$

Therefore, $V(t)$ is bounded. So, each solution of the system (7.2.1)–(7.2.3) is bounded. □

7.4 Dynamical Behavior of the System

In this section, we analyze the system for the asymptotic stability at all the feasible equilibrium states and obtain the conditions for the existence of Hopf bifurcation at the disease-free equilibrium and endemic equilibrium states.

The system (7.2.1)–(7.2.3) has the following non-negative equilibrium points:

(i) Trivial equilibrium $E_0(0,0,0)$ always exists.

(ii) Boundary equilibrium $E_1(k,0,0)$ exists.

(iii) Prey-free equilibrium $E_2(0,0,\frac{c}{d})$ exists.

(iv) Predator-free equilibrium $E_3(S_3,I_3,0)$ exists, if $(\mathbf{H_1})$ holds, where

$$S_3 = \frac{d_0}{\beta}, \quad I_3 = \frac{a(\beta k - d_0)}{\beta(\beta k + a)}$$

and

$$(\mathbf{H_1}) : \beta k - d_0 > 0.$$

(v) Disease-free equilibrium (DFE) $E_4(S_4,0,P_4)$ exists, where S_4, P_4 is given by

$$\begin{cases} a\left(1-\frac{S}{k}\right) - \frac{bP}{S+l} = 0, \\ c + \frac{mbS}{S+l} - dP = 0. \end{cases} \tag{7.4.1}$$

(vi) Endemic equilibrium (EE) $E^*(S^*,I^*,P^*)$ exists, where S^*, I^*, P^* is given by

$$\begin{cases} a\left(1-\frac{S+I}{k}\right) - \frac{bP}{S+l} - \beta I = 0, \\ \beta S - b_0 P - d_0 = 0, \\ c - hI + \frac{mbS}{S+l} - dP = 0. \end{cases} \tag{7.4.2}$$

Now, we will discuss the local behavior of non-negative equilibria of the system (7.2.1)–(7.2.3).

Theorem 7.4.1. *The local behavior of different equilibria of the system (7.2.1)–(7.2.3) is as follows;*

(i) The trivial equilibrium $E_0(0,0,0)$ *is unstable.*

(ii) The boundary equilibrium $E_1(k,0,0)$ is unstable.

(iii) The prey-free equilibrium $E_2(0,0,\frac{c}{d})$ is locally asymptotically stable for all τ, if (H_2) holds, otherwise it is unstable.

Proof. (i) The characteristic equation for $E_0(0,0,0)$ is

$$(\lambda - a)(\lambda + d_0)(\lambda - c) = 0. \qquad (7.4.3)$$

The eigenvalues are $\lambda = a$, $\lambda = -d_0$, $\lambda = c$. The equilibrium $E_0(0,0,0)$ is unstable, because two of the eigenvalues of (7.4.3) are positive.

(ii) The characteristic equation for $E_1(k,0,0)$ is

$$(\lambda + a)(\lambda + d_0 - \beta k)\left(\lambda - c - \frac{mbk}{k+l}e^{-\lambda\tau}\right) = 0. \qquad (7.4.4)$$

The eigenvalues are $\lambda = -a$, $\lambda = -(d_0 - \beta k)$, $\lambda = c + \frac{mbk}{k+l}e^{-\lambda\tau}$. The equilibrium $E_1(k,0,0)$ is unstable because one eigenvalue of (7.4.4) is positive.

(iii) The characteristic equation for $E_2(0,0,\frac{c}{d})$ is

$$\left(\lambda - a + \frac{bc}{dl}\right)\left(\lambda + d_0 + \frac{b_0 c}{d}\right)(\lambda + c) = 0. \qquad (7.4.5)$$

The eigenvalues are $\lambda = a - \frac{bc}{dl}$, $\lambda = -(d_0 + \frac{b_0 c}{d})$, $\lambda = -c$. The equilibrium $E_2(0,0,\frac{c}{d})$ is locally asymptotically stable if $(\mathbf{H_2})$: $adl \leq bc$ holds and it is unstable otherwise.

□

Now, similar to Ref. [186], we will discuss the transcendental polynomial equation of the first degree

$$\lambda + r + qe^{-\lambda\tau} = 0 \qquad (7.4.6)$$

for the following cases:

(A1) $q + r > 0$;

(A2) $r^2 - q^2 > 0$;

(A3) $r^2 - q^2 < 0$.

Lemma 7.4.2. *For equation (7.4.6);*

(i) If (A1)–(A2) holds, then all the roots of (7.4.6) have negative real parts for all $\tau \geq 0$.

(ii) If (A1) and (A3) hold and $\tau = \tau_j^+$, then equation (7.4.6) has a pair of purely imaginary roots $\pm iw_+$. When $\tau = \tau_j^+$ then all roots of (7.4.6) except $\pm iw_+$ have negative real parts.

Proof. If $\tau = 0$, then (7.4.6) can be written as

$$\lambda + r + q = 0. \tag{7.4.7}$$

Now the root of (7.4.7) is negative if and only if $(\mathbf{A_1})$: $q + r > 0$ holds. If $\lambda = iw$, then from (7.4.6), we get

$$iw + r + qe^{-iw\tau} = 0. \tag{7.4.8}$$

Equating real and imaginary parts from (7.4.8), we get

$$q\cos w\tau = r, \tag{7.4.9}$$

$$q\sin w\tau = w. \tag{7.4.10}$$

Solving (7.4.9)–(7.4.10), we get

$$w^2 + (r^2 - q^2) = 0. \tag{7.4.11}$$

If $(\mathbf{A_2})$: $r^2 - q^2 > 0$ holds, then (7.4.11) does not have positive roots and hence (7.4.6) does not have purely imaginary roots. Since (A_1) ensure that the root of (7.4.7) is negative, by Rouche's theorem, it follows that the roots of (7.4.6) have negative real parts. Therefore, if (A_1) and (A_2) holds, then the roots of (7.4.6) have negative real parts for all $\tau \geq 0$.

On the other hand, if $(\mathbf{A_3})$: $r^2 - q^2 < 0$, then the equation (7.4.11) has a positive root. In this case the characteristic equation (7.4.6) has purely imaginary roots, when τ take certain values. The critical value of τ is given by

$$\tau_k^+ = \frac{1}{w_0}\left[\cos^{-1}\left(-\frac{r}{q}\right) + 2k\pi\right],$$

where $k = 0, 1, 2, \ldots$.

Therefore, if (A_1) and (A_3) holds and $\tau = \tau_k^+$, then the roots of (7.4.6) have a pair of purely imaginary roots. □

Theorem 7.4.3. *If (H_1), (H_3)-(H_5) holds, then predator-free equilibrium $E_3(S_3, I_3, 0)$ is locally asymptotically stable for all τ, otherwise it is unstable.*

Proof. The characteristic equation of the Jacobian matrix at the equilibrium point $E_3(S_3, I_3, 0)$ can be written as:

$$F(\lambda)\left[\lambda^2 - (a_1 + b_2)\lambda + (a_1 b_2 - a_2 b_1)\right] = 0, \tag{7.4.12}$$

where

$$F(\lambda) = \lambda - (d_3 + c_3 e^{-\lambda\tau}),$$

and

$$\begin{aligned}
a_1 &= a - \frac{2aS_3}{k} - \frac{aI_3}{k} - \beta I_3, \\
b_1 &= -\frac{aS_3}{k} - \beta S_3, \\
a_2 &= \beta I_3, \\
b_2 &= \beta S_3 - d_0, \\
c_3 &= \frac{mbS_3}{S_3 + l}, \\
d_3 &= c - hI_3.
\end{aligned}$$

When

$$\lambda^2 - (a_1 + b_2)\lambda + (a_1 b_2 - a_2 b_1) = 0, \tag{7.4.13}$$

then by Routh-Hurwitz criteria, the eigen values of (7.4.13) have negative real parts if $(\mathbf{H_3})$: $(a_1 + b_2) < 0$ and $(\mathbf{H_4})$: $(a_1 b_2 - a_2 b_1) > 0$ holds.

If $F(\lambda) = 0$, then

$$\lambda - (d_3 + c_3 e^{-\lambda\tau}) = 0. \tag{7.4.14}$$

Now (7.4.14) can be written as

$$\lambda + r + q e^{-\lambda\tau} = 0, \tag{7.4.15}$$

where $r = -d_3$, $q = -c_3$. Here q is always negative because c_3 is positive.

Using Lemma (7.4.2), $F(\lambda) = 0$ have roots with negative real parts if $q + r > 0$, that is, if $(\mathbf{H_5}) : c_3 + d_3 < 0$ holds. Thus the equilibrium $E_3(S_3, I_3, 0)$ is locally asymptotically stable if (H_1), (H_3)–(H_5) holds.

Now, $F(\lambda) = 0$ have a pair of purely imaginary roots by Lemma (7.4.2), if $-q < r < q$, which is impossible because q is negative. Therefore, Hopf bifurcation does not exists for the predator-free equilibrium $E_3(S_3, I_3, 0)$. □

Assume, the transcendental polynomial equation of the second degree

$$\lambda^2 + p\lambda + r + (s\lambda + q)e^{-\lambda\tau} = 0 \tag{7.4.16}$$

and this equation has been studied by Ref. [186] and discussed the following results:

(B1) $p + s > 0$;

(B2) $q + r > 0$;

(B3) *either* $s^2 - p^2 + 2r < 0$ *and* $r^2 - q^2 > 0$ *or* $(s^2 - p^2 + 2r)^2 < 4(r^2 - q^2)$;

(B4) *either* $r^2 - q^2 < 0$ *or* $s^2 - p^2 + 2r > 0$ *and* $(s^2 - p^2 + 2r)^2 = 4(r^2 - q^2)$;

(B5) *either* $r^2 - q^2 > 0, s^2 - p^2 + 2r > 0$ *and* $(s^2 - p^2 + 2r)^2 > 4(r^2 - q^2)$.

Lemma 7.4.4. *For equation (7.4.16) [186];*

(i) If (B1)–(B3) holds, then all the roots of (7.4.16) have negative real parts for all $\tau \geq 0$.

(ii) *If (B1), (B2) and (B4) hold and* $\tau = \tau_j^+$, *then equation (7.4.16) has a pair of purely imaginary roots* $\pm iw_+$. *When* $\tau = \tau_j^+$ *then all roots of (7.4.16) except* $\pm iw_+$ *have negative real parts.*

(iii) *If (B1), (B2) and (B5) hold and* $\tau = \tau_j^+ (\tau = \tau_j^-$ *respectively) then equation (7.4.16) has a pair of purely imaginary roots* $\pm iw_+$ ($\pm iw_-$, *respectively). Furthermore* $\tau = \tau_j^+$ (τ_j^-, *respectively), then all roots of (7.4.16) except* $\pm iw_+$ ($\pm iw_-$, *respectively) have negative real parts.*

Theorem 7.4.5. *Let* (H_6) *holds. For the system (7.2.1)–(7.2.3), we have;*

(i) *If* (H_7), (H_8) *and* (H_9) *holds, then the disease-free equilibrium* $E_4(S_4, 0, P_4)$ *is locally asymptotically stable for all* τ.

(ii) *If* (H_7), (H_8) *and* (H_{10}) *holds, then the equilibrium* $E_4(S_4, 0, P_4)$ *is locally asymptotically stable for all* $\tau \in [0, \tau_0^+)$, *and unstable when* $\tau \geq \tau_0^+$.

Proof. The characteristic equation of the Jacobian matrix at the equilibrium point $E_4(S_4, 0, P_4)$ can be written as:

$$(\lambda - b_2)F(\lambda) = 0, \tag{7.4.17}$$

where

$$F(\lambda) = \lambda^2 - (a_1 + d_3)\lambda + a_1 d_3 + (a_1 c_3 - a_3 c_1 - c_3 \lambda)e^{-\lambda\tau},$$

and

$$\begin{aligned}
a_1 &= a - \frac{2aS_4}{k} - \frac{bP_4}{S_4 + l} + \frac{bS_4P_4}{(S_4 + l)^2}, \\
c_1 &= -\frac{bS_4}{S_4 + l}, \\
b_2 &= \beta S_4 - b_0 P_4 - d_0, \\
a_3 &= \frac{mbP_4}{S_4 + l} - \frac{mbS_4P_4}{(S_4 + l)^2}, \\
c_3 &= \frac{mbS_4}{S_4 + l}, \\
d_3 &= c - 2dP_4.
\end{aligned}$$

Assume $(\mathbf{H_6})$: $b_2 < 0$ holds.

If $F(\lambda) = 0$, then we have

$$\lambda^2 - (a_1 + d_3)\lambda + a_1 d_3 + (a_1 c_3 - a_3 c_1 - c_3\lambda)e^{-\lambda\tau} = 0. \qquad (7.4.18)$$

Equation (7.4.18) can be written as

$$\lambda^2 + p\lambda + r + (s\lambda + q)e^{-\lambda\tau} = 0, \qquad (7.4.19)$$

where

$$\begin{aligned} p &= -(a_1 + d_3), \\ r &= a_1 d_3, \\ s &= -c_3, \\ q &= a_1 c_3 - a_3 c_1. \end{aligned}$$

Case I: In the absence of delay $\tau_2 = 0$, we get

$$\lambda^2 + (p+s)\lambda + (q+r) = 0. \qquad (7.4.20)$$

If $(\mathbf{H_7})$: $p+s>0$ and $(\mathbf{H_8})$: $q+r>0$ holds, then the roots of the characteristic equation (7.4.18) have negative real parts. Hence the equilibrium $E_4(S_4, 0, P_4)$ is locally asymptotically stable.

Case II: If $\tau > 0$, then we get

$$\lambda^2 + p\lambda + r + (s\lambda + q)e^{-\lambda\tau} = 0. \qquad (7.4.21)$$

Assume

$(\mathbf{H_9})$: either $s^2 - p^2 + 2r < 0$ and $r^2 - q^2 > 0$ or $(s^2 - p^2 + 2r)^2 < 4(r^2 - q^2)$;

$(\mathbf{H_{10}})$: either $r^2 - q^2 < 0$ or $s^2 - p^2 + 2r > 0$ and $(s^2 - p^2 + 2r)^2 = 4(r^2 - q^2)$.

Using Lemma 7.4.4, if (H_7), (H_8) and (H_9) holds, then all the roots of (7.2.1)–(7.2.3) have negative real parts for all τ and hence the system is locally asymptotically stable.

Further, using Lemma 7.4.4, if (H_7), (H_8) and (H_{10}) holds, then the system (7.2.1)–(7.2.3) has a pair of purely imaginary roots.

Put $\lambda = iw$ in (7.4.21), we get

$$(iw)^2 + p(iw) + r + (iws + q)e^{-iw\tau} = 0. \tag{7.4.22}$$

Equating real and imaginary parts from (7.4.22), we get

$$-w^2 + r + sw\sin w\tau + q\cos w\tau = 0, \tag{7.4.23}$$

$$pw + sw\cos w\tau - q\sin w\tau = 0. \tag{7.4.24}$$

Solving (7.4.23) and (7.4.24), we get

$$\sin w\tau = \frac{sw^3 + (pq - rs)w}{s^2w^2 + q^2}, \tag{7.4.25}$$

$$\cos w\tau = \frac{(q - ps)w^2 - qr}{s^2w^2 + q^2}, \tag{7.4.26}$$

and

$$w^4 + (p^2 - 2r - s^2)w^2 + (r^2 - q^2) = 0. \tag{7.4.27}$$

We define

$$F(w) = w^4 + (p^2 - 2r - s^2)w^2 + (r^2 - q^2) = 0.$$

By Descart's rule of sign, there is at least one positive root of $F(w) = 0$. Let w_0 is the positive root of $F(w) = 0$. From (7.4.26), we get

$$\tau_k^+ = \frac{1}{w_0}\left[\cos^{-1}\left(\frac{(q - ps)w_0{}^2 - qr}{s^2w_0{}^2 + q^2}\right) + 2k\pi\right],$$

where $k = 0, 1, 2, \ldots$.

Since for the existence of Hopf bifurcation at τ_0^+, it is required that the transversality condition $Re\left[\left(\frac{d\lambda}{d\tau}\right)^{-1}\right]_{\tau=\tau_0^+} \neq 0$ should hold, therefore taking the derivative of λ with respect to τ in (7.4.21), we get

$$\frac{d\lambda}{d\tau} = \frac{\lambda(s\lambda + q)e^{-\lambda\tau}}{2\lambda + p + se^{-\lambda\tau} - (s\lambda + q)\tau e^{-\lambda\tau}}.$$

At $\lambda = iw_0$ and $\tau = \tau_0^+$, we have

$$Re\left(\frac{d\lambda}{d\tau}\right)^{-1} = \frac{qG - sw_0H}{w_0(q^2 + s^2w_0^2)}, \tag{7.4.28}$$

where $G = psinw_0\tau_0 + 2w_0cosw_0\tau_0$ and $H = s + pcosw_0\tau_0 - 2w_0sinw_0\tau_0$.

Simplifying (7.4.28), we have

$$Re\left[\left(\frac{d\lambda}{d\tau}\right)^{-1}\right]_{\tau=\tau_0^+} \neq 0, \text{ if } qG \neq sw_0H. \qquad \square$$

Now, we state a lemma as similar as given in Ref. [187].

Lemma 7.4.6. *For the polynomial equation* $z^3+pz^2+qz+r=0$,

(i) If $r<0$, *then the equation has at least one positive root;*

(ii) If $r \geq 0$ *and* $\triangle = p^2-3q \leq 0$, *the equation has no positive root;*

(iii) If $r \geq 0$ *and* $\triangle = p^2-3q > 0$, *the equation has positive roots iff* $z_1^* = \frac{-p+\sqrt{\triangle}}{3}$ *and* $h(z_1^*) \leq 0$, *where* $h(z) = z^3+pz^2+qz+r$.

Theorem 7.4.7. *Let* (H_{11}) *holds. For the system (7.2.1)–(7.2.3),*

(i) The endemic equilibrium $E^*(S^*,I^*,P^*)$ *is locally asymptotically stable for all* $\tau \in [0, \tau_0^+)$.

(ii) If $\tau \geq \tau_0^+$, *then the endemic equilibrium* $E^*(S^*,I^*,P^*)$ *is unstable and the system undergoes Hopf bifurcation around* E^*.

Proof. The characteristic equation of the Jacobian matrix at the equilibrium point $E^*(S^*,I^*,P^*)$ can be written as:

$$\lambda^3 + A\lambda^2 + B\lambda + C + (F\lambda^2 + E\lambda + D)e^{-\lambda\tau} = 0, \qquad (7.4.29)$$

where

$$\begin{aligned}
A &= -(a_1+b_2+d_3),\\
B &= b_2d_3 - b_3c_2 - a_2b_1 + a_1d_3 + a_1b_2,\\
C &= a_2b_1d_3 + a_1b_3c_2 - a_1b_2d_3 - a_2b_3c_1,\\
D &= a_2b_1c_3 - a_1b_2c_3 - a_3b_1c_2 + a_3b_2c_1,\\
E &= b_2c_3 + a_1c_3 - a_3c_1,\\
F &= -c_3,
\end{aligned}$$

and

$$
\begin{aligned}
a_1 &= a - \frac{2aS^*}{k} - \frac{aI^*}{k} - \frac{bP^*}{S^*+l} + \frac{bS^*P^*}{(S^*+l)^2} - \beta I^*,\\
b_1 &= -\frac{aS^*}{k} - \beta S^*,\\
c_1 &= -\frac{bS^*}{S^*+l},\\
a_2 &= \beta I^*,\\
b_2 &= \beta S^* - b_0 P^* - d_0,\\
c_2 &= -b_0 I^*,\\
a_3 &= \frac{mbP^*}{S^*+l} - \frac{mbS^*P^*}{(S^*+l)^2},\\
b_3 &= -hP^*,\\
c_3 &= \frac{mbS^*}{S^*+l},\\
d_3 &= c - hI^* - 2dP^*.
\end{aligned}
$$

In the absence of delay ($\tau = 0$), the transcendental equation (7.4.29) reduces to

$$\lambda^3 + (A+F)\lambda^2 + (B+E)\lambda + (C+D) = 0, \tag{7.4.30}$$

where

$$
\begin{aligned}
&A+F = -(a_1+b_2+c_3+d_3),\\
&B+E = b_2d_3 - b_3c_2 - a_2b_1 + a_1d_3 + a_1b_2 + b_2c_3 + a_1c_3 - a_3c_1,\\
&C+D = a_2b_1d_3 + a_1b_3c_2 - a_1b_2d_3 - a_2b_3c_1\\
&\qquad +a_2b_1c_3 - a_1b_2c_3 - a_3b_1c_2 + a_3b_2c_1.
\end{aligned}
$$

By Routh-Hurwitz criterion, all the roots of equation (7.4.30) have negative real parts and the equilibrium E^* is locally asymptotically stable if $(\mathbf{H_{11}}) : A+F, B+E, C+D > 0$ and $(A+F)(B+E)-(C+D) > 0$ holds.

Assume that for some $\tau > 0$, $\lambda = iw$ is root of (7.4.29), therefore we have

$$(iw)^3 + A(iw)^2 + B(iw) + C + (F(iw)^2 + E(iw) + D)e^{-iw\tau} = 0. \tag{7.4.31}$$

Equating real and imaginary parts from (7.4.31), it can be obtained

$$Ew\sin w\tau + (D - Fw^2)\cos w\tau = Aw^2 - C, \tag{7.4.32}$$
$$Ew\cos w\tau - (D - Fw^2)\sin w\tau = w^3 - Bw. \tag{7.4.33}$$

Solving (7.4.32) and (7.4.33), we get

$$w^6 + pw^4 + qw^2 + r = 0, \tag{7.4.34}$$

where

$$p = A^2 - 2B - F^2,$$
$$q = B^2 - 2AC + 2DF - E^2,$$
$$r = C^2 - D^2.$$

By substituting $w^2 = z$ in equation (7.4.34), we define

$$F(z) = z^3 + pz^2 + qz + r.$$

By Lemma 7.4.6, there exists at least one positive root $w = w_0$ of equation (7.4.34) satisfying (7.4.32) and (7.4.33), which implies characteristic equation (7.4.29) has a pair of purely imaginary roots of the form $\pm iw_0$. Solving (7.4.32) and (7.4.33) for τ and substituting the value of $w = w_0$, the corresponding $\tau_k > 0$ is given by

$$\tau_k^+ = \frac{1}{w_0}\left[\cos^{-1}\left(\frac{(E - AF)w_0^4 + (AD + CF - BE)w_0^2 - CD}{E^2 w_0^2 + (D - Fw_0^2)^2}\right) + 2k\pi\right],$$

where $k = 0, 1, 2, ...$

Taking the derivative of λ with respect to τ in (7.4.29), we get

$$\left(\frac{d\lambda}{d\tau}\right)^{-1} = \frac{(3\lambda^2 + 2A\lambda + B)e^{\lambda\tau} + (2F\lambda + E)}{\lambda(F\lambda^2 + E\lambda + D)} - \frac{\tau}{\lambda}.$$

At $\lambda = iw$ and $\tau = \tau_0^+$, we have

$$Re\left[\left(\frac{d\lambda}{d\tau}\right)^{-1}\right] = \frac{MQ - NR}{w_0(L^2 + M^2)},$$

where $K = -3w_0^2 + B$, $L = 2Aw_0$, $M = D - Fw_0^2$, $N = Ew_0$, $Q = Ksinw_0\tau_0 + Lcosw_0\tau_0 + 2Fw_0$ and $R = Kcosw_0\tau_0 - Lsinw_0\tau_0 + E$.

Now, we have

$Re\left[\left(\frac{d\lambda}{d\tau}\right)^{-1}\right]_{\tau=\tau_0^+} \neq 0$, if $MQ \neq NR$. □

7.5 Sensitivity Analysis

In this section, we perform the sensitivity analysis of state variables of the system (7.2.1)–(7.2.3) with respect to the model parameters at the endemic equilibrium state. The respective sensitive parameters of the state variables at the endemic equilibrium are shown in the Table 7.2 using parameter values $a = 0.5$; $k = 5$; $b = 0.4$; $l = 2$; $\beta = 0.8$; $b_0 = 0.1$; $d_0 = 0.5$; $c = 0.9$; $h = 0.04$; $m = 0.6$; $d = 0.5$. We observe that b, b_0, d_0, c, m have a positive impact on the S^* and the rest of the parameters have a negative impact. Moreover β is the most sensitive parameter to S^*. Again a, b, l, β, c and d are more sensitive parameter to I^* than other parameters. Further c and d are the most sensitive parameter to P^* and all the other parameters are less sensitive to P^*.

TABLE 7.2 The Sensitivity Indices $\gamma_{y_j}^{x_i} = \frac{\partial x_i}{\partial y_j} \times \frac{y_j}{x_i}$ of the State Variables of the System (7.2.1)–(7.2.3) to the Parameters y_j for the Parameter Values $a = 0.5$; $k = 5$; $b = 0.4$; $l = 2$; $\beta = 0.8$; $b_0 = 0.1$; $d_0 = 0.5$; $c = 0.9$; $h = 0.04$; $m = 0.6$; $d = 0.5$

Parameter (y_j)	$\gamma_{y_j}^{S^*}$	$\gamma_{y_j}^{I^*}$	$\gamma_{y_j}^{P^*}$
a	–0.00560234	2.45514	–0.0201201
k	–0.000987291	0.432665	–0.00354573
b	0.0250564	–1.6707	0.0899869
l	–0.0174842	1.1658	–0.0627921
β	–1.01115	–1.60952	–0.0400482
b_0	0.282529	0.0192823	0.0146659
d_0	0.732137	0.0499677	0.0380049
c	0.26688	–1.43287	0.958466
h	–0.00231018	0.0124033	–0.00829674
m	0.0215076	–0.115474	0.0772417
d	–0.286077	1.53595	–1.02741

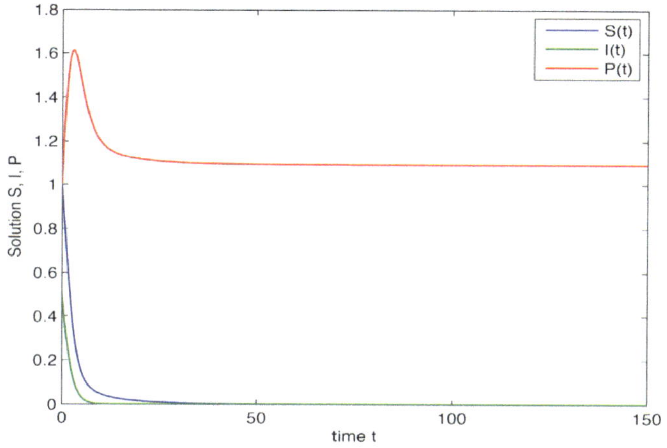

FIGURE 7.2 The prey-free equilibrium E_2 is stable for parametric values $a = 0.8$; $k = 3$; $b = 1.6$; $l = 2$; $\beta = 0.2$; $b_0 = 0.1$; $d_0 = 0.5$; $c = 0.6$; $h = 0.04$; $m = 0.9$; $d = 0.55$.

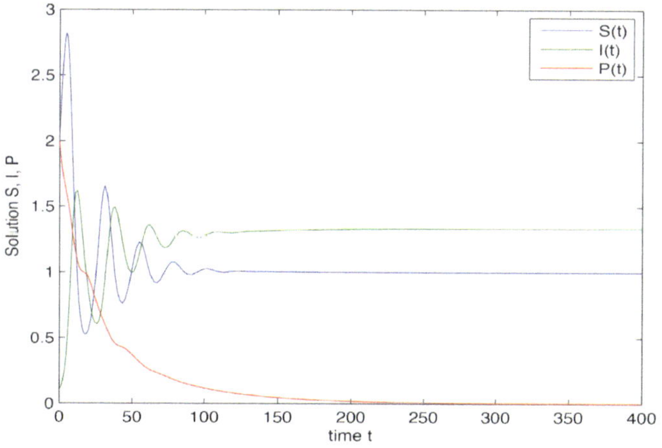

FIGURE 7.3 The predator-free equilibrium E_3 is stable for parametric values $a = 0.5$; $k = 5$; $b = 0.25$; $l = 1.25$; $\beta = 0.2$; $b_0 = 0.01$; $d_0 = 0.2$; $c = 0.01$; $h = 0.1$; $m = 0.8$; $d = 0.1$.

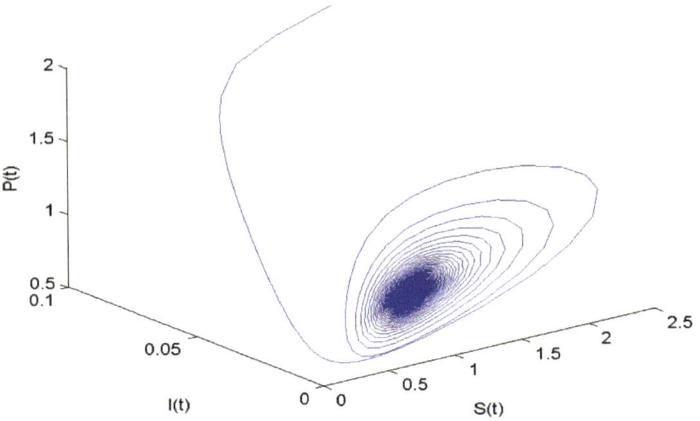

FIGURE 7.4 The disease-free equilibrium E_4 is stable for parametric values $a = 0.8$; $k = 10$; $b = 2$; $l = 2$; $\beta = 0.2$; $b_0 = 0.1$; $d_0 = 0.2$; $c = 0.1$; $h = 0.1$; $m = 0.8$; $d = 0.5$; $\tau = 1.44 < \tau_0^+ = 1.5$.

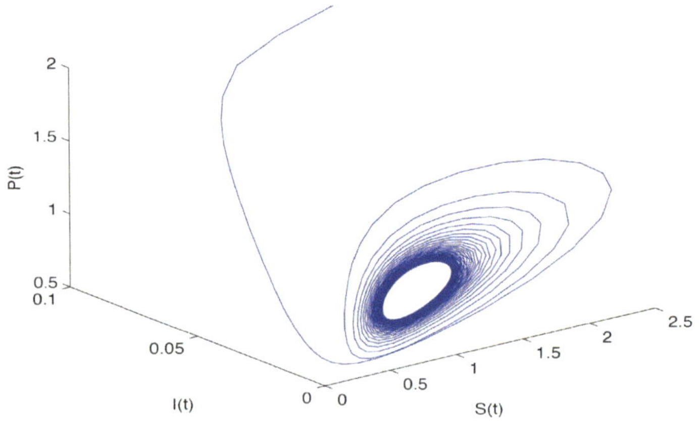

FIGURE 7.5 The disease-free equilibrium E_4 is unstable and Hopf bifurcation appears for the parametric values $a = 0.8$; $k = 10$; $b = 2$; $l = 2$; $\beta = 0.2$; $b_0 = 0.1$; $d_0 = 0.2$; $c = 0.1$; $h = 0.1$; $m = 0.8$; $d = 0.5$; $\tau = 1.52 > \tau_0^+ = 1.5$.

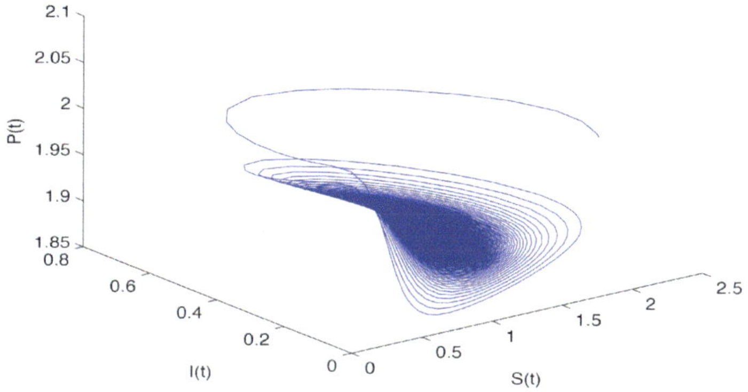

FIGURE 7.6 The endemic equilibrium E^* is stable for parametric values $a = 0.5$; $k = 5$; $b = 0.4$; $l = 2$; $\beta = 0.8$; $b_0 = 0.1$; $d_0 = 0.5$; $c = 0.9$; $h = 0.04$; $m = 0.6$; $d = 0.5$; $\tau = 6.6 < \tau_0^+ = 6.7$.

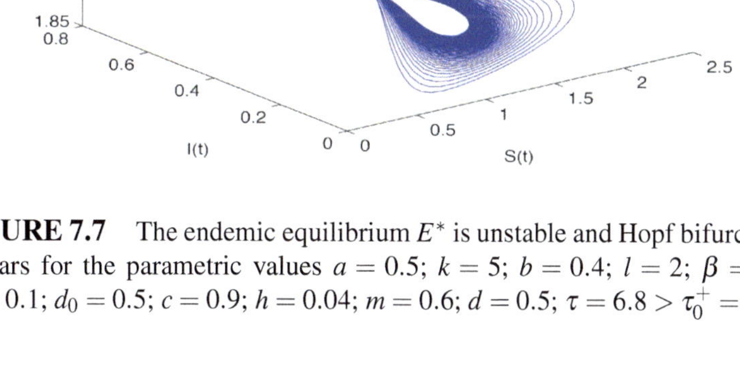

FIGURE 7.7 The endemic equilibrium E^* is unstable and Hopf bifurcation appears for the parametric values $a = 0.5$; $k = 5$; $b = 0.4$; $l = 2$; $\beta = 0.8$; $b_0 = 0.1$; $d_0 = 0.5$; $c = 0.9$; $h = 0.04$; $m = 0.6$; $d = 0.5$; $\tau = 6.8 > \tau_0^+ = 6.7$.

7.6 Numerical Simulations

We perform the numerical simulations of the model (7.2.1)–(7.2.3) to justify the analytic findings. We use initial population sizes as $S_0 = 2,\ I_0 = 0.1,\ P_0 = 2$. From Figure 7.2, we observe that the prey-free equilibrium $E_2(0,0,1.09)$ is stable for parameter values $a = 0.8$; $k = 3$; $b = 1.6$; $l = 2$; $\beta = 0.2$; $b_0 = 0.1$; $d_0 = 0.5$; $c = 0.6$; $h = 0.04$; $m = 0.9$; $d = 0.55$, which establish the Theorem 7.4.1. It is observed from Figure 7.3 that the predator-free equilibrium $E_3(1,1.33,0)$ is stable for parameter values $a = 0.5$; $k = 5$; $b = 0.25$; $l = 1.25$; $\beta = 0.2$; $b_0 = 0.01$; $d_0 = 0.2$; $c = 0.01$; $h = 0.1$; $m = 0.8$; $d = 0.1$, which results that the Theorem 7.4.3 holds good.

The endemic equilibrium $E_4(0.66,0,0.99)$ is stable for parameter values $a = 0.8$; $k = 10$; $b = 2$; $l = 2$; $\beta = 0.2$; $b_0 = 0.1$; $d_0 = 0.2$; $c = 0.1$; $h = 0.1$; $m = 0.8$; $d = 0.5$; $\tau = 1.44 < \tau_0^+ = 1.5$ (see Figure 7.4) and Hopf bifurcation exists for $\tau = 1.52 > \tau_0^+ = 1.5$ (see Figure 7.5), which shows that the Theorem 7.4.5 is true. The endemic equilibrium point E^* is stable for parameter values $a = 0.5$; $k = 5$; $b = 0.4$; $l = 2$; $\beta = 0.8$; $b_0 = 0.1$; $d_0 = 0.5$; $c = 0.9$; $h = 0.04$; $m = 0.6$; $d = 0.5$; $\tau = 6.6 < \tau_0^+ = 6.7$ (see Figure 7.6) and the equilibrium is unstable and Hopf bifurcation appears for $\tau = 6.8 > \tau_0^+ = 6.7$ (see Figure 7.7), which is in accordance with the results stated in the Theorem 7.4.7.

7.7 Summary

In this chapter, we proposed a prey-predator model with predator depends on alternative resources, disease in the prey and maturation delay for predator. We investigated the asymptotic stability of the model for all the feasible equilibrium states. The existence of Hopf bifurcation is explored at the equilibrium states. It is established that the disease-free equilibrium E_4 as well as endemic equilibrium E^*, both exhibit Hopf bifurcation, when the gestation delay for predator (τ) is greater than or equal to their corresponding critical value (τ_0^+) under certain respective conditions. Finally, the normalized forward sensitivity indices are calculated for the endemic equilibrium to the various parameters. Numerical simulations of the system are performed with a particular set of parameters to justify our analytic findings.

Chapter 8

An Epidemic Model of Childhood Disease Dynamics with Maturation Delay and Latent Period of Infection

8.1 Introduction

There are a number of diseases, which affects mostly the children, for example, Rubella, Measles, Chickenpox, Polio, Mumps, etc., because pre-mature (child) population is more prone to the diseases than the mature (adult) population [91, 92]. Rubella is a disease that occurs worldwide, mostly affecting children up to the age of 10 years old [91] and Measles is a highly contagious viral infection that is most common among children [92]. Therefore, in disease dynamics the population can be divided into two major categories: pre-mature population and mature population, and the pre-mature population takes a constant time to become mature. Also, in disease dynamics, the spread of a disease is not instantaneous, it will take some time in the host body before the outbreak and this time period is known as the latent period of a particular disease.

In the present chapter, we proposed and analyzed an epidemic model of childhood disease, incorporating maturation delay and latent period of infection. This chapter is organized as follows. In Section 8.2, formulation of epidemic model is presented. In Section 8.3, positivity and boundedness of the system has been obtained. In Section 8.4, the system is analyzed for the asymptotic stability at all the feasible equilibrium states and obtained the conditions for the existence of Hopf bifurcation at the endemic equilibrium state. In Section 8.5, the sensitivity analysis of the state variables at endemic equilibrium state with respect to model parameters, is performed. In Section 8.6, we presented some numerical simulations to support our analytical findings and in the last section, a brief conclusion is given.

8.2 Formulation of Mathematical Model

Keeping in view, the childhood disease dynamics, a mathematical model is developed with the following assumptions:

(i) The population exhibit age structure and the total population at time t is divided into three mutually exclusive compartments, namely, pre-mature (P), mature (M) and infected (I).

(ii) τ_1 is maturation delay (i.e. the pre-mature period) and d_1 is the death rate of pre-mature population. The transformation from pre-mature to mature population is $\gamma e^{-d_1\tau_1}M(t-\tau_1)$, where γ is the birth rate of pre-mature, who was born at time $t-\tau_1$ and survive at time t.

(iii) τ_2 is a latent period of infection.

(iv) No vertical transmission of the disease from mature to pre-mature compartment.

(v) Treatment limitation is shown as the overcrowding in disease compartment.

(vi) Resource limitation is shown as the overcrowding in mature compartment.

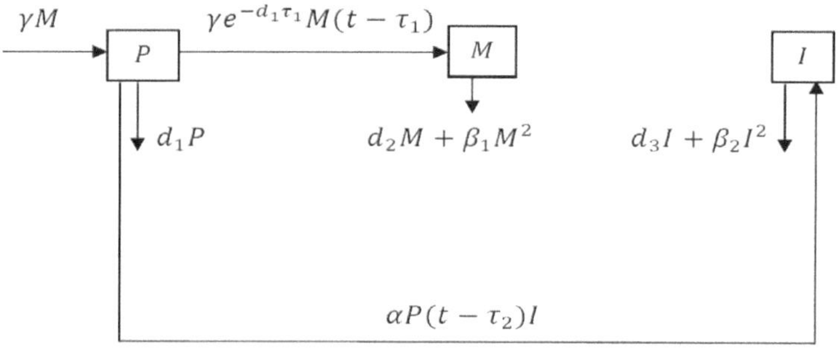

FIGURE 8.1 The schematic diagram of the model.

The proposed system is of the form:

$$\frac{dP}{dt} = \gamma M - d_1 P - \gamma e^{-d_1\tau_1} M(t-\tau_1) - \alpha P(t-\tau_2) I, \quad (8.2.1)$$

$$\frac{dM}{dt} = \gamma e^{-d_1\tau_1} M(t-\tau_1) - d_2 M - \beta_1 M^2, \quad (8.2.2)$$

$$\frac{dI}{dt} = \alpha P(t-\tau_2) I - d_3 I - \beta_2 I^2, \quad (8.2.3)$$

with initial conditions:

$$P(\theta) = \phi_1(\theta),\ M(\theta) = \phi_2(\theta),\ I(\theta) = \phi_3(\theta),$$

$$\phi_1(0) > 0,\ \phi_2(0) > 0,\ \phi_3(0) > 0,$$

where $\theta \in [-\tau, 0]$ and $\phi_1(\theta), \phi_2(\theta), \phi_3(\theta) \in \mathscr{C}([-\tau, 0], R^3_+)$, the Banach space of continuous functions mapping the interval $[-\tau, 0]$ into R^3_+, where $R^3_+ = \{(x_1, x_2, x_3) : x_i \geq 0, i = 1, 2, 3\}$. The details of the parameters of the proposed system is given in Table 8.1.

8.3 Positivity and Boundedness of the System

We state and prove the following lemmas for the positivity and boundedness of the solution of the system (8.2.1)–(8.2.3):

Lemma 8.3.1. *The solution of the system (8.2.1)–(8.2.3) with initial conditions are positive, for all $t \geq 0$.*

TABLE 8.1 Description of Parameters for the System (8.2.1)–(8.2.3)

Parameter	Description	Unit
γ	Birth rate of pre-mature individuals	days^{-1}
α	Rate of infection to the pre-mature individuals	days^{-1}
d_1	Death rates of pre-mature individuals	days^{-1}
d_2	Death rates of mature individuals	days^{-1}
d_3	Death rates of infected individuals	days^{-1}
β_1	Overcrowding rates of mature individuals	days^{-1}
β_2	Overcrowding rates of infected individuals	days^{-1}
τ_1	Maturation delay	days
τ_2	Latent period of infection	days

Proof. Let $(P(t), M(t), I(t))$ be a solution of the system (8.2.1)–(8.2.3) with initial conditions. Let us consider $I(t)$ for $t \in [0, \tau^*]$, where $\tau^* = min\{\tau_1, \tau_2\}$. We obtain from the equation (8.2.3) that

$$\frac{dI}{dt} \geq -d_3 I - \beta_2 I^2,$$

it follows that

$$I(t) \geq \frac{d_3 I(0)}{\beta_2 I(0)(e^{d_3 t} - 1) + d_3 e^{d_3 t}} > 0.$$

For $t \in [0, \tau^*]$, the equation (8.2.2) can be rewritten as

$$\frac{dM}{dt} \geq -d_2 M - \beta_1 M^2,$$

which implies that

$$M(t) \geq \frac{d_2 M(0)}{\beta_1 M(0)(e^{d_2 t} - 1) + d_2 e^{d_2 t}} > 0.$$

The equation (8.2.1) for $t \in [0, \tau^*]$ can be rewritten as

$$\frac{dP}{dt} \geq -d_1 P - \gamma e^{-d_1 \tau_1} M(t-\tau_1) - \alpha P(t-\tau_2) I,$$

which evidences that

$$P(t) = e^{-\tilde{I}} \left[P(0) - \int_0^t \gamma e^{-d_1 \tau_1} M(r-\tau_1) e^{\tilde{I}} dr \right] > 0,$$

where $\tilde{I} = \int_0^t (d_1 + \alpha I(s)) ds$.

In the similar way, we can treat the intervals $[\tau^*, 2\tau^*], \ldots, [n\tau^*, (n+1)\tau^*], n \in N$. Thus by induction, we establish that $P(t) > 0, M(t) > 0$ and $I(t) > 0$ for all $t \geq 0$. □

Lemma 8.3.2. *The solution of the system of equations (8.2.1)–(8.2.3) with initial conditions is uniformly bounded in* Ω*, where*

$$\Omega = \{(P, M, I) : 0 \leq P(t) + M(t) + I(t) \leq \frac{k_2}{k_1}\},$$

$k_1 = min\{d_1, d_2, d_3\}$ *and* $k_2 = \frac{\gamma^2}{4\beta_1}$.

Proof. Let $V(t) = P(t) + M(t) + I(t)$. Calculating the derivative of $V(t)$ with respect to t, we have

$$\begin{aligned} \frac{dV(t)}{dt} &= \gamma M - d_1 P - d_2 M - \beta_1 M^2 - d_3 I - \beta_2 I^2 \\ &\leq \gamma M - d_1 P - d_2 M - \beta_1 M^2 - d_3 I. \end{aligned}$$

Taking $k_1 = min\{d_1, d_2, d_3\}$, we obtain that

$$\frac{dV(t)}{dt} + k_1 V \leq \gamma M - \beta_1 M^2.$$

There exists a positive constant $k_2 = \frac{\gamma^2}{4\beta_1}$, such that

$$\frac{dV(t)}{dt} + k_1 V \leq k_2.$$

Thus we get

$$0 < V(t) \leq V(0) e^{-k_1 t} + \frac{k_2}{k_1}.$$

As $t \to \infty$, we have

$$0 \leq V(t) \leq \frac{k_2}{k_1}.$$

Therefore, $V(t)$ is bounded. So, each solution of the system (8.2.1)–(8.2.3) is bounded. □

8.4 Dynamical Behavior of the System

In this section, we analyze the system for the asymptotic stability at all the feasible equilibrium states and obtain the conditions for the existence of Hopf bifurcation at the endemic equilibrium state.

The system (8.2.1)–(8.2.3) has three non-negative equilibrium points:

(i) The trivial equilibrium $E_0(0,0,0)$ always exists.

(ii) The disease-free equilibrium (DFE) $E_1(P_1, M_1, 0)$ exists, if (H_1) holds, where

$P_1 = \frac{\gamma\left(1-e^{-d_1\tau_1}\right)\left(\gamma e^{-d_1\tau_1}-d_2\right)}{\beta_1 d_1}$, $M_1 = \frac{\left(\gamma e^{-d_1\tau_1}-d_2\right)}{\beta_1}$ and

$$(\mathbf{H_1}) : \tau_1 < \frac{1}{d_1}\ln\left(\frac{\gamma}{d_2}\right) := \tau_{10}.$$

(iii) The endemic equilibrium (EE) $E^*(P^*, M^*, I^*)$ exists, if $(\mathbf{H_1})$, $(\mathbf{H_2})$ and $(\mathbf{H_3})$ holds, where $M^* = \frac{\gamma e^{-d_1\tau_1}-d_2}{\beta_1}$, $I^* = \frac{\alpha P^*-d_3}{\beta_2}$ and P^* satisfy

$$AP^{*2} - BP^* - C = 0$$

and

$$\begin{aligned} A &= \alpha^2\beta_1, \\ B &= \alpha\beta_1 d_3 - d_1\beta_1\beta_2, \\ C &= \beta_2\gamma\left(1-e^{-d_1\tau_1}\right)\left(\gamma e^{-d_1\tau_1}-d_2\right). \end{aligned}$$

Here

$$(\mathbf{H_2}) : B^2 + 4AC \geq 0, \quad (\mathbf{H_3}) : P^* > \tfrac{d_3}{\alpha}.$$

Now, if (H_1) holds, then M^*, P^* are positive and P^* is uniquely defined by $P^* = \frac{B+\sqrt{B^2+4AC}}{2A}$. Also P^* is real if (H_2) holds. Further I^* is positive if (H_3) holds.

Now, we will discuss the local behavior of non-negative equilibria of the system (8.2.1)–(8.2.3).

Theorem 8.4.1. *The local behavior of different equilibria of the system (8.2.1)–(8.2.3) is as follows;*

(i) If $\tau_1 \geq \tau_{10}$, then trivial equilibrium E_0 is locally asymptotically stable for all τ_2 and if $\tau_1 < \tau_{10}$, then it is unstable.

(ii) If (H_1) and (H_4) holds, then disease-free equilibrium E_1 is locally asymptotically stable for all τ_2, otherwise it is unstable.

(iii) If (H_1)-(H_3) and (H_5) holds, then the endemic equilibrium E^* is locally asymptotically stable for all τ_2, otherwise it is unstable.

Proof. (i) The characteristic equation for $E_0(0,0,0)$ is

$$(\lambda + d_1)(\lambda - \gamma e^{-d_1\tau_1} e^{-\lambda\tau_1} + d_2)(\lambda + d_3) = 0. \qquad (8.4.1)$$

Clearly $\lambda = -d_1, \lambda = -d_3$ are negative eigenvalues. If $\gamma e^{-d_1\tau_1} \leq d_2$, then all the eigenvalues of (8.4.1) have negative real part. Therefore, the equilibrium $E_0(0,0,0)$ is locally asymptotically stable, if $\gamma e^{-d_1\tau_1} \leq d_2$, that is, if

$$\tau_1 \geq \frac{1}{d_1} \ln\left(\frac{\gamma}{d_2}\right) = \tau_{10}.$$

Thus, if $\tau_1 \geq \tau_{10}$, then the equilibrium $E_0(0,0,0)$ is locally asymptotically stable for all τ_2. Moreover, $E_0(0,0,0)$ is unstable for all $\tau_1 < \tau_{10}$, because one of the eigenvalues of (8.4.1) has positive real part.

(ii) The characteristic equation for $E_1(P_1, M_1, 0)$ is

$$(\lambda + d_1)F_1(\lambda)F_2(\lambda) = 0, \qquad (8.4.2)$$

where $F_1(\lambda) = \lambda - \alpha P_1 + d_3$, $F_2(\lambda) = \lambda - \gamma e^{-d_1\tau_1} e^{-\lambda\tau_1} + d_2 + 2\beta_1 M_1$. Now $d_2 + 2\beta_1 M_1 - \gamma e^{-d_1\tau_1} e^{-\lambda\tau_1} > 0$, if (H_1) holds. Further $d_3 - \alpha P_1 > 0$, if (H_4) holds, where

$$(\mathbf{H_4}) : \alpha P_1 < d_3.$$

Thus, if (H_1) and (H_4) holds, than all the eigen values of (8.4.2) have negative real parts and hence non-negative equilibrium

$E_1(P_1, M_1, 0)$ is locally asymptotically stable for all τ_2, otherwise it is unstable.

(iii) The characteristic equation of the Jacobian matrix at the equilibrium point $E^*(P^*, M^*, I^*)$ can be written as:

$$(\lambda + A)F(\lambda) = 0, \tag{8.4.3}$$

where

$$F(\lambda) = (\lambda + \beta_2 I^*)(\lambda + d_1 + \alpha e^{-\lambda \tau_2} I^*) + \alpha^2 I^* P^* e^{-\lambda \tau_2}$$

and

$$A = \gamma e^{-d_1 \tau_1}(2 - e^{-\lambda \tau_1}) - d_2.$$

Here $A > 0$ if (H_1) holds.

From (8.4.3), we obtain that $\lambda = -A$ or $F(\lambda) = 0$. If $F(\lambda) = 0$, then we have

$$(\lambda + \beta_2 I^*)(\lambda + d_1 + \alpha e^{-\lambda \tau_2} I^*) + \alpha^2 I^* P^* e^{-\lambda \tau_2} = 0. \tag{8.4.4}$$

Substituting $\lambda = \xi + i\omega$ into (8.4.4) and separating real and imaginary parts, we get

$$\begin{aligned} G_1 G_2 - \omega H &= -\alpha^2 I^* P^* e^{-\xi \tau_2} cos \omega \tau_2, \\ G_1 H + \omega G_2 &= \alpha^2 I^* P^* e^{-\xi \tau_2} sin \omega \tau_2, \end{aligned}$$

where

$$\begin{aligned} G_1 &= \xi + \beta_2 I^*, \\ G_2 &= \xi + d_1 + \alpha I^* e^{-\xi \tau_2} cos \omega \tau_2, \\ H &= \omega - \alpha I^* e^{-\xi \tau_2} sin \omega \tau_2. \end{aligned}$$

Thus we have

$$(G_1 G_2)^2 + (\omega H)^2 + (G_1 H)^2 + (\omega G_2)^2 = (\alpha^2 I^* P^*)^2 e^{-2\xi \tau_2}. \tag{8.4.5}$$

Now we assume that $(\mathbf{H_5})$: $\beta_2 d_1 > \alpha^2 P^*$. We have to show that $\xi < 0$.
If possible, suppose that $\xi \geq 0$. We have

$$G_1 = \xi + \beta_2 I^*, G_2 = \xi + d_1 + \alpha I^* e^{-\xi\tau_2} cos\omega\tau_2 > \xi + d_1.$$

Therefore

$$(G_1 G_2)^2 > (\alpha^2 I^* P^*)^2 e^{-2\xi\tau_2},$$

which is a contradiction of (8.4.5). Therefore, $\xi < 0$ if (H_5) holds. Thus, all the solutions of (8.4.4) have negative real parts, if (H_5) holds.

Therefore, the endemic equilibrium $E^*(P^*, M^*, I^*)$ is locally asymptotically stable if (H_1)-(H_3) and (H_5) holds for all τ_2.

□

Next, we will discuss the behavior of (8.2.1)–(8.2.3) taken all possible cases of τ_1 and τ_2. From (8.4.4), we have

$$\lambda^2 + A_1\lambda + A_2 + (B_1\lambda + B_2)e^{-\lambda\tau_2} + Ce^{-\lambda\tau_1} = 0, \qquad (8.4.6)$$

where

$$\begin{aligned} A_1 &= d_1 + \beta_2 I^*, \\ A_2 &= \beta_2 d_1 I^*, \\ B_1 &= \alpha I^*, \\ B_2 &= \alpha\beta_2 I^{*2} + \alpha^2 I^* P^*, \\ C &= 0. \end{aligned}$$

Case I: If $\tau_2 = 0$, then we get

$$\lambda^2 + (A_1 + B_1)\lambda + (A_2 + B_2) = 0. \qquad (8.4.7)$$

Thus the roots of characteristic equation have negative real parts. Hence the endemic equilibrium $E^*(P^*, M^*, I^*)$ is locally asymptotically stable.

Case II: If $\tau_2 > 0$, then we get

$$\lambda^2 + p\lambda + r + (s\lambda + q)e^{-\lambda\tau_2} = 0, \tag{8.4.8}$$

where

$$\begin{aligned} p &= d_1 + \beta_2 I^*, \\ r &= \beta_2 d_1 I^*, \\ s &= \alpha I^*, \\ q &= \alpha\beta_2 I^{*2} + \alpha^2 I^* P^*. \end{aligned}$$

We have

$$q + r = \alpha\beta_2 I^{*2} + \alpha^2 I^* P^* + \beta_2 d_1 I^* > 0,$$

$$p + s = d_1 + \beta_2 I^* + \alpha I^* > 0,$$

$$s^2 - p^2 + 2r = -d_1^2 - (\beta_2^2 - \alpha^2)I^{*2},$$

$$r^2 - q^2 = (\beta_2 d_1 I^*)^2 - (\alpha\beta_2 I^{*2} + \alpha^2 I^* P^*)^2.$$

We have $s^2 - p^2 + 2r < 0$, if (H_6) holds and $r^2 - q^2 > 0$, if (H_7) holds, where

$$(\mathbf{H_6}) : (\alpha^2 - \beta_2^2)I^{*2} < d_1^2,$$

$$(\mathbf{H_7}) : \frac{d_3}{\alpha} < P^* < \frac{1}{2\alpha}(d_3 + \frac{\beta_2 d_1}{\alpha}).$$

Using Lemma 7.4.4 stated in Chapter 7, if (H_6) and (H_7) holds, then all the roots of (8.2.1)–(8.2.3) have negative real parts for all τ_2 and hence $E^*(P^*, M^*, I^*)$ is locally asymptotically stable.

Further $r^2 - q^2 < 0$, if $(\mathbf{H_8})$: $P^* > \frac{1}{2\alpha}(d_3 + \frac{\beta_2 d_1}{\alpha})$ holds.

Using Lemma 7.4.4 given in Chapter 7, if (H_8) holds, then the system (8.2.1)–(8.2.3) has a pair of purely imaginary roots.

Put $\lambda = iw$ in (8.4.8), we get

$$(iw)^2 + p(iw) + r + (iws + q)e^{-iw\tau_2} = 0.$$

Equating real and imaginary parts, we get

$$-w^2 + r + sw\sin w\tau_2 + q\cos w\tau_2 = 0, \tag{8.4.9}$$

$$pw + sw\cos w\tau_2 - q\sin w\tau_2 = 0. \tag{8.4.10}$$

Solving (8.4.9) and (8.4.10), we get

$$\sin w\tau_2 = \frac{sw^3 + (pq - rs)w}{s^2w^2 + q^2}, \tag{8.4.11}$$

$$\cos w\tau_2 = \frac{(q - ps)w^2 - qr}{s^2w^2 + q^2}, \tag{8.4.12}$$

and

$$w^4 + (p^2 - 2r - s^2)w^2 + (r^2 - q^2) = 0. \tag{8.4.13}$$

We define

$$F(w) = w^4 + (p^2 - 2r - s^2)w^2 + (r^2 - q^2) = 0.$$

Now, $F(0) = (r^2 - q^2) < 0$, if (H_8) holds. By Descartes' rule of sign, there is at least one positive root of $F(w) = 0$. Let w_0 is the positive root of $F(w) = 0$.

From (8.4.12), we get

$$\tau_{2k}^{+} = \frac{1}{w_0}\left[\cos^{-1}\left(\frac{(q - ps)w_0{}^2 - qr}{s^2 w_0{}^2 + q^2}\right) + 2k\pi\right],$$

where $k = 0, 1, 2, \ldots$.

Since for the existence of Hopf bifurcation at τ_{20}^{+}, it is required that the transversality condition $Re\left[\left(\frac{d\lambda}{d\tau_2}\right)^{-1}\right]_{\tau_2=\tau_{20}^{+}} \neq 0$ should hold, therefore taking the derivative of λ with respect to τ_2 in (8.4.8), we get

$$\frac{d\lambda}{d\tau_2} = \frac{\lambda(s\lambda + q)e^{-\lambda\tau_2}}{2\lambda + p - (s\lambda + q)\tau_2 e^{-\lambda\tau_2} + se^{-\lambda\tau_2}}.$$

At $\lambda = iw_0$ and $\tau_2 = \tau_{20}^{+}$, we have

$$Re\left(\frac{d\lambda}{d\tau_2}\right)^{-1} = \frac{(sw_0p + 2w_0q)cosw_0\tau_2 + (pq - 2sw_0^2)sinw_0\tau_2 + s^2w_0}{w_0(q^2 + s^2w_0^2)}. \tag{8.4.14}$$

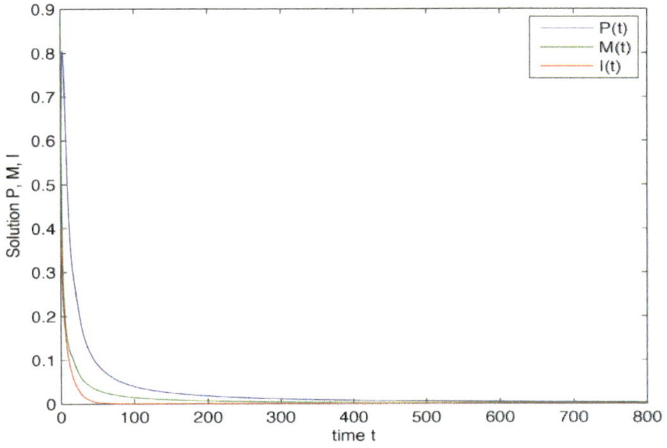

FIGURE 8.2 The trivial equilibrium E_0 is stable for parameter values $\gamma = 0.8, \alpha = 0.04, \beta_1 = 0.8, \beta_2 = 0.3, d_1 = 0.3, d_2 = 0.01, d_3 = 0.09, \tau_1 = 15 > \bar{\tau}_{10} = 14.6$ and $\tau_2 = 7.2$.

Simplifying (8.4.14), we have

$$Re\left[\left(\frac{d\lambda}{d\tau_2}\right)^{-1}\right]_{\tau_2=\tau_{20}^{+}} \neq 0,$$

for $pq > 2sw_0^2$, which is one of the sufficient condition.

Theorem 8.4.2. *Let* (H_1)*-*(H_3) *holds. For the system (8.2.1)–(8.2.3), we have*

(i) If (H_6) *and* (H_7) *holds, then the endemic equilibrium* $E^*(P^*, M^*, I^*)$ *is locally asymptotically stable for all* τ_2.

(ii) If (H_8) *holds, then the endemic equilibrium* $E^*(P^*, M^*, I^*)$ *is locally asymptotically stable for all* $\tau_2 \in [0, \tau_{20}^{+})$*, and unstable when* $\tau_2 \geq \tau_{20}^{+}$.

8.5 Sensitivity Analysis

In this section, we perform the sensitivity analysis of the endemic equilibrium with respect to model parameters, for a particular set of parameters $\gamma = 0.8$, $\alpha = 0.09$, $\beta_1 = 0.2$, $\beta_2 = 0.3$, $d_1 = 0.05$, $d_2 = 0.01$, $d_3 = 0.01$, $\tau_1 = 12.2$ and $\tau_2 = 7.23$. The normalized sensitive indices of the endemic equilibrium with respect to parameters are shown in Table 8.2. From the Table 8.2, it is observed that γ, β_2, d_3 have a positive impact on the P^* and rest of the parameters have a negative impact. Moreover γ and α are most sensitive parameter to P^*, hence, the significant change in P^* is observed by small changes in these parameters. Again γ and β_1 are most sensitive parameters to both M^* and I^*.

TABLE 8.2 The Sensitivity Indices $\gamma_{y_j}^{x_i} = \frac{\partial x_i}{\partial y_j} \times \frac{y_j}{x_i}$ of the State Variables of the System (8.2.1)–(8.2.3) to the Parameters y_j for the Parameter Values $\gamma = 0.8, \alpha = 0.09, \beta_1 = 0.2, \beta_2 = 0.3, d_1 = 0.05, d_2 = 0.01, d_3 = 0.01, \tau_1 = 12.2, \tau_2 = 7.2$

Parameter (y_j)	$\gamma_{y_j}^{P^*}$	$\gamma_{y_j}^{M^*}$	$\gamma_{y_j}^{I^*}$
γ	1.17394	1.02355	1.20326
α	–0.829488	0	0.17477
β_1	–0.58014	–1	–1.59463
β_2	0.409629	0	0.41986
d_1	–0.111654	–0.624364	–0.114443
d_2	–0.0136606	–0.0235471	–0.0140018
d_3	0.0102307	0	–0.0144893

8.6 Numerical Simulations

We perform the numerical simulations of the system (8.2.1)–(8.2.3) keeping the parameters $\gamma = 0.8$, $\alpha = 0.04$, $\beta_1 = 0.8$, $\beta_2 = 0.3$ as fixed and varying the parameters d_1, d_2 and d_3. We use initial population sizes as $P_0 = 0.3$, $M_0 = 0.9$ and $I_0 = 0.4$.

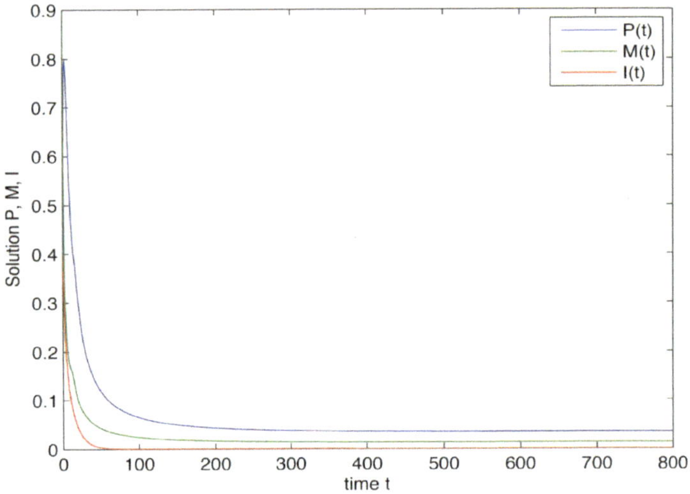

FIGURE 8.3 The disease-free equilibrium E_1 is stable for parameter values $\gamma = 0.8, \alpha = 0.04, \beta_1 = 0.8, \beta_2 = 0.3, d_1 = 0.3, d_2 = 0.01, d_3 = 0.09, \tau_1 = 12.2 < \bar{\tau}_{10} = 14.6$ and $\tau_2 = 7.2$.

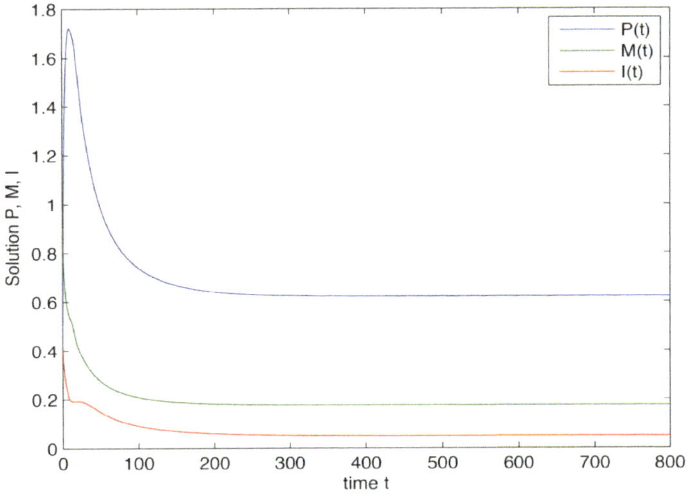

FIGURE 8.4 The endemic equilibrium E^* is stable for parameter values $\gamma = 0.8, \alpha = 0.04, \beta_1 = 0.2, \beta_2 = 0.3, d_1 = 0.2, d_2 = 0.05, d_3 = 0.01, \tau_1 = 11.2 < \bar{\tau}_{10} = 13.86$ and $\tau_2 = 7.2$.

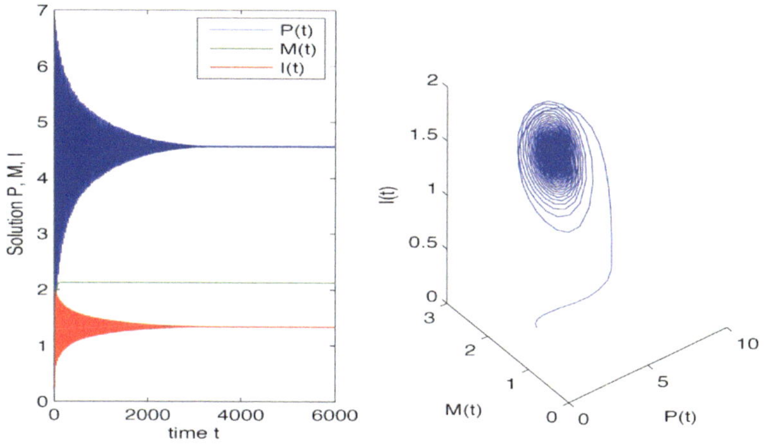

FIGURE 8.5 The endemic equilibrium E^* is stable for parameter values $\gamma = 0.8, \alpha = 0.09, \beta_1 = 0.2, \beta_2 = 0.3, d_1 = 0.05, d_2 = 0.01, d_3 = 0.01, \tau_1 = 12.2, \tau_2 = 7.2 < \tau_{20}^{+} = 7.25$.

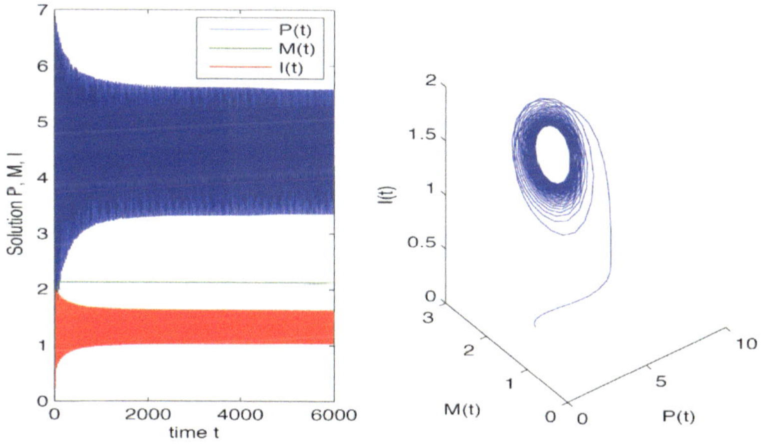

FIGURE 8.6 The endemic equilibrium E^* is unstable for parameter values $\gamma = 0.8, \alpha = 0.09, \beta_1 = 0.2, \beta_2 = 0.3, d_1 = 0.05, d_2 = 0.01, d_3 = 0.01, \tau_1 = 12.2, \tau_2 = 7.35 > \tau_{20}^{+} = 7.25$.

The trivial equilibrium $E_0(0,0,0)$ is locally asymptotically stable for the parameter values $d_1 = 0.3$, $d_2 = 0.01$ and $d_3 = 0.09$, when $\tau_1 = 15 \geq \bar{\tau}_{10} = 14.6$ and $\tau_2 = 7.2$ (see Figure 8.2). For the same set of parameter values the DFE $E_1(P_1, M_1, 0)$ is locally asymptotically stable when $\tau_1 = 12.2 < \bar{\tau}_{10} = 14.6$ and $\tau_2 = 7.2$ as shown in Figure 8.3. Further, EE $E^*(P^*, M^*, I^*)$ is locally asymptotically stable when $\tau_1 = 11.2 < \bar{\tau}_{10} = 13.86$ and $\tau_2 = 7.2$ for parameter values $d_1 = 0.2$, $d_2 = 0.05$ and $d_3 = 0.01$ (see Figure 8.4). These results show that the Theorem 8.4.1 is true.

Again, we take parameter values as $d_1 = 0.05$, $d_2 = 0.01$, $d_3 = 0.01$ and $\tau_1 = 12.2$. The EE $E^*(P^*, M^*, I^*)$ is stable when $\tau_2 = 7.2 < \tau_{20}^+ = 7.25$ as shown in Figure 8.5. Further, $E^*(P^*, M^*, I^*)$ is unstable and Hopf bifurcation appears when $\tau_2 = 7.35 \geq \tau_{20}^+ = 7.25$ as shown in Figure 8.6, which is in accordance with the results stated in Theorem 8.4.2.

8.7 Summary

In this chapter, we proposed a model for childhood disease dynamics with maturation delay and latent period of infection and investigated the asymptotic stability of the model for all the feasible equilibrium states, namely, E_0, E_1, and E^*. The conditions are obtained under which the equilibriums are locally asymptotically stable. The existence of Hopf bifurcation at the endemic equilibrium state (E^*) is explored and it is locally asymptotically stable for all $\tau_2 \in [0, \tau_{20}^+)$, and exhibits Hopf bifurcation, when the latent period (τ_2) is greater than or equal to some critical value (τ_{20}^+) under specific conditions. Finally, the normalized forward sensitivity indices are calculated for endemic equilibrium to various model parameters. Numerical simulations of the system are performed with a particular set of parameters to justify our analytic findings.

Chapter 9

Bifurcation in Disease Dynamics with Latent Period of Infection and Media Awareness

9.1 Introduction

Many emerging diseases spread rapidly due to the cross-borders movement of millions of people per day taking place internationally [1]. To control the spread of diseases, the health officials may have various pharmaceutical and non-pharmaceutical options in terms of wearing masks, closing schools, isolation and staying at home etc. [129]. Media plays a very important role to communicate awareness in public for use of non-pharmaceutical interventions (NPIs) to control the epidemics [130, 136–141].

In the modeling of infectious diseases, the incidence function plays a pivotal role [188]. The standard incidence rate $\beta\tilde{S}\tilde{I}/\tilde{N}$ is frequently used in many epidemic models, where β is the contact transmission rate, $\tilde{S}$ is the susceptible population, $\tilde{I}$ is the infected population and $\tilde{N}$ is total population at any time. Further, the spread of disease is not an instantaneous process and susceptible population takes a constant time to become infective, when it comes in contact with an infected person and this constant time is called the latent period of infection (τ).

Therefore, we modify the incidence rate as $\beta\tilde{S}(t-\tau)\tilde{I}/\tilde{N}$. However, this incidence function does not consider the impact of media coverage to control the spread of epidemics. Liu et al. [137] and Cui et al. [138] used media induced transmission rate of the form $\beta(\tilde{I}) = \beta e^{-m\tilde{I}}$ which has a major limitation, because $\beta e^{-m\tilde{I}} \to 0$ as $\tilde{I} \to \infty$, independent of the value of m. Since the media awareness is not the intrinsic deterministic factor responsible for the transmission, hence the transmission rate cannot be reduced below a certain level merely through media awareness. We consider media induced transmission rate as $\beta(\tilde{I}) = \beta\left(1 - m\frac{\tilde{I}}{\tilde{N}}\right)$ in the proposed model which is more reasonable because $\beta(\tilde{I}) \to \beta(1-m) \neq 0$ as $\tilde{I} \to \infty$ and it depends on coefficient of media awareness m. Further, as the value of m increases, the transmission rate decreases and therefore growth rate of infected population also decreases.

In the present chapter, we proposed and analyzed an SIS epidemic model in the absence of the disease induced immunity with the consideration of latent period and media awareness in controlling the epidemics using stability theory of ordinary differential equations. This chapter is organized as follows. In Section 9.2, formulation of epidemic model is presented and discussed the boundedness and positivity of the solution in the Section 9.3. In Section 9.4, the dynamical behavior of the system is studied and obtained the conditions for locally asymptotically stability in case of disease-free equilibrium and endemic equilibrium. Further, we obtained the specific conditions for the existence of Hopf bifurcation at the endemic equilibrium state. In Section 9.5, the sensitivity analysis of the basic reproduction number and state variables at endemic steady state with respect to model parameters is performed. Finally, in Section 9.6, we presented some numerical simulations to support our analytical findings and in the last section, a brief conclusion is given.

9.2 Formulation of Mathematical Model

Most of the contagious disease not only affect the pre-mature population, but can spread among the mature population also. Therefore, for that class of diseases, the susceptible population has no restriction on age. Further, there are certain diseases like influenza for which immunity is developed for a very short period, even sometimes the period is negligible. Therefore a person after recovery from the disease will rejoin the susceptible class almost instantaneously. In this chapter, we proposed an SIS model in the absence of disease-induced immunity and the awareness through the media as a control strategy. We have also considered latent period of infection and the assumptions of the model are:

(i) The population $\tilde{N}(\tilde{t})$ at ant time $\tilde{t}$ is divided into two mutually exclusive compartments; susceptible($\tilde{S}$) and infected($\tilde{I}$).

(ii) Newborn join to susceptible class with a fixed recruitment rate Λ and they die naturally at a rate $\tilde{\mu}$.

(iii) The population is mixed and interacting homogeneously.

(iv) Disease transmission is horizontal, not vertical.

(v) Media awareness reduces the disease burden and the transmission rate decreases with increase in infection.

(vi) Media induced transmission rate is of the form $\tilde{\beta}\left(1-m\frac{\tilde{I}}{\tilde{N}}\right)$, where $\tilde{\beta}$ and m are contact rate and coefficient of media awareness.

(vii) The disease acquired immunity is negligible. Therefore a person after recovery from the disease will rejoin the susceptible class almost instantaneously.

(viii) τ is the latent period of infection.

Our proposed SIS epidemic system is given below:

$$\frac{d\tilde{S}}{d\tilde{t}} = \Lambda - \tilde{\beta}\left(1-m\frac{\tilde{I}}{\tilde{N}}\right)\frac{\tilde{S}(t-\tau)\tilde{I}}{\tilde{N}} - \tilde{\mu}\tilde{S} + \tilde{\gamma}\tilde{I}, \tag{9.2.1}$$

$$\frac{d\tilde{I}}{d\tilde{t}} = \tilde{\beta}\left(1-m\frac{\tilde{I}}{\tilde{N}}\right)\frac{\tilde{S}(t-\tau)\tilde{I}}{\tilde{N}} - \tilde{\mu}\tilde{I} - \tilde{\delta}\tilde{I} - \tilde{\gamma}\tilde{I}, \tag{9.2.2}$$

with initial conditions:

$$\tilde{S}(\theta) = \phi_1(\theta),\ \tilde{I}(\theta) = \phi_2(\theta), \qquad \phi_1(0) > 0, \phi_2(0) > 0,$$

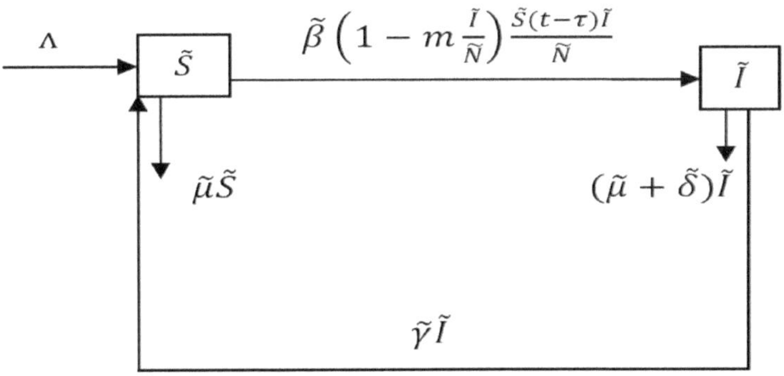

FIGURE 9.1 The schematic diagram of the model.

where $\theta \in [-\tau, 0]$ and $\phi_1(\theta)$, $\phi_2(\theta) \in \mathscr{C}([-\tau, 0], R^2_+)$, the Banach space of continuous functions mapping the interval $[-\tau, 0]$ into R^2_+, where $R^2_+ = \{(x_1, x_2) : x_i \geq 0, i = 1, 2\}$. The description of the parameters of the system is given in Table 9.1.

Since $\tilde{N}(\tilde{t}) = \tilde{S}(\tilde{t}) + \tilde{I}(\tilde{t})$. Therefore

$$\frac{d\tilde{N}}{d\tilde{t}} = \Lambda - \tilde{\mu}\tilde{N} - \tilde{\delta}\tilde{I}. \tag{9.2.3}$$

TABLE 9.1 Description of Parameters for the System (9.2.1)–(9.2.2)

Parameter	Description	Unit
Λ	Recruitment rate	days^{-1}
$\tilde{\delta}$	Disease-induced death rate	days^{-1}
$1/\tilde{\mu}$	Average life-span	days
$\tilde{\beta}$	Contact rate (in absence of NPIs through media awareness)	days^{-1}
m	Coefficient of media awareness	–
τ	latent period of Infection	days
$1/\tilde{\gamma}$	Average length of infection	days

9.3 Positivity and Boundedness of the System

We state and prove the following lemmas for the positivity and boundedness of the solution of the system (9.2.1)–(9.2.2):

Lemma 9.3.1. *All the solution trajectories of system (9.2.1)–(9.2.2) initiating inside* Γ, *will stay within the interior of* Γ, *where*

$$\Gamma = \left\{ (\tilde{S},\tilde{I}) : 0 \leq \tilde{S},\tilde{I} \leq \frac{\Lambda}{\tilde{\mu}} \right\}.$$

Proof. Let $R_+^2 = \left\{ (\tilde{S},\tilde{I}) \in R^2 : \tilde{S} \geq 0, \tilde{I} \geq 0 \right\}$ be the two dimensional space. Equation (9.2.3) can be rewritten as

$$\frac{d\tilde{N}}{dt} < \Lambda - \tilde{\mu}\tilde{N},$$

which implies that $0 \leq \tilde{N}(\tilde{t}) \leq \frac{\Lambda}{\tilde{\mu}} = \tilde{N}^0$ as $\tilde{t} \to \infty$.

Therefore the system (9.2.1)–(9.2.2) is bounded and any solution of the system originates from Γ remains in Γ. □

To reduce the number of parameter in proposed system, we non-dimensionalize the equations (9.2.1)–(9.2.3) using

$$S = \frac{\tilde{S}}{\tilde{N}}, I = \frac{\tilde{I}}{\tilde{N}}, N = \frac{\tilde{N}}{\tilde{N^0}}, \tilde{N^0} = \frac{\Lambda}{\tilde{\mu}}, t = \tilde{\mu}\tilde{t}.$$

The rescaled equations are:

$$\begin{aligned}
\frac{dS}{dt} &= \frac{1}{N} - \beta(1-mI)S(t-\tau)I + \gamma I - \frac{S}{N} + \delta SI := f_1, &(9.3.1)\\
\frac{dI}{dt} &= \beta(1-mI)S(t-\tau)I - \delta I - \gamma I - \frac{I}{N} + \delta I^2 := f_2, &(9.3.2)\\
\frac{dN}{dt} &= 1 - N - \delta NI := f_3, &(9.3.3)
\end{aligned}$$

where

$$\beta = \frac{\tilde{\beta}}{\tilde{\mu}}, \gamma = \frac{\tilde{\gamma}}{\tilde{\mu}}, \delta = \frac{\tilde{\delta}}{\tilde{\mu}}.$$

Lemma 9.3.2. *The solution of the system (9.3.1)–(9.3.3) are positive, for all* $t \geq 0$.

Proof. Let $(S(t), I(t), N(t))$ be a solution of the system (9.3.1)–(9.3.3). The equation (9.3.1) can be rewritten as

$$\begin{aligned}\frac{dS}{dt} &\geq -\beta(1-mI)S(t-\tau)I - \frac{S}{N}.\\ &\geq -\beta(1-m)S(t-\tau) - S.\end{aligned}$$

Solving, we get

$$S(t) \geq S(0)e^{-(1+\beta(1-m))t},$$

which evidences that $S(t) \geq 0$ as $t \to \infty$.

The equation (9.3.2) can be rewritten as

$$\begin{aligned}\frac{dI}{dt} &\geq -\delta I - \gamma I - \frac{I}{N}.\\ &\geq -\delta I - \gamma I - I.\end{aligned}$$

Solving, we get

$$I(t) \geq I(0)e^{-(1+\delta+\gamma)t},$$

which implies that $I(t) \geq 0$ as $t \to \infty$.

The equation (9.3.3) can be rewritten as

$$\begin{aligned}\frac{dN}{dt} &\geq -\delta NI - N.\\ &\geq -\delta N - N.\end{aligned}$$

Solving, we get

$$N(t) \geq N(0)e^{-(1+\delta)t},$$

which implies that $N(t) \geq 0$ as $t \to \infty$.

Therefore $S(t), I(t), N(t)$ are positive for all $t \geq 0$. □

9.4 Dynamical Behavior of the System

Now, we will calculate the basic reproduction number, analyze the local stability at all the feasible equilibrium states and explore the possibility for existence of Hopf bifurcation at the endemic equilibrium state for the system (9.3.1)–(9.3.3).

The system (9.3.1)–(9.3.3) has the disease-free equilibrium (DFE) $E_0 = (1,0,1)$. Now, we calculate the basic reproduction number R_0. Let $x = (S,I)$. Therefore

$$\frac{dx}{dt} = f - v,$$

where

$$f = \begin{pmatrix} -\beta(1-mI)S(t-\tau)I + \delta SI \\ \beta(1-mI)S(t-\tau)I + \delta I^2 \end{pmatrix}$$

and

$$v = \begin{pmatrix} -\frac{1}{N} - \gamma I + \frac{S}{N} \\ \delta I + \gamma I + \frac{I}{N} \end{pmatrix}.$$

We have

$$F = Df|_{E_0} = \begin{pmatrix} 0 & -\beta + \delta \\ 0 & \beta \end{pmatrix}$$

and

$$V = Dv|_{E_0} = \begin{pmatrix} 1 & -\gamma \\ 0 & \delta + \gamma + 1 \end{pmatrix}.$$

The next generation matrix for the model is given by

$$K = FV^{-1} = \begin{pmatrix} 0 & \frac{-\beta+\delta}{\delta+\gamma+1} \\ 0 & \frac{\beta}{\delta+\gamma+1} \end{pmatrix}.$$

The basic reproduction number is given by $R_0 = \rho(FV^{-1})$. Therefore

$$R_0 = \frac{\beta}{\delta + \gamma + 1}. \tag{9.4.1}$$

Further the system (9.3.1)–(9.3.3) also has endemic equilibrium (EE) given by

$$E^* = (S^*, I^*, N^*),$$

where $N^* = \frac{1}{1+\delta I^*}$, $S^* = 1 - I^*$ and the value I^* is given by

$$\frac{1}{R_0(1-mI^*)} = 1 - I^*.$$

If there is no media effect, then

$$I^* = 1 - \frac{1}{R_0}.$$

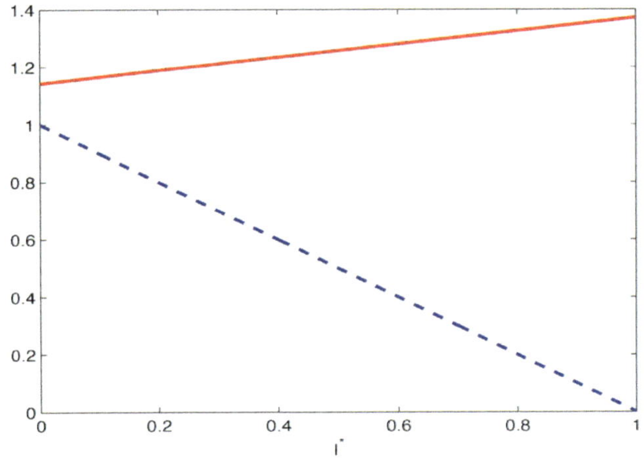

FIGURE 9.2 Non-existence of endemic equilibrium for parameteric values $\tilde{\beta} = 0.07$, $m = 0.2$, $\tilde{\gamma} = 0.05$, $\tilde{\delta} = 0.01$, $\tilde{\mu} = 0.02$, $R_0 = 0.875 < 1$, where the red curve represents $\frac{1}{R_0(1-mI^*)}$ and blue dotted curve represents $1 - I^*$.

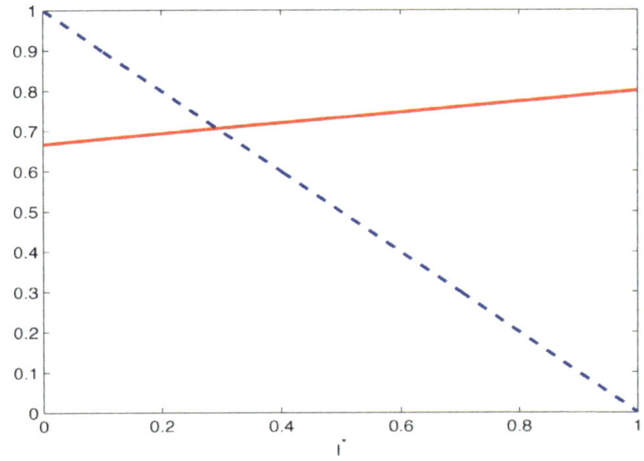

FIGURE 9.3 Existence of endemic equilibrium for parameteric values $\tilde{\beta} = 0.12$, $m = 0.2$, $\tilde{\gamma} = 0.05$, $\tilde{\delta} = 0.01$, $\tilde{\mu} = 0.02$, $R_0 = 1.5 > 1$, where the red curve represents $\frac{1}{R_0(1-mI^*)}$ and blue dotted curve represents $1 - I^*$.

Clearly, in the absence of media effect, I^* exists if and only if $R_0 > 1$. The EE does not exists for $R_0 \leq 1$ (no point of intersection, see Figure 9.2) but, EE exists for $R_0 > 1$ (see Figure 9.3). In the both Figures the red curve represents $\frac{1}{R_0(1-mI^*)}$ and blue dotted curve represents $1 - I^*$ at $m = 0.2$.

Theorem 9.4.1. *The system (9.3.1)–(9.3.3) has*

(i) the disease-free equilibrium (DFE) $E_0 = (1,0,1)$ *that exists for all the parameter values;*

(ii) no endemic equilibrium (EE), if $R_0 \leq 1$*;*

(iii) unique endemic equilibrium, if $R_0 > 1$.

Theorem 9.4.2. *The disease-free equilibrium (DFE)* E_0 *is*

(i) locally asymptotically stable for all τ*, if* $R_0 < 1$ *and*

(ii) unstable, if $R_0 > 1$.

Proof. The variational matrix at the DFE is given by

$$J_0 = \begin{pmatrix} -1 & -\beta+\gamma+\delta & 0 \\ 0 & \beta-\delta-\gamma-1 & 0 \\ 0 & -\delta & -1 \end{pmatrix}.$$

The characteristic equation of J_0 is given by

$$(\lambda+1)(\lambda-\beta+\delta+\gamma+1)(\lambda+1) = 0.$$

The roots of characteristic equation are

$$\lambda = -1, -1, \beta-(1+\delta+\gamma).$$

Now, if $R_0 < 1$, then there exists three negative real eigen values of J_0 and if $R_0 > 1$, then there exists one positive real eigen value. Therefore, if $R_0 < 1$, then the disease-free equilibrium is locally asymptotically stable for all τ and it is unstable, if $R_0 > 1$. □

Theorem 9.4.3. *The endemic equilibrium (EE) is locally asymptotically stable for* $R_0 > 1$*, but close to 1.*

Proof. Here, we use the method based on central manifold theory to establish the local stability of endemic equilibrium taking β as bifurcation parameter. The critical value of the bifurcation parameter at $R_0 = 1$ is $\beta^* = 1+\gamma+\delta$. It can be easily verified that the Jacobian J_0 at $\beta = \beta^*$ has right eigen vector given by $W = (w_1, w_2, w_3)^T$ such that $J_0 W = 0$, where

$$w_1 = [\gamma - \beta + \delta]\sigma, \;\; w_2 = \sigma, \;\; w_3 = -\delta\sigma.$$

The left eigen vector is given by $V = (v_1, v_2, v_3)$ which satisfy $V.J_0 = 0$ and $V.W = 1$, where

$$v_1 = 0, \;\; v_2 = \frac{1}{\sigma}, \;\; v_3 = 0.$$

The associated non-zero partial derivatives of $F = (f_1, f_2, f_3)^T$ at the DFE and $\beta = \beta^*$ are given by

$$\frac{\partial^2 f_1}{\partial S \partial I} = -\beta e^{-\lambda\tau} + \delta, \;\; \frac{\partial^2 f_1}{\partial S \partial N} = 1, \;\; \frac{\partial^2 f_1}{\partial I^2} = 2\beta m,$$

$$\frac{\partial^2 f_2}{\partial S \partial I} = \beta e^{-\lambda\tau}, \;\; \frac{\partial^2 f_2}{\partial I^2} = -2\beta m + 2\delta, \;\; \frac{\partial^2 f_2}{\partial I \partial N} = 1,$$

$$\frac{\partial^2 f_3}{\partial I \partial N} = -\delta, \;\; \frac{\partial^2 f_2}{\partial I \partial \beta} = 1.$$

Here we use notations $x_1 = S, x_2 = I, x_3 = N$. We have

$$a = \sum_{k,i,j=1}^{3} v_k w_i w_j \frac{\partial^2 f_k}{\partial x_i \partial x_j}$$

and

$$b = \sum_{k,i=1}^{3} v_k w_i \frac{\partial^2 f_k}{\partial x_i \partial \phi}.$$

By simple calculations, we get

$$a = -\sigma\beta[\beta - (1+\gamma+\delta)]e^{-\lambda\tau} - 2\sigma[\beta m - \delta] - \sigma\beta e^{-\lambda\tau} - \sigma\delta$$

and

$$b = 1.$$

Now $a < 0$ if $\beta > 1+\gamma+\delta$ and $\beta m > \delta$. Using (9.4.1), we get $a < 0$ if $R_0 > 1$ and $\beta m > \delta$, which is one of the sufficient condition.

Since $a < 0$ and $b > 0$ at $\beta = \beta^*$, a transcritical bifurcation occurs at $R_0 = 1$ and unique endemic equilibrium is locally asymptotically stable for $R_0 > 1$. □

Now, we will discuss the asymptotical stability of the endemic equilibrium point with respect to the latent period of infection.

The characteristic equation of the Jacobian matrix at the equilibrium point $E^*(S^*, I^*, N^*)$ can be written as:

$$\lambda^3 + A\lambda^2 + B\lambda + C + (F\lambda^2 + E\lambda + D)e^{-\lambda\tau} = 0, \tag{9.4.2}$$

where

$$\begin{aligned}
A &= -(b_2 + c_3 + d_1),\\
B &= b_2c_3 - b_3c_2 + c_3d_1 + b_2d_1,\\
C &= -(b_2c_3d_1 - b_3c_2d_1),\\
D &= a_2b_1c_3 + a_2b_3c_1 - a_1b_2c_3 + a_1b_3c_2,\\
E &= a_1c_3 + a_1b_2 - a_2b_1,\\
F &= -a_1
\end{aligned}$$

and

$$\begin{aligned}
a_1 &= -\beta(1 - mI^*)I^*,\\
b_1 &= -\beta(1 - 2mI^*)S^* + \gamma + \delta S^*,\\
c_1 &= -\tfrac{1}{N^{*2}} + \tfrac{S^*}{N^{*2}},\\
d_1 &= -\tfrac{1}{N^*} + \delta I^*,\\
a_2 &= -a_1,\\
b_2 &= \beta(1 - 2mI^*)S^* - \delta - \gamma - \tfrac{1}{N^*} + 2\delta I^*,\\
c_2 &= \tfrac{I^*}{N^{*2}},\\
b_3 &= -\delta N^*,\\
c_3 &= -1 - \delta I^*.
\end{aligned}$$

In the absence of delay ($\tau = 0$), the transcendental equation (9.4.2) reduces to

$$\lambda^3 + (A + F)\lambda^2 + (B + E)\lambda + (C + D) = 0. \tag{9.4.3}$$

We have

$$\begin{aligned}
A + F &= -(a_1 + b_2 + c_3 + d_1),\\
B + E &= b_2c_3 - b_3c_2 + c_3d_1 + b_2d_1 + a_1c_3 + a_1b_2 - a_2b_1,\\
C + D &= -b_2c_3d_1 + b_3c_2d_1 + a_2b_1c_3 + a_2b_3c_1 - a_1b_2c_3 + a_1b_3c_2.
\end{aligned}$$

By Routh-Hurwitz criterion, all the roots of equation (9.4.3) have negative real parts that is the equilibrium E^* is locally asymptotically stable if

$(\mathbf{H_1}): A+F,\ B+E,\ C+D>0$ and $(A+F)(B+E)-(C+D)>0$ holds.

Assume that for some $\tau>0$, $\lambda = iw$ is root of (9.4.2), therefore we have

$$(iw)^3+A(iw)^2+B(iw)+C+(F(iw)^2+E(iw)+D)e^{-iw\tau}=0.$$

Equating real and imaginary parts, it can be obtained

$$Ew\sin w\tau+(D-Fw^2)\cos w\tau = Aw^2-C, \quad (9.4.4)$$
$$Ew\cos w\tau-(D-Fw^2)\sin w\tau = w^3-Bw. \quad (9.4.5)$$

Solving (9.4.4) and (9.4.5), we get

$$w^6+pw^4+qw^2+r=0, \quad (9.4.6)$$

where

$$\begin{aligned} p &= A^2-2B-F^2,\\ q &= B^2-2AC+2DF-E^2,\\ r &= C^2-D^2. \end{aligned}$$

By substituting $w^2=z$ in equation (9.4.6), we define

$$F(z)=z^3+pz^2+qz+r.$$

By Lemma 7.4.6 stated in Chapter 7, there exists at least one positive root $w=w_0$ of equation (9.4.6) satisfying (9.4.4) and (9.4.5), which implies characteristic equation (9.4.2) has a pair of purely imaginary roots of the form $\pm iw_0$. Solving (9.4.4) and (9.4.5) for τ and substituting the value of $w=w_0$, the corresponding $\tau_k>0$ is given by

$$\tau_k^+=\frac{1}{w_0}\left[\cos^{-1}\left(\frac{(E-AF)w_0^4+(AD+CF-BE)w_0^2-CD}{E^2w_0^2+(D-Fw_0^2)^2}\right)+2k\pi\right],$$

where $k=0,1,2,\ldots$.

Since the existence of Hopf bifurcation at τ_0^+, it is required that the transversality condition $Re\left[\left(\frac{d\lambda}{d\tau}\right)^{-1}\right]_{\tau=\tau_0^+} \neq 0$ should hold, therefore taking the derivative of λ with respect to τ in (9.4.2), we get

$$\left(\frac{d\lambda}{d\tau}\right)^{-1} = \frac{(3\lambda^2+2A\lambda+B)e^{\lambda\tau}+(2F\lambda+E)}{\lambda(F\lambda^2+E\lambda+D)} - \frac{\tau}{\lambda}.$$

At $\lambda = iw$ and $\tau = \tau_0^+$, we have

$$Re\left[\left(\frac{d\lambda}{d\tau}\right)^{-1}\right] = \frac{MP-NR}{w_0(L^2+M^2)},$$

where $K = -3w_0^2+B,\ L = 2Aw_0,\ M = D-Fw_0^2,\ N = Ew_0,\ P = Ksinw_0\tau_0+Lcosw_0\tau_0+2Fw_0$ and $R = Kcosw_0\tau_0-Lsinw_0\tau_0+E$.

Therefor, $Re\left[\left(\frac{d\lambda}{d\tau}\right)^{-1}\right]_{\tau=\tau_0^+} \neq 0$, if $MP \neq NR$.

Theorem 9.4.4. *Let $R_0 > 1$ and (H_1) holds. For the system (9.3.1)–(9.3.3),*

(i) The endemic equilibrium $E^*(S^*,I^*,N^*)$ is locally asymptotically stable for all $\tau \in [0, \tau_0^+)$.

(ii) If $\tau \geq \tau_0^+$, then the endemic equilibrium $E^*(S^*,I^*,N^*)$ is unstable and the system undergoes Hopf bifurcation around E^*.

TABLE 9.2 Parametric Values Used for Simulation

Parameter	Value	References
Λ	5.0	[136, 138]
$\tilde{\delta}$	0.01	[136, 138]
$\tilde{\mu}$	0.02	[136, 138]
$\tilde{\beta}$	[0.07,0.12]	Variable
m	[0,0.9]	Variable
$\tilde{\gamma}$	0.05	[136, 138]

9.5 Sensitivity Analysis

In this section, we perform the sensitivity analysis of the basic reproduction number R_0 and endemic equilibrium with respect to model parameters, for a particular set of parameters that are given in the Table 9.2. The normalized sensitivity indices of the basic reproduction number R_0 with respect to parameters are shown in Table 9.3. From the table, we observe that β has a positive impact on R_0 and δ, γ have a negative impact on R_0. For example 10% increase (decrease) in β resulting in 10% increase (decrease) in R_0 and on the other hand 10% increase (decrease) in δ resulting in 1.25% decrease (increase) in R_0. Moreover β is most sensitive to R_0, hence we observe significant changes in R_0 by a small change in this parameter.

TABLE 9.3 The Sensitivity Indices $\gamma_{y_j}^{R_0} = \frac{\partial R_0}{\partial y_j} \times \frac{y_j}{R_0}$ of the Basic Reproduction Number R_0 to the Parameters y_j for the Parameter Values Given in Table 9.2

Parameter (y_j)	Sensitivity index of R_0 w.r.t. y_j $(\gamma_{y_j}^{R_0})$
β	1
δ	–0.125
γ	–0.625
m	0

We perform the sensitivity analysis of state variables of the system (9.3.1)–(9.3.3) at endemic steady state with respect to model parameters. Sensitivity indices of the state variables at the endemic equilibrium are shown in the Table 9.4 using parameter values given in the Table 9.2. We observe that β has a negative impact and the rest of the parameters have a positive impact on the S^*. Further, β has a positive impact and the rest of the parameters have a negative impact on the I^*. Moreover β and γ are most sensitive parameter to I^*, hence we observe significant changes in I^* by small changes in these parameters. It is further observed that all the parameters are less sensitive to N^*.

TABLE 9.4 The Sensitivity Indices $\gamma_{y_j}^{x_i} = \frac{\partial x_i}{\partial y_j} \times \frac{y_j}{x_i}$ of the State Variables of the System (9.3.1)–(9.3.3) to the Parameters y_j for the Parameter Values Given in Table 9.2

Parameter (y_j)	$\gamma_{y_j}^{S^*}$	$\gamma_{y_j}^{I^*}$	$\gamma_{y_j}^{N^*}$
β	–0.529412	4.23529	–0.22291
δ	0.0661765	–0.529412	–0.0247678
γ	0.330882	–2.64706	0.139319
m	0.0588235	–0.470588	0.0247678

9.6 Numerical Simulations

We perform the numerical simulations of the model (9.3.1)–(9.3.3) to justify the analytic findings. The parameter used for simulation of the system are listed in Table (9.2) taking a time unit in days. We use initial population sizes as $S_0 = 0.8$, $I_0 = 0.2$, $N_0 = 0.9$, parameter value $m = 0.2$ fixed and varying only $\tilde{\beta}$ parameter.

We observe that, when $\tilde{\beta} = 0.07$ and $\tau = 0.4$ then $R_0 = 0.875 < 1$ and the DFE E_0 is locally asymptotically stable for all τ as shown in Figure 9.4, which is in accordance with the results stated in Theorem 9.4.2. When $\tilde{\beta} = 0.12$ and $\tau = 0.4$ then $R_0 = 1.5 > 1$ and EE E^* is locally asymptotically stable as shown in Figure 9.5, which is in accordance with the result stated in Theorem 9.4.3.

Further for $R_0 = 1.5 > 1$, the EE E^* is locally asymptotically stable when $\tau = 0.95 < \tau_0^+ = 0.96$ (see Figure 9.6), whereas the EE E^* is unstable and Hopf bifurcation appears when $\tau = 0.974 > \tau_0^+ = 0.96$ (see Figure 9.7), which are in accordance with the results stated in Theorem 9.4.4.

The effect of m on the fraction of infectious population is shown in Figures 9.8 and 9.9 with different values of m. We observe that the endemic equilibrium is significantly influenced by media coefficient m.

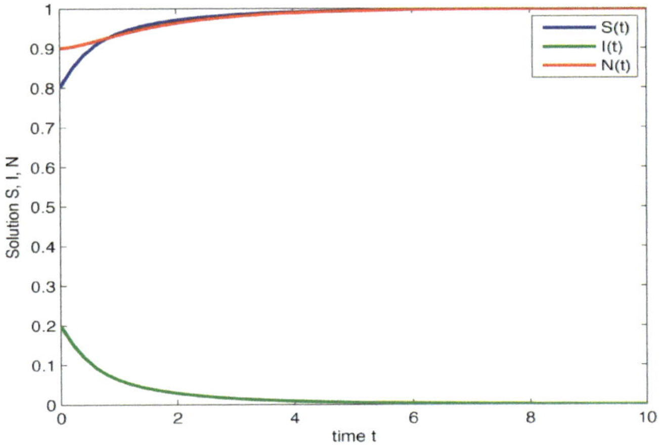

FIGURE 9.4 The variation of scaled population in scaled time for parameteric values $\tilde{\beta} = 0.07$, $m = 0.2$, $\tilde{\gamma} = 0.05$, $\tilde{\delta} = 0.01$, $\tilde{\mu} = 0.02$, $\tau = 0.4$ and $R_0 = 0.875 < 1$.

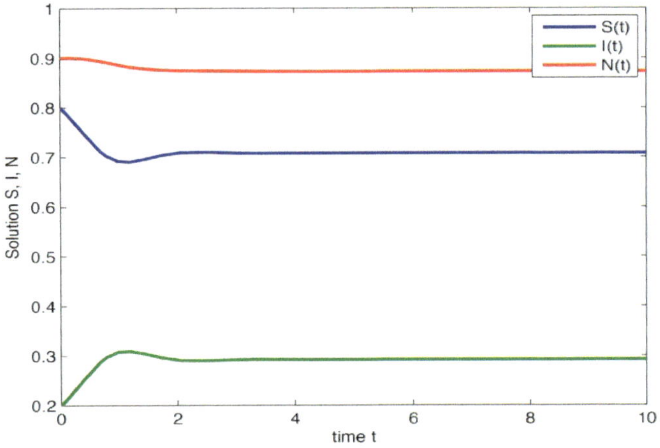

FIGURE 9.5 The variation of scaled population in scaled time for parameteric values $\tilde{\beta} = 0.12$, $m = 0.2$, $\tilde{\gamma} = 0.05$, $\tilde{\delta} = 0.01$, $\tilde{\mu} = 0.02$, $\tau = 0.4$ and $R_0 = 1.5 > 1$.

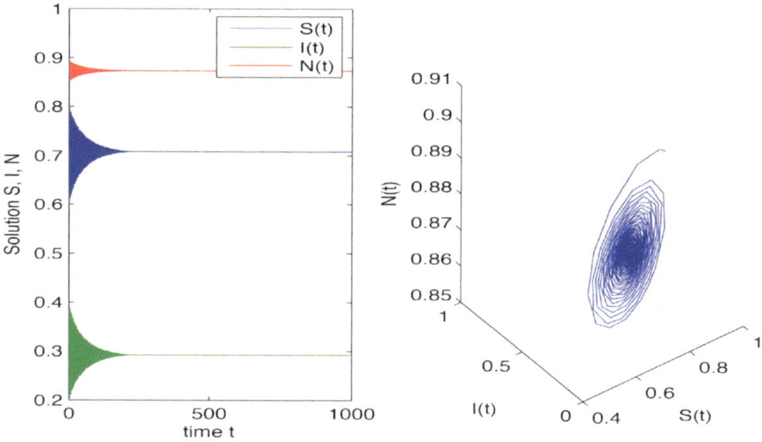

FIGURE 9.6 The endemic equilibrium E^* is stable for parameteric values $\tilde{\beta} = 0.12$, $m = 0.2$, $\tilde{\gamma} = 0.05$, $\tilde{\delta} = 0.01$, $\tilde{\mu} = 0.02$, $R_0 = 1.5$ and $\tau = 0.95 < \tau_0^+ = 0.96$.

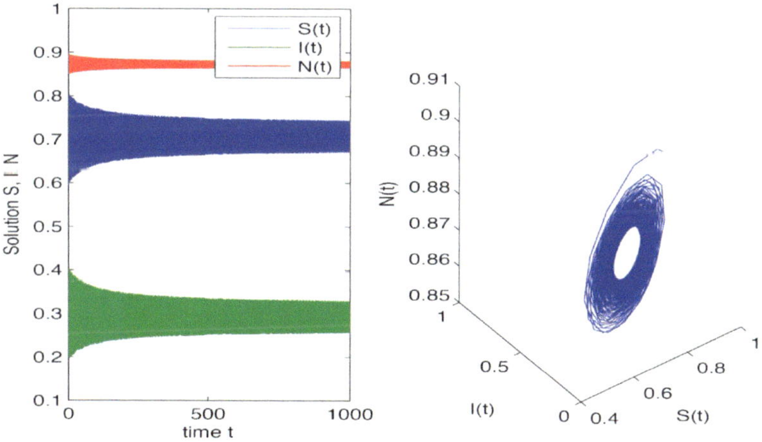

FIGURE 9.7 The endemic equilibrium E^* is unstable and Hopf bifurcation appears for the parameteric values $\tilde{\beta} = 0.12$, $m = 0.2$, $\tilde{\gamma} = 0.05$, $\tilde{\delta} = 0.01$, $\tilde{\mu} = 0.02$, $R_0 = 1.5$ and $\tau = 0.974 > \tau_0^+ = 0.96$.

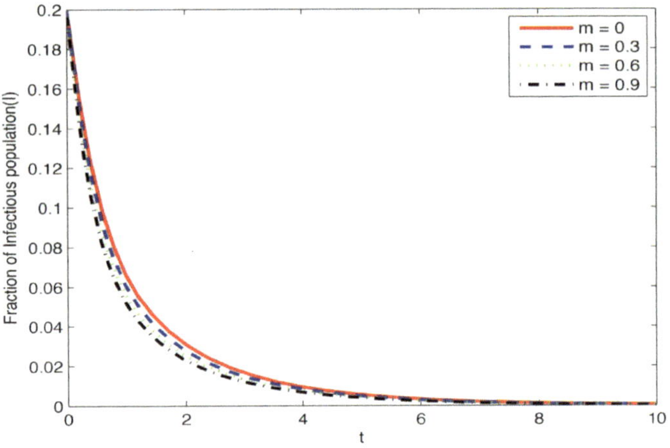

FIGURE 9.8 The effect of m on I for parameteric values $\tilde{\beta} = 0.07$, $\tilde{\gamma} = 0.05$, $\tilde{\delta} = 0.01$, $\tilde{\mu} = 0.02$, $\tau = 0.4$ and $R_0 = 0.875 < 1$.

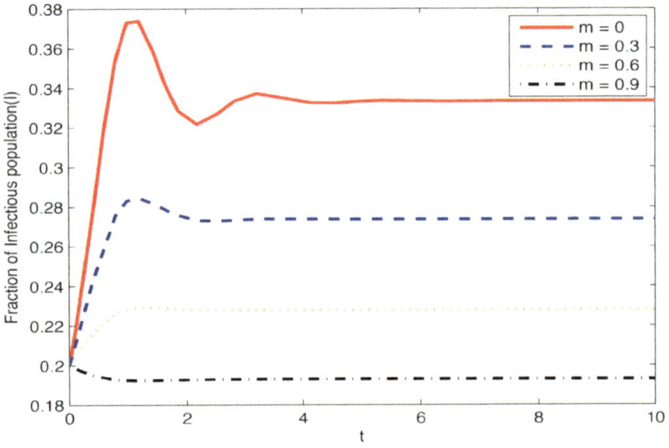

FIGURE 9.9 The effect of m on I for parameteric values $\tilde{\beta} = 0.12$, $\tilde{\gamma} = 0.05$, $\tilde{\delta} = 0.01$, $\tilde{\mu} = 0.02$, $\tau = 0.4$ and $R_0 = 1.5 > 1$.

9.7 Summary

In this chapter, we proposed an SIS epidemic model in the absence of disease induced immunity incorporating latent period of infection and media awareness. We observed that the coefficient of media awareness m does not affect the basic reproduction number R_0. We investigated the asymptotic stability of the model at all the equilibrium states. If $R_0 < 1$, then the disease-fee state exists and is locally asymptotically stable for all τ (i.e., stability of disease-free equilibrium is independent of the latent period of infection). A transcritical bifurcation occurs at $R_0 = 1$ and a locally asymptotically stable endemic equilibrium exists for $R_0 > 1$. It is observed that the endemic state is locally asymptotically stable, when the latent period of infection is less than some critical value τ_0^+, whereas endemic equilibrium is unstable and Hopf bifurcation appears, when the latent period is greater than or equal to some critical value τ_0^+ under certain specific conditions.

We calculated sensitivity indices of the reproduction number and endemic equilibrium to various parameters and identified respective sensitive parameters. Numerical simulations of the system justify the analytic findings and we also observed that endemic equilibrium state is greatly influenced by media coefficient m.

Chapter 10

Continuous and Discrete Dynamics of SIRS Epidemic Model with Media Awareness

10.1 Introduction

As, we have already discussed in last chapter, that non-pharmaceutical interventions (NPIs) through media awareness are found useful in reducing the burden of certain infectious diseases from the particular environment [189]. In the present chapter, we proposed and analyzed a SIRS epidemic model incorporating disease induced immunity and media awareness to control the epidemics. Here, we consider the media induced transmission rate as $\beta(\tilde{I}) = \beta e^{-m\frac{I}{N}}$ and $\min\{\beta(\tilde{I})\} = \beta e^{-m}$ remains unchanged with respect to the total population size. Also, the movement of the population is instantaneous from one compartment to another.

This chapter is organized as follows. In Section 10.2, formulation of a SIRS epidemic model incorporating media awareness as control strategy is presented. In Section 10.3, the dynamical behavior of the system is studied and obtained the conditions for locally asymptotically stability in case of disease-free equilibrium and endemic equilibrium. In Section 10.4, SIRS system is reduced to SI and discrete-time behavior is explored. In Section 10.5, stability conditions of the discrete-time system are discussed at the fixed points and obtained the existence conditions for flip bifurcation and Hopf bifurcation by using bifurcation theory. In Section 10.6, the sensitivity analysis of the reproduction number and endemic steady state with respect to model parameters is performed. In Section 10.7, we presented some numerical simulations to support our analytical findings. Finally a brief conclusion is given in the last section.

10.2 Formulation of Mathematical Model

We proposed a SIRS epidemic model considering media awareness, as a control strategy with the assumptions (ii)–(v) of the model proposed in Chapter 9 and including the following new assumptions:

(i) The population $\tilde{N}(\tilde{t})$ at ant time $\tilde{t}$ is divided into various mutually exclusive compartments, namely, susceptible($\tilde{S}$), infected($\tilde{I}$) and recovered($\tilde{R}$).

(ii) Media induced effective transmission rate is proposed as $\beta(\tilde{I}) = \beta e^{-\frac{m\tilde{I}}{\tilde{N}}}$.

(iii) Recovered individuals develop disease-acquired temporary immunity that wanes at rate $\tilde{\theta}$.

(iv) The movement of population is instantaneous from one compartment to other.

The proposed SIRS epidemic system with a media induced transmission rate is of the form:

$$\frac{d\tilde{S}}{d\tilde{t}} = \Lambda - \tilde{\beta} e^{-m\frac{I}{N}} \frac{\tilde{S}\tilde{I}}{\tilde{N}} + \tilde{\theta}\tilde{R} - \tilde{\mu}\tilde{S}, \tag{10.2.1}$$

$$\frac{d\tilde{I}}{d\tilde{t}} = \tilde{\beta} e^{-m\frac{I}{N}} \frac{\tilde{S}\tilde{I}}{\tilde{N}} - \tilde{\mu}\tilde{I} - \tilde{\delta}\tilde{I} - \tilde{\gamma}\tilde{I}, \tag{10.2.2}$$

$$\frac{d\tilde{R}}{d\tilde{t}} = \tilde{\gamma}\tilde{I} - \tilde{\theta}\tilde{R} - \tilde{\mu}\tilde{R}, \tag{10.2.3}$$

with initial conditions:

$$\tilde{S}(0) = \tilde{S}_0 > 0, \tilde{I}(0) = \tilde{I}_0 > 0, \tilde{R}(0) = \tilde{R}_0 > 0 \tag{10.2.4}$$

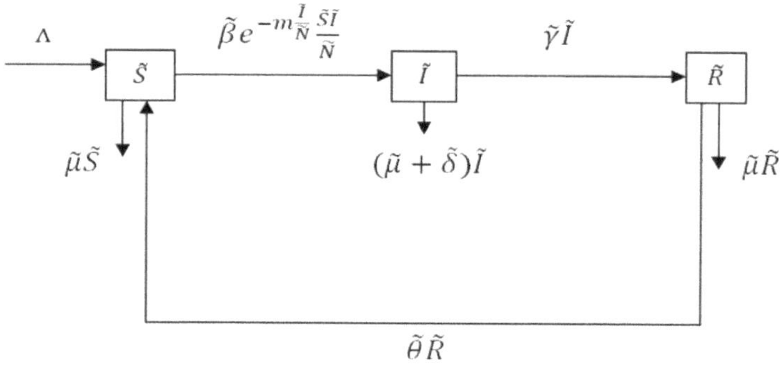

FIGURE 10.1 The schematic diagram of the model.

and the description of the parameters of the proposed system is mentioned in the Table 10.1.

Also $\tilde{N}(\tilde{t}) = \tilde{S}(\tilde{t}) + \tilde{I}(\tilde{t}) + \tilde{R}(\tilde{t})$. Therefore

$$\frac{d\tilde{N}}{d\tilde{t}} = \Lambda - \tilde{\mu}\tilde{N} - \tilde{\delta}\tilde{I}. \tag{10.2.5}$$

Consider the three dimensional region

$$\Gamma = \left\{ (\tilde{S}, \tilde{I}, \tilde{R}) : 0 \leq \tilde{S}, \tilde{I}, \tilde{R} \leq \frac{\Lambda}{\tilde{\mu}} \right\}.$$

Proposition 10.2.1. *All the solution trajectories of system (10.2.1)–(10.2.4) initiating inside Γ, will stay within the interior of Γ.*

Proof. Let $R^3_+ = \left\{(\tilde{S}, \tilde{I}, \tilde{R}) \in R^3 : \tilde{S} \geq 0, \tilde{I} \geq 0, \tilde{R} \geq 0\right\}$ be the three dimensional space. From the system (10.2.1)–(10.2.4), we observe that

$$\frac{d\tilde{S}}{d\tilde{t}}\Big|_{\tilde{S}=0} = \Lambda + \tilde{\theta}\tilde{R} > 0,$$

$$\frac{d\tilde{I}}{d\tilde{t}}\Big|_{\tilde{I}=0} = 0,$$

$$\frac{d\tilde{R}}{d\tilde{t}}\Big|_{\tilde{R}=0} = \tilde{\gamma}\tilde{I} > 0$$

and $\tilde{S}(\tilde{t}), \tilde{I}(\tilde{t}), \tilde{R}(\tilde{t})$ are continuous function of $\tilde{t}$. Thus the vector field initiating in R^3_+ will remain inside R^3_+ for all the time. Also the total

TABLE 10.1 Description of Parameters for the System (10.2.1)–(10.2.4)

Parameter	Description	Unit
Λ	Recruitment rate	days^{-1}
$\tilde{\delta}$	Disease-induced death rate	days^{-1}
$1/\tilde{\mu}$	Average life-span	days
$\tilde{\beta}$	Contact rate (in absence of NPI's through media awareness)	days^{-1}
m	Coefficient of media awareness	–
$1/\tilde{\gamma}$	Average length of infection	days
$\tilde{\theta}$	Rate at which disease-induced immunity wanes	days^{-1}

population $\tilde{N}(\tilde{t}) = \tilde{S}(\tilde{t}) + \tilde{I}(\tilde{t}) + \tilde{R}(\tilde{t})$ satisfies $\frac{d\tilde{N}}{dt} = \Lambda - \tilde{\mu}\tilde{N} - \tilde{\delta}\tilde{I}$. Then $\frac{d\tilde{N}}{dt} < \Lambda - \tilde{\mu}\tilde{N}$ as $\tilde{t} \to \infty$ implies that $0 \leq \tilde{N}(\tilde{t}) \leq \frac{\Lambda}{\tilde{\mu}} = \tilde{N}^0$. Therefore the system (10.2.1)–(10.2.4) is bounded and any solution of the system originates from Γ remains in Γ. □

We non dimensionalize the above system using

$$S = \frac{\tilde{S}}{\tilde{N}}, I = \frac{\tilde{I}}{\tilde{N}}, R = \frac{\tilde{R}}{\tilde{N}}, N = \frac{\tilde{N}}{\tilde{N^0}}, \tilde{N^0} = \frac{\Lambda}{\tilde{\mu}}, t = \tilde{\mu}\tilde{t}.$$

The rescaled equations are

$$\frac{dS}{dt} = \frac{1}{N} - \beta e^{-mI} SI + \theta R - \frac{S}{N} + \delta SI := f_1, \quad (10.2.6)$$

$$\frac{dI}{dt} = \beta e^{-mI} SI - \delta I - \gamma I - \frac{I}{N} + \delta I^2 := f_2, \quad (10.2.7)$$

$$\frac{dR}{dt} = \gamma I - \theta R - \frac{R}{N} + \delta RI := f_3, \quad (10.2.8)$$

$$\frac{dN}{dt} = 1 - N - \delta NI := f_4, \quad (10.2.9)$$

where

$$\beta = \frac{\tilde{\beta}}{\tilde{\mu}}, \theta = \frac{\tilde{\theta}}{\tilde{\mu}}, \gamma = \frac{\tilde{\gamma}}{\tilde{\mu}}, \delta = \frac{\tilde{\delta}}{\tilde{\mu}}$$

and with the initial conditions:

$$S(0) = S_0 > 0, I(0) = I_0 > 0, R(0) = R_0 > 0, N(0) = N_0 > 0. \quad (10.2.10)$$

In the following section, we will study the dynamical behavior of the system (10.2.6)–(10.2.9) with the initial condition (10.2.10).

10.3 Dynamical Behavior of the System

In this section, we calculate the basic reproduction number, feasible steady states and analyze the local stability of the equilibria for the proposed system. The biological feasible region for the non-dimensional system is

$$\Omega = \{(S, I, R, N) : 0 \leq S, I, R, N \leq 1\}.$$

The system (10.2.6)–(10.2.9) has the disease free equilibrium (DFE) $E^0 = (1, 0, 0, 1)$. Now, we calculate the basic reproduction number R_0. Let $x = (S, I)$. Therefore

$$\frac{dx}{dt} = f - v,$$

where

$$f = \begin{pmatrix} -\beta e^{-mI} SI + \delta SI \\ \beta e^{-mI} SI + \delta I^2 \end{pmatrix}$$

and

$$v = \begin{pmatrix} -\frac{1}{N} - \theta R + \frac{S}{N} \\ \delta I + \gamma I + \frac{I}{N} \end{pmatrix}.$$

We have

$$F = Df|_{E^0} = \begin{pmatrix} 0 & -\beta + \delta \\ 0 & \beta \end{pmatrix}$$

and

$$V = Dv|_{E^0} = \begin{pmatrix} 1 & 0 \\ 0 & \delta + \gamma + 1 \end{pmatrix}.$$

The next generation matrix for the model is given by

$$K = FV^{-1} = \begin{pmatrix} 0 & \frac{-\beta+\delta}{\delta+\gamma+1} \\ 0 & \frac{\beta}{\delta+\gamma+1} \end{pmatrix}.$$

The basic reproduction number is given by $R_0 = \rho(FV^{-1})$. Therefore

$$R_0 = \frac{\beta}{\delta + \gamma + 1}.$$

Further the system (10.2.6)–(10.2.9) also has endemic equilibrium (EE) given by

$$\bar{E} = (S^*, I^*, R^*, N^*),$$

where $R^* = \frac{\gamma I^*}{1+\theta}$, $N^* = \frac{1}{1+\delta I^*}$, $S^* = 1 - I^* - R^*$ and the value I^* is given by

$$\frac{e^{mI^*}}{R_0} = 1 - \left(1 + \frac{\gamma}{1+\theta}\right) I^*.$$

If there is no media effect, i.e. $m = 0$, then

$$I^* = \frac{1 - \frac{1}{R_0}}{\left(1 + \frac{\gamma}{1+\theta}\right)}.$$

Clearly, in the absence of media effect, I^* exists if and only if $R_0 > 1$. The EE does not exists for $R_0 \leq 1$ (no point of intersection, see Fig. 10.2) but, EE exists for $R_0 > 1$ (see Fig. 10.3). In the both Figures the red curve represents $\frac{e^{mI^*}}{R_0}$ and blue dotted curve represents $1 - \left(1 + \frac{\gamma}{1+\theta}\right) I^*$ at $m = 2.3$.

Theorem 10.3.1. *The system (10.2.6)–(10.2.9) has*

(i) the disease free equilibrium (DFE) $E^0 = (1, 0, 0, 1)$ *that exists for all the parameter values;*

(ii) no endemic equilibrium (EE), if $R_0 \leq 1$;

(iii) unique endemic equilibrium if $R_0 > 1$.

Theorem 10.3.2. *The disease free equilibrium (DFE)* E^0 *is*

(i) locally asymptotically stable, if $R_0 < 1$ *and*

(ii) unstable, if $R_0 > 1$.

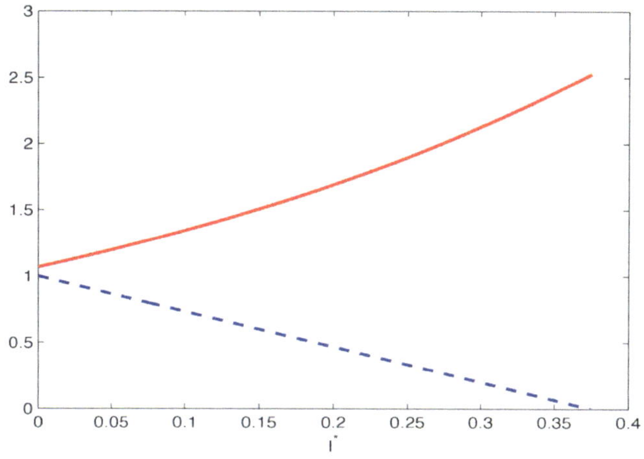

FIGURE 10.2 Non-existence of endemic equilibrium for parametric values $\tilde{\beta} = 0.075$, $m = 2.3$, $\tilde{\theta} = 0.01$, $\tilde{\gamma} = 0.05$, $\tilde{\delta} = 0.01$, $\tilde{\mu} = 0.02$, $R_0 = 0.9375 < 1$, where red curve represents $\frac{e^{mI^*}}{R_0}$ and blue dotted curve represents $1 - \left(1 + \frac{\gamma}{1+\theta}\right) I^*$.

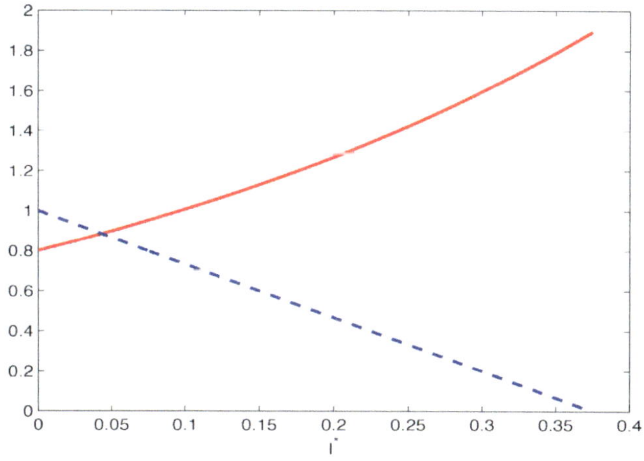

FIGURE 10.3 Existence of endemic equilibrium for parametric values $\tilde{\beta} = 0.1$, $m = 2.3$, $\tilde{\theta} = 0.01$, $\tilde{\gamma} = 0.05$, $\tilde{\delta} = 0.01$, $\tilde{\mu} = 0.02$, $R_0 = 1.25 > 1$, where red curve represents $\frac{e^{mI^*}}{R_0}$ and blue dotted curve represents $1 - \left(1 + \frac{\gamma}{1+\theta}\right) I^*$.

Proof. The variational matrix at the DFE is given by

$$J_0 = \begin{pmatrix} -1 & -\beta+\delta & \theta & 0 \\ 0 & \beta-\delta-\gamma-1 & 0 & 0 \\ 0 & \gamma & -\theta-1 & 0 \\ 0 & -\delta & 0 & -1 \end{pmatrix}.$$

The characteristic equation of J_0 is given by

$$\lambda^4 + [(3+\theta)+(1+\gamma+\delta)(1-R_0)]\lambda^3 + [(3+2\theta)+(3+\theta)(1+\gamma+\delta)(1-R_0)]\lambda^2$$

$$+[(1+\theta)+(3+2\theta)(1+\gamma+\delta)(1-R_0)]\lambda + (1+\theta)(1+\gamma+\delta)(1-R_0) = 0.$$

If $R_0 < 1$, then there exists: (i) four negative real eigen values of J_0 or (ii) two negative real eigen values and one pair of complex conjugate eigen values with negative real parts of J_0 or (iii) two pair of complex conjugate eigen values with negative real parts of J_0. Further, if $R_0 > 1$, then there exists at least one positive real eigen value. Therefore, disease free equilibrium is locally asymptotically stable, if $R_0 < 1$ and unstable, if $R_0 > 1$. □

Theorem 10.3.3. *The endemic equilibrium (EE) is locally asymptotically stable for $R_0 > 1$, but close to 1.*

Proof. Here, we use the method based on central manifold theory to establish the local stability of endemic equilibrium taking β as bifurcation parameter. The critical value of the bifurcation parameter at $R_0 = 1$ is $\beta^* = 1+\gamma+\delta$. It can be easily verified that the Jacobian J_0 at $\beta = \beta^*$ has right eigen vector given by $W = (w_1, w_2, w_3, w_4)^T$ such that $J_0 W = 0$, where

$$w_1 = \left[\frac{\theta\gamma}{\theta+1} - \beta + \delta\right]\sigma, \quad w_2 = \sigma, \quad w_3 = \frac{\gamma\sigma}{\theta+1}, \quad w_4 = -\delta\sigma.$$

The left eigen vector is given by $V = (v_1, v_2, v_3, v_4)$ which satisfy $V.J_0 = 0$ and $V.W = 1$, where

$$v_1 = 0, \quad v_2 = \frac{1}{\sigma}, \quad v_3 = 0, \quad v_4 = 0.$$

The associated non-zero partial derivatives of $F = (f_1, f_2, f_3, f_4)^T$ at the DFE and $\beta = \beta^*$ are given by

$$\frac{\partial^2 f_1}{\partial S \partial I} = -\beta + \delta, \quad \frac{\partial^2 f_1}{\partial S \partial N} = 1, \quad \frac{\partial^2 f_1}{\partial I^2} = 2\beta m,$$

$$\frac{\partial^2 f_2}{\partial S \partial I} = \beta, \quad \frac{\partial^2 f_2}{\partial I^2} = -2\beta m + 2\delta, \quad \frac{\partial^2 f_2}{\partial I \partial N} = 1,$$

$$\frac{\partial^2 f_3}{\partial I \partial R} = \delta, \quad \frac{\partial^2 f_3}{\partial R \partial N} = 1, \quad \frac{\partial^2 f_4}{\partial I \partial N} = -\delta, \quad \frac{\partial^2 f_2}{\partial I \partial \beta} = 1.$$

Here we use notations $x_1 = S, x_2 = I, x_3 = R, x_4 = N$. We have

$$a = \sum_{k,i,j=1}^{4} v_k w_i w_j \frac{\partial^2 f_k}{\partial x_i \partial x_j}$$

and

$$b = \sum_{k,i=1}^{4} v_k w_i \frac{\partial^2 f_k}{\partial x_i \partial h}.$$

By simple calculations we get

$$a = -\frac{\sigma(\theta + \gamma + 1)(1 + \gamma + \delta)}{\theta + 1} - 2\sigma[m(1 + \gamma + \delta) - \delta] - \delta\sigma$$

and $b = 1$.

Since $a < 0$ and $b > 0$ at $\beta = \beta^*$, a transcritical bifurcation occurs at $R_0 = 1$ and unique endemic equilibrium is locally asymptotically stable for $R_0 > 1$. □

In the following section, we will reduce the system (10.2.6)–(10.2.9) to the discrete-time SI system and explore the possibility of flip and Hopf bifurcation.

10.4 Discrete-Time System

In the limiting case, i.e., at the steady state $\frac{dN}{dt} = 0$, which implies $max\, N = 1$. Therefore the system of equations (10.2.6)–(10.2.9) reduces to

$$\frac{dS}{dt} = 1 - \beta e^{-mI} SI + \theta R - S + \delta SI, \quad (10.4.1)$$

$$\frac{dI}{dt} = \beta e^{-mI} SI - \delta I - \gamma I - I + \delta I^2, \quad (10.4.2)$$

$$\frac{dR}{dt} = \gamma I - \theta R - R + \delta RI. \quad (10.4.3)$$

Here $S+I+R=N$ and $maxN = 1$. In the limiting case $S+I+R=1$, the system of equations (10.4.1)–(10.4.3) further reduces to

$$\frac{dS}{dt} = 1 - \beta e^{-mI} SI + \theta(1-S-I) - S + \delta SI, \quad (10.4.4)$$

$$\frac{dI}{dt} = \beta e^{-mI} SI - \delta I - \gamma I - I + \delta I^2. \quad (10.4.5)$$

Applying forward Euler's scheme to the system of equations (10.4.4)–(10.4.5), we obtain the following discrete-time system:

$$S \rightarrow S + h\left[1 - \beta e^{-mI} SI + \theta(1-S-I) - S + \delta SI\right], \quad (10.4.6)$$

$$I \rightarrow I + h\left[\beta e^{-mI} SI - \delta I - \gamma I - I + \delta I^2\right]. \quad (10.4.7)$$

where h is the step size. Shrinking the step size in Euler's method will yield numerical solutions that more accurately approximate the true solution. Numerical solution to the initial-value problem obtained from Euler's method with step size h and total number of steps M satisfies $0 < h \leq \frac{L}{M}$, where L is the length of the interval.

10.5 Discrete Dynamical Behavior of the System

The fixed points of the system (10.4.6)–(10.4.7) are $A(1,0)$ and $B(S^*, I^*)$, where I^*, S^* satisfy

$$1 - \beta e^{-mI} SI + \theta(1-S-I) - S + \delta SI = 0, \quad (10.5.1)$$

$$\beta e^{-mI} S - \delta - \gamma - 1 + \delta I = 0. \quad (10.5.2)$$

The Jacobian matrix of system of equations (10.4.6)–(10.4.7) at the fixed point (S,I) is given by

$$J = \begin{bmatrix} 1+ha & hb \\ hc & 1+hd \end{bmatrix},$$

where

$$a = -\beta e^{-mI} I - \theta - 1 + \delta I,$$

$$b = -\beta e^{-mI} S + \beta m e^{-mI} SI - \theta + \delta S,$$

$$c = \beta e^{-mI} I,$$

$$d = \beta e^{-mI} S - \beta m e^{-mI} SI - \delta - \gamma - 1 + 2\delta I.$$

The characteristic equation of the Jacobian matrix at the fixed point (S,I) can be written as:

$$\lambda^2 + p(S,I)\lambda + q(S,I) = 0, \tag{10.5.3}$$

where

$$p(S,I) = -trJ = -2 - h(a+d),$$

$$q(S,I) = detJ = 1 + h(a+d) + h^2(ad - bc).$$

Proposition 10.5.1. *There exist different topological types of $A(1,0)$ for possible parameters.*

(i) *$A(1,0)$ is sink if $1+\gamma+\delta > \beta$ and $0 < h < min\left\{\frac{2}{1+\theta}, \frac{2}{1+\gamma+\delta-\beta}\right\}$.*

(ii) *$A(1,0)$ is source if $1+\gamma+\delta > \beta$ and $h > max\left\{\frac{2}{1+\theta}, \frac{2}{1+\gamma+\delta-\beta}\right\}$.*

(iii) *$A(1,0)$ is non-hyperbolic if $h = \frac{2}{1+\theta}$ or $h = \frac{2}{1+\gamma+\delta-\beta}$ and $1+\gamma+\delta > \beta$.*

(iv) *$A(1,0)$ is saddle for all values of the parameters, except for that values which lies in (i) to (iii).*

The term *(iii)* of Proposition 10.5.1 implies that the parameters lie in the set

$$\begin{aligned} F_A = \ & \{(\beta, m, \theta, \gamma, \delta, h),\ h = \tfrac{2}{1+\theta},\ h \neq \tfrac{2}{1+\gamma+\delta-\beta}, \\ & 1+\gamma+\delta > \beta \text{ and } \beta, m, \theta, \gamma, \delta, h > 0\}. \end{aligned}$$

If the term *(iii)* of Proposition 10.5.1 holds, then one of the eigen values of the fixed point $A(1,0)$ is -1 and magnitude of the other is not equal to 1. The point $A(1,0)$ undergoes flip bifurcation when the parameter changes in limited neighborhood of F_A.

The characteristic equation of the Jacobian matrix J of the system (10.4.6)–(10.4.7) at the fixed point $B(S^*, I^*)$ can be written as

$$\lambda^2 + p(S^*, I^*)\lambda + q(S^*, I^*) = 0, \qquad (10.5.4)$$

where

$$p(S^*, I^*) = -2 - Gh,$$

$$q(S^*, I^*) = 1 + Gh + Hh^2,$$

$$\begin{aligned} G = \ & -\beta e^{-mI^*} I^* - \theta - 1 + \delta I^* + \beta e^{-mI^*} S^* \\ & -\beta m e^{-mI^*} S^* I^* - \delta - \gamma - 1 + 2\delta I^*, \end{aligned}$$

$$\begin{aligned} H = \ & \left[-\beta e^{-mI^*} I^* - \theta - 1 + \delta I^*\right] \\ & \times \left[\beta e^{-mI^*} S^* - \beta m e^{-mI^*} S^* I^* - \delta - \gamma - 1 + 2\delta I^*\right] \\ & -\beta e^{-mI^*} I^* [-\beta e^{-mI^*} S^* + \beta m e^{-mI^*} S^* I^* - \theta + \delta S^*]. \end{aligned}$$

Now

$$F(\lambda) = \lambda^2 - (2 + Gh)\lambda + (1 + Gh + Hh^2).$$

Therefore

$$F(1) = Hh^2,\ F(-1) = 4 + 2Gh + Hh^2.$$

Using Lemma 2.3.1 stated in Chapter 2, we get the following proposition:

Proposition 10.5.2. *There exist different topological types of $B(S^*, I^*)$ for all possible parameters.*

(i) $B(S^*,I^*)$ *is sink if either condition (i.1) or (i.2) holds:*

(i.1) $G < -2\sqrt{H}$ *and* $0 < h < \frac{-G-\sqrt{G^2-4H}}{H}$,

(i.2) $-2\sqrt{H} \leq G < 0$ *and* $0 < h < -\frac{G}{H}$.

(ii) $B(S^*,I^*)$ *is source if either condition (ii.1) or (ii.2) holds:*

(ii.1) $G < -2\sqrt{H}$ *and* $h > \frac{-G+\sqrt{G^2-4H}}{H}$,

(ii.2) $-2\sqrt{H} \leq G < 0$ *and* $h > -\frac{G}{H}$.

(iii) $B(S^*,I^*)$ *is non-hyperbolic if either condition (iii.1) or (iii.2) holds:*

(iii.1) $G < -2\sqrt{H}$ *and* $h = \frac{-G\pm\sqrt{G^2-4H}}{H}$,

(iii.2) $-2\sqrt{H} \leq G < 0$ *and* $h = -\frac{G}{H}$.

(iv) $B(S^*,I^*)$ *is saddle for all values of the parameters, except for that values which lies in (i) to (iii).*

If the term *(iii.1)* of Proposition 10.5.2 holds, then one of the eigen values of the fixed point $B(S^*,I^*)$ is -1 and magnitude of the other is not equal to 1. The term *(iii.1)* of Proposition 10.5.2 may be written as follows:

$$\begin{aligned} F_{B1} = \quad & \{(\beta,m,\theta,\gamma,\delta,h) : \ h = \tfrac{-G-\sqrt{G^2-4H}}{H}, \ G < -2\sqrt{H} \text{ and} \\ & \qquad \beta,m,\theta,\gamma,\delta,h > 0\}, \\ F_{B2} = \quad & \{(\beta,m,\theta,\gamma,\delta,h) : \ h = \tfrac{-G+\sqrt{G^2-4H}}{H}, \ G < -2\sqrt{H} \text{ and} \\ & \qquad \beta,m,\theta,\gamma,\delta,h > 0\}. \end{aligned}$$

If the term *(iii.2)* of Proposition 10.5.2 holds, then the eigen values of the fixed point $B(S^*,I^*)$ are a pair of conjugate complex numbers with modulus 1. The term *(iii.2)* of Proposition 10.5.2 may be written as follows:

$$\begin{aligned} H_B = \quad & \{(\beta,m,\theta,\gamma,\delta,h) : \ h = -\tfrac{G}{H}, -2\sqrt{H} \leq G < 0 \text{ and} \\ & \qquad \beta,m,\theta,\gamma,\delta,h > 0\}, \end{aligned}$$

where

$$\beta = \frac{\tilde{\beta}}{\tilde{\mu}}, \theta = \frac{\tilde{\theta}}{\tilde{\mu}}, \gamma = \frac{\tilde{\gamma}}{\tilde{\mu}}, \delta = \frac{\tilde{\delta}}{\tilde{\mu}}.$$

In this section, we study the flip bifurcation and Hopf bifurcation of the system (10.4.6)–(10.4.7) at the fixed point $B(S^*, I^*)$.

10.5.1 Flip Bifurcation

Consider the system (10.4.6)–(10.4.7) with arbitrary parameter $(\beta, m, \theta, \gamma, \delta, h_1) \in F_{B1}$, which is described as follows:

$$\begin{aligned} S &\rightarrow S + h_1\left[1 - \beta e^{-mI}SI + \theta(1 - S - I) - S + \delta SI\right], && (10.5.5)\\ I &\rightarrow I + h_1\left[\beta e^{-mI}SI - \delta I - \gamma I - I + \delta I^2\right]. && (10.5.6)\end{aligned}$$

System of equations (10.5.5)–(10.5.6) has fixed point $B(S^*, I^*)$, where S^*, I^* satisfy (10.5.1)–(10.5.2) and

$$h_1 = \frac{-G - \sqrt{G^2 - 4H}}{H}.$$

The eigen values of $B(S^*, I^*)$ are $\lambda_1 = -1$, $\lambda_2 = 3 + Gh_1$ with $|\lambda_2| \neq 1$ by Proposition 10.5.2.

Consider the perturbation of (10.5.5)–(10.5.6) as below:

$$\begin{aligned} S \rightarrow S &+ (h_1 + h_1^*)\\ &\times\left[1 - \beta e^{-mI}SI + \theta(1 - S - I) - S + \delta SI\right], \end{aligned} \qquad (10.5.7)$$

$$I \rightarrow I + (h_1 + h_1^*)\left[\beta e^{-mI}SI - \delta I - \gamma I - I + \delta I^2\right], \qquad (10.5.8)$$

where $|h_1^*| \ll 1$ is a limited perturbation parameter.

Let $u = S - S^*$ and $v = I - I^*$.

After transformation of the fixed point $B(S^*, I^*)$ of map (10.5.7)–(10.5.8) to the point $(0, 0)$, we obtain

$$\begin{pmatrix} u \\ v \end{pmatrix} \rightarrow \begin{pmatrix} a_{11}u + a_{12}v + a_{13}uv + a_{14}v^2 + b_{11}h_1^*u + b_{12}h_1^*v \\ +b_{13}h_1^*uv + b_{14}h_1^*v^2 + O(|u|, |v|, |h_1^*|)^3 \\ a_{21}u + a_{22}v + a_{23}uv + a_{24}v^2 + b_{21}h_1^*u + b_{22}h_1^*v \\ +b_{23}h_1^*uv + b_{24}h_1^*v^2 + O(|u|, |v|, |h_1^*|)^3 \end{pmatrix}, \qquad (10.5.9)$$

where

$$a_{11} = 1 - \frac{h_1}{S^*}(1 + \theta - \theta I^*),$$

$$a_{12} = h_1 \left[m(1+\theta-\theta S^* - \theta I^* - S^* + \delta S^* I^*) - \frac{1}{I^*}(1+\theta-\theta S^* - S^*) \right],$$

$$a_{13} = h_1 \left[\frac{m}{S^*}(1+\theta-\theta S^* - \theta I^* - S^* + \delta S^* I^*) - \frac{1}{S^* I^*}(1+\theta-\theta S^* - \theta I^* - S^*) \right],$$

$$a_{14} = h_1 \left(\frac{m}{I^*} - \frac{m^2}{2} \right) (1+\theta-\theta S^* - \theta I^* - S^* + \delta S^* I^*),$$

$$b_{11} = -\frac{1}{S^*}(1+\theta-\theta I^*),$$

$$b_{12} = \left[m(1+\theta-\theta S^* - \theta I^* - S^* + \delta S^* I^*) - \frac{1}{I^*}(1+\theta-\theta S^* - S^*) \right],$$

$$b_{13} = \left[\frac{m}{S^*}(1+\theta-\theta S^* - \theta I^* - S^* + \delta S^* I^*) - \frac{1}{S^* I^*}(1+\theta-\theta S^* - \theta I^* - S^*) \right],$$

$$b_{14} = \left(\frac{m}{I^*} - \frac{m^2}{2} \right) (1+\theta-\theta S^* - \theta I^* - S^* + \delta S^* I^*),$$

$$a_{21} = \frac{h_1}{S^*}\left(I^* + \gamma I^* + \delta I^* - \delta I^{*2} \right), \tag{10.5.10}$$

$$a_{22} = 1 + h_1 \delta I^* - m h_1 (I^* + \gamma I^* + \delta I^* - \delta I^{*2}),$$

$$a_{23} = \frac{h_1}{S^*}\left(\frac{1}{I^*} - m \right)(I^* + \gamma I^* + \delta I^* - \delta I^{*2}),$$

$$a_{24} = h_1 \delta + h_1 m \left(\frac{m}{2} - \frac{1}{I^*} \right)(I^* + \gamma I^* + \delta I^* - \delta I^{*2}),$$

$$b_{21} = \frac{1}{S^*}\left(I^* + \gamma I^* + \delta I^* - \delta I^{*2} \right),$$

$$b_{22} = \delta I^* - m(I^* + \gamma I^* + \delta I^* - \delta I^{*2}),$$

$$b_{23} = \frac{1}{S^*}\left(\frac{1}{I^*} - m \right)(I^* + \gamma I^* + \delta I^* - \delta I^{*2}),$$

$$b_{24} = \delta + m \left(\frac{m}{2} - \frac{1}{I^*} \right)(I^* + \gamma I^* + \delta I^* - \delta I^{*2}).$$

Consider the following translation:

$$\begin{pmatrix} u \\ v \end{pmatrix} = T \begin{pmatrix} \tilde{S} \\ \tilde{I} \end{pmatrix},$$

where

$$T=\begin{pmatrix} a_{12} & a_{12} \\ -1-a_{11} & \lambda_2-a_{11} \end{pmatrix}.$$

Taking T^{-1} on both sides of equation (10.5.9), we get

$$\begin{pmatrix} \tilde{S} \\ \tilde{I} \end{pmatrix} \to \begin{pmatrix} -1 & 0 \\ 0 & \lambda_2 \end{pmatrix} \begin{pmatrix} \tilde{S} \\ \tilde{I} \end{pmatrix} + \begin{pmatrix} f(u,v,h_1^*) \\ g(u,v,h_1^*) \end{pmatrix}, \qquad (10.5.11)$$

where

$$\begin{aligned} f(u,v,h_1^*) = & \frac{[a_{13}(\lambda_2-a_{11})-a_{12}a_{23}]uv}{a_{12}(\lambda_2+1)} + \frac{[a_{14}(\lambda_2-a_{11})-a_{12}a_{24}]v^2}{a_{12}(\lambda_2+1)} \\ & + \frac{[b_{11}(\lambda_2-a_{11})-a_{12}b_{21}]h_1^*u}{a_{12}(\lambda_2+1)} + \frac{[b_{12}(\lambda_2-a_{11})-a_{12}b_{22}]h_1^*v}{a_{12}(\lambda_2+1)} \\ & + \frac{[b_{13}(\lambda_2-a_{11})-a_{12}b_{23}]h_1^*uv}{a_{12}(\lambda_2+1)} + \frac{[b_{14}(\lambda_2-a_{11})-a_{12}b_{24}]h_1^*v^2}{a_{12}(\lambda_2+1)} \\ & + O(|u|,|v|,|h_1^*|)^3, \end{aligned}$$

$$\begin{aligned} g(u,v,h_1^*) = & \frac{[a_{13}(1+a_{11})+a_{12}a_{23}]uv}{a_{12}(\lambda_2+1)} + \frac{[a_{14}(1+a_{11})+a_{12}a_{24}]v^2}{a_{12}(\lambda_2+1)} \\ & + \frac{[b_{11}(1+a_{11})+a_{12}b_{21}]h_1^*u}{a_{12}(\lambda_2+1)} + \frac{[b_{12}(1+a_{11})+a_{12}b_{22}]h_1^*v}{a_{12}(\lambda_2+1)} \\ & + \frac{[b_{13}(1+a_{11})+a_{12}b_{23}]h_1^*uv}{a_{12}(\lambda_2+1)} + \frac{[b_{14}(1+a_{11})+a_{12}b_{24}]h_1^*v^2}{a_{12}(\lambda_2+1)} \\ & + O(|u|,|v|,|h_1^*|)^3, \end{aligned}$$

$$u = a_{12}(\tilde{S}+\tilde{I}),$$

$$v = -(1+a_{11})\tilde{S} + (\lambda_2-a_{11})\tilde{I}.$$

Applying center manifold theorem to equation (10.5.11) at the origin in the limited neighborhood of $h_1^*=0$. The center manifold $W^c(0,0)$ can be approximately presented as:

$$W^c(0,0) = \left\{ (\tilde{S},\tilde{I}) : \tilde{I} = a_0h_1^* + a_1\tilde{S}^2 + a_2\tilde{S}h_1^* + a_3h_1^{*2} + O\left((|\tilde{S}|+|h_1^*|)^3 \right) \right\},$$

where $O\left((|\tilde{S}|+|h_1^*|)^3 \right)$ is a function with at least third order in variables $(\tilde{S},\ h_1^*)$.

By simple calculations for center manifold, we have

$$a_0 = 0,$$

$$a_1 = \frac{[a_{13}(1+a_{11})+a_{12}a_{23}]a_{12}(1+a_{11}) - [a_{14}(1+a_{11})+a_{12}a_{24}](1+a_{11})^2}{a_{12}(\lambda_2^2 - 1)},$$

$$a_2 = \frac{-[b_{11}(1+a_{11})+a_{12}b_{21}]a_{12} + [b_{12}(1+a_{11})+a_{12}b_{22}](1+a_{11})}{a_{12}(\lambda_2+1)^2},$$

$$a_3 = 0.$$

Now, consider the map restricted to the center manifold $W^c(0,0)$ as below:

$$K : \tilde{S} \to -\tilde{S} + k_1\tilde{S}^2 + k_2\tilde{S}h_1^* + k_3\tilde{S}^2h_1^* + k_4\tilde{S}h_1^{*2} + k_5\tilde{S}^3 + O\left((|\tilde{S}| + |h_1^*|)^4\right),$$

where

$$k_1 = -\frac{[a_{13}(\lambda_2-a_{11})-a_{12}a_{23}](1+a_{11})}{(\lambda_2+1)} + \frac{[a_{14}(\lambda_2-a_{11})-a_{12}a_{24}](1+a_{11})^2}{a_{12}(\lambda_2+1)},$$

$$k_2 = \frac{[b_{11}(\lambda_2-a_{11})-a_{12}b_{21}]}{(\lambda_2+1)} - \frac{[b_{12}(\lambda_2-a_{11})-a_{12}b_{22}](1+a_{11})}{a_{12}(\lambda_2+1)},$$

$$\begin{aligned} k_3 = {} & \frac{[a_{13}(\lambda_2-a_{11})-a_{12}a_{23}](\lambda_2-1-2a_{11})a_2}{(\lambda_2+1)} + \frac{[a_{14}(\lambda_2-a_{11})-a_{12}a_{24}][-2(1+a_{11})(\lambda-a_{11})a_2]}{a_{12}(\lambda_2+1)} \\ & + \frac{[b_{11}(\lambda_2-a_{11})-a_{12}b_{21}]a_1}{(\lambda_2+1)} + \frac{[b_{12}(\lambda_2-a_{11})-a_{12}b_{22}](\lambda_2-a_{11})a_1}{a_{12}(\lambda_2+1)} \\ & - \frac{[b_{13}(\lambda_2-a_{11})-a_{12}b_{23}](1+a_{11})}{(\lambda_2+1)} + \frac{[b_{14}(\lambda_2-a_{11})-a_{12}b_{24}](1+a_{11})^2}{a_{12}(\lambda_2+1)}, \end{aligned}$$

$$k_4 = \frac{[b_{11}(\lambda_2-a_{11})-a_{12}b_{21}]a_2}{(\lambda_2+1)} + \frac{[b_{12}(\lambda_2-a_{11})-a_{12}b_{22}](\lambda_2-a_{11})a_2}{a_{12}(\lambda_2+1)},$$

$$k_5 = \frac{[a_{13}(\lambda_2-a_{11})-a_{12}a_{23}](\lambda_2-1-2a_{11})a_1}{(\lambda_2+1)} - \frac{[a_{14}(\lambda_2-a_{11})-a_{12}a_{24}](1+a_{11})(\lambda_2-a_{11})2a_1}{a_{12}(\lambda_2+1)}.$$

According to Flip bifurcation, the discriminatory quantities γ_1 and γ_2 are given by:

$$\gamma_1 = \left(\frac{\partial^2 K}{\partial\tilde{S}\partial h_1^*} + \frac{1}{2}\frac{\partial K}{\partial h_1^*}\frac{\partial^2 K}{\partial\tilde{S}^2}\right)\Bigg|_{(0,0)},$$

$$\gamma_2 = \left(\frac{1}{6}\frac{\partial^3 K}{\partial\tilde{S}^3} + \left(\frac{1}{2}\frac{\partial^2 K}{\partial\tilde{S}^2}\right)^2\right)\Bigg|_{(0,0)}.$$

After simple calculations, we obtain $\gamma_1 = k_2$ and $\gamma_2 = k_5 + k_1^2$.

Analyzing above and the flip bifurcation conditions discussed in [149], we write the following theorem:

Theorem 10.5.3. *If $\gamma_2 \neq 0$, and the parameter h_1^* alters in the limiting region of the point (0,0), then the system (10.5.7)–(10.5.8) passes through flip bifurcation at the point $B(S^*, I^*)$. Also, the period-2 points that bifurcate from fixed point $B(S^*, I^*)$ are stable (resp., unstable) if $\gamma_2 > 0$ (resp., $\gamma_2 < 0$).*

10.5.2 Hopf Bifurcation

Consider the system (10.4.6)–(10.4.7) with arbitrary parameter $(\beta, m, \theta, \gamma, \delta, h_2) \in H_B$, which is described as follows:

$$S \rightarrow S + h_2\left[1 - \beta e^{-mI}SI + \theta(1 - S - I) - S + \delta SI\right], \tag{10.5.12}$$

$$I \rightarrow I + h_2\left[\beta e^{-mI}SI - \delta I - \gamma I - I + \delta I^2\right]. \tag{10.5.13}$$

Equation (10.5.12)–(10.5.13) has fixed point $B(S^*, I^*)$, where S^*, I^* is given by (10.5.1)–(10.5.2) and

$$h_2 = -\frac{G}{H}.$$

Consider the perturbation of (10.5.12)–(10.5.13) as follows:

$$S \rightarrow S + (h_2 + h_2^*)\left[1 - \beta e^{-mI}SI + \theta(1 - S - I) - S + \delta SI\right], \tag{10.5.14}$$

$$I \rightarrow I + (h_2 + h_2^*)\left[\beta e^{-mI}SI - \delta I - \gamma I - I + \delta I^2\right], \tag{10.5.15}$$

where $|h_2^*| \ll 1$ is small perturbation parameter.

The characteristic equation of map (10.5.14)–(10.5.15) at $B(S^*, I^*)$ is given by

$$\lambda^2 + p(h_2^*)\lambda + q(h_2^*) = 0,$$

where

$$p(h_2^*) = -2 - G(h_2 + h_2^*),$$
$$q(h_2^*) = 1 + G(h_2 + h_2^*) + H(h_2 + h_2^*)^2.$$

Since the parameter $(\beta, m, \theta, \gamma, \delta, h_2) \in H_B$, the eigen values of $B(S^*, I^*)$ are a pair of complex conjugate numbers $\overline{\lambda}$ and λ with modulus 1 by Proposition 10.5.2, where

$$\overline{\lambda},\, \lambda = \frac{-p(h_2^*) \mp i\sqrt{4q(h_2^*) - p^2(h_2^*)}}{2}.$$

Therefore

$$\overline{\lambda},\ \lambda = 1 + \frac{G(h_2+h_2^*)}{2} \mp \frac{i(h_2+h_2^*)\sqrt{4H-G^2}}{2}.$$

Now we have

$$|\lambda| = (q(h_2^*))^{1/2},\ l = \left.\frac{d|\lambda|}{dh_2^*}\right|_{h_2^*=0} = -\frac{G}{2} > 0.$$

When h_2^* varies in small neighborhood of $h_2^* = 0$, then $\overline{\lambda}$, $\lambda = a \mp ib$, where

$$a = 1 + \frac{h_2 G}{2},\ b = \frac{h_2\sqrt{4H-G^2}}{2}.$$

Hopf bifurcation requires that when $h_2^* = 0$, then $\overline{\lambda}^n, \lambda^n \neq 1$ $(n = 1,\ 2,\ 3,\ 4)$ which is equivalent to $p(0) \neq -2,\ 0,\ 1,\ 2$.

Since the parameter $(\beta, m, \theta, \gamma, \delta, h_2) \in H_B$, therefore $p(0) \neq -2,\ 2$. It is the only requirement that $p(0) \neq 0,\ 1$, which follows that

$$G^2 \neq 2H,\ 3H. \tag{10.5.16}$$

Let $u = S - S^*$ and $v = I - I^*$.

After transformation of the fixed point $B(S^*, I^*)$ of system (10.5.14)–(10.5.15) to the point $(0,0)$, we have

$$\begin{pmatrix} u \\ v \end{pmatrix} \to \begin{pmatrix} a_{11}u + a_{12}v + a_{13}uv + a_{14}v^2 + O(|u|,|v|)^3 \\ a_{21}u + a_{22}v + a_{23}uv + a_{24}v^2 + O(|u|,|v|)^3 \end{pmatrix}, \tag{10.5.17}$$

where $a_{11},\ a_{12},\ a_{13},\ a_{14},\ a_{21},\ a_{22},\ a_{23},\ a_{24}$ are given in (10.5.10) by substituting h_2 for $h_2 + h_2^*$.

Next, we discuss the normal form of (10.5.17) when $h_2^* = 0$.

Consider the following translation:

$$\begin{pmatrix} u \\ v \end{pmatrix} = T \begin{pmatrix} \hat{S} \\ \hat{I} \end{pmatrix},$$

where

$$T = \begin{pmatrix} a_{12} & 0 \\ a - a_{11} & -b \end{pmatrix}.$$

Taking T^{-1} on both sides of (10.5.17), we get

$$\begin{pmatrix} \hat{S} \\ \hat{I} \end{pmatrix} \to \begin{pmatrix} a & -b \\ b & a \end{pmatrix} \begin{pmatrix} \hat{S} \\ \hat{I} \end{pmatrix} + \begin{pmatrix} \hat{f}(\hat{S},\hat{I}) \\ \hat{g}(\hat{S},\hat{I}) \end{pmatrix},$$

where

$$\hat{f}\left(\hat{S},\hat{I}\right) = \frac{a_{13}}{a_{12}} uv + \frac{a_{14}}{a_{12}} v^2 + O(|u|,|v|)^3,$$

$$\begin{aligned} \hat{g}\left(\hat{S},\hat{I}\right) &= \frac{\left[a_{13}\left(a-a_{11}\right)-a_{12}a_{23}\right]}{a_{12}b} uv \\ &+ \frac{\left[a_{14}\left(a-a_{11}\right)-a_{12}a_{24}\right]}{a_{12}b} v^2 + O(|u|,|v|)^3, \end{aligned}$$

$$u = a_{12}\hat{S},$$

and

$$v = \left(a-a_{11}\right)\hat{S} - b\hat{I}.$$

Now

$$\hat{f}_{\hat{S}\hat{S}} = 2a_{13}(a-a_{11}) + \frac{2a_{14}}{a_{12}}(a-a_{11})^2,$$

$$\hat{f}_{\hat{S}\hat{I}} = -a_{13}b - \frac{2a_{14}}{a_{12}}(a-a_{11})b, \quad \hat{f}_{\hat{I}\hat{I}} = \frac{2a_{14}}{a_{12}} b^2,$$

$$\hat{f}_{\hat{S}\hat{S}\hat{S}} = 0, \quad \hat{f}_{\hat{S}\hat{S}\hat{I}} = 0, \quad \hat{f}_{\hat{S}\hat{I}\hat{I}} = 0, \quad \hat{f}_{\hat{I}\hat{I}\hat{I}} = 0,$$

$$\begin{aligned} \hat{g}_{\hat{S}\hat{S}} &= \frac{2(a-a_{11})}{b}\left[a_{13}\left(a-a_{11}\right)-a_{12}a_{23}\right] \\ &+ \frac{2(a-a_{11})^2}{a_{12}b}\left[a_{14}\left(a-a_{11}\right)-a_{12}a_{24}\right] \end{aligned}$$

$$\begin{aligned} \hat{g}_{\hat{S}\hat{I}} &= -\left[a_{13}\left(a-a_{11}\right)-a_{12}a_{23}\right] \\ &- \frac{2(a-a_{11})}{a_{12}}\left[a_{14}\left(a-a_{11}\right)-a_{12}a_{24}\right], \end{aligned}$$

$$\hat{g}_{\hat{I}\hat{I}} = \frac{2b}{a_{12}}\left[a_{14}\left(a-a_{11}\right)-a_{12}a_{24}\right],$$

$$\hat{g}_{\hat{S}\hat{S}\hat{S}} = 0, \quad \hat{g}_{\hat{S}\hat{S}\hat{I}} = 0, \quad \hat{g}_{\hat{S}\hat{I}\hat{I}} = 0, \quad \hat{g}_{\hat{I}\hat{I}\hat{I}} = 0.$$

According to Hopf bifurcation, the discriminatory quantity s is given by

$$s = -Re\left[\frac{(1-2\overline{\lambda})\overline{\lambda}^2}{1-\lambda}\varphi_{11}\varphi_{20}\right] - \frac{1}{2}||\varphi_{11}||^2 - ||\varphi_{02}||^2 + Re(\overline{\lambda}\varphi_{21}), \tag{10.5.18}$$

where

$$\varphi_{20} = \frac{1}{8}\left[(\hat{f}_{\hat{S}\hat{S}} - \hat{f}_{\hat{I}\hat{I}} + 2\hat{g}_{\hat{S}\hat{I}}) + i\,(\hat{g}_{\hat{S}\hat{S}} - \hat{g}_{\hat{I}\hat{I}} - 2\hat{f}_{\hat{S}\hat{I}})\right],$$

$$\varphi_{11} = \frac{1}{4}\left[(\hat{f}_{\hat{S}\hat{S}} + \hat{f}_{\hat{I}\hat{I}}) + i\,(\hat{g}_{\hat{S}\hat{S}} + \hat{g}_{\hat{I}\hat{I}})\right],$$

$$\varphi_{02} = \frac{1}{8}\left[(\hat{f}_{\hat{S}\hat{S}} - \hat{f}_{\hat{I}\hat{I}} - 2\hat{g}_{\hat{S}\hat{I}}) + i\,(\hat{g}_{\hat{S}\hat{S}} - \hat{g}_{\hat{I}\hat{I}} + 2\hat{f}_{\hat{S}\hat{I}})\right],$$

$$\varphi_{21} = \frac{1}{16}\left[(\hat{f}_{\hat{S}\hat{S}\hat{S}} + \hat{f}_{\hat{S}\hat{I}\hat{I}} + \hat{g}_{\hat{S}\hat{S}\hat{I}} + \hat{g}_{\hat{I}\hat{I}\hat{I}}) + i\,(\hat{g}_{\hat{S}\hat{S}\hat{S}} + \hat{g}_{\hat{S}\hat{I}\hat{I}} - \hat{f}_{\hat{S}\hat{S}\hat{I}} - \hat{f}_{\hat{I}\hat{I}\hat{I}})\right].$$

Analyzing above and Hopf bifurcation conditions discussed given in [149], we write the following theorem:

Theorem 10.5.4. *If the condition (10.5.16) holds, $s \neq 0$ and the parameter h_2^* alters in the limited region of the point (0,0), then the system (10.5.14)–(10.5.15) passes through Hopf bifurcation at the point $B(S^*, I^*)$. Moreover, if $s < 0$ (resp., $s > 0$), then an attracting (resp., repelling) invariant closed curve bifurcates from the fixed point $B(S^*, I^*)$ for $h_2^* > 0$ (resp., $h_2^* < 0$).*

10.6 Sensitivity Analysis

In this section, we perform the sensitivity analysis of the basic reproduction number R_0 and endemic equilibrium with respect to model parameters, for a particular set of parameters is given in the Table 10.2. The sensitive indices of the basic reproduction number R_0 with respect to parameters are shown in Table 10.3. From the table, we observe that β has a positive impact on R_0 and δ, γ have a negative impact on R_0. Moreover β and γ are most sensitive to R_0, hence we observe large changes in

TABLE 10.2 Parametric Values Used for Simulation of the System (10.2.6)–(10.2.9)

Parameter	Value	References
Λ	5.0	[136, 138]
$\tilde{\delta}$	0.01	[136, 138]
$\tilde{\mu}$	0.02	[136, 138]
$\tilde{\beta}$	[0.05,1.5]	variable
m	[0,2.3]	variable
$\tilde{\gamma}$	0.05	[136, 138]
$\tilde{\theta}$	0.01	[136, 138]

TABLE 10.3 The Sensitivity Indices $\gamma_{y_j}^{R_0} = \frac{\partial R_0}{\partial y_j} \times \frac{y_j}{R_0}$ of the Basic Reproduction Number R_0 to the Parameters y_j for the Parameter Values Given in Table 10.2

Parameter (y_j)	Sensitivity index of R_0 w.r.t. y_j $(\gamma_{y_j}^{R_0})$
β	1
δ	–0.125
θ	0
γ	–0.625
m	0

TABLE 10.4 The Sensitivity Indices $\gamma_{y_j}^{x_i} = \frac{\partial x_i}{\partial y_j} \times \frac{y_j}{x_i}$ of the State Variables to the Parameters y_j for the Parameter Values Given in Table 10.2

Parameter (y_j)	$\gamma_{y_j}^{S^*}$	$\gamma_{y_j}^{I^*}$	$\gamma_{y_j}^{R^*}$	$\gamma_{y_j}^{N^*}$
β	–0.625469	1.42029	1.42029	–0.0770053
δ	0.0781837	–0.177536	–0.177536	–0.0445924
θ	0.0343618	0.130306	–0.203027	–0.00706494
γ	0.287833	–1.2786	–0.278599	0.0693231
m	0.164937	–0.374531	–0.374531	0.0203063

R_0 by small changes in these parameters. Again, we perform the sensitivity analysis of endemic steady state (shown in the Table 10.4) with respect to model parameters, using parameter values given in the Table 10.2. We observe that β has a negative impact on the S^* and the rest of the parameters have a positive impact. Moreover β is the most sensitive parameter to S^*, hence we observe significant changes in S^* by a small change in this parameter. Similarly, β and γ are most sensitive parameter to I^*. Further, β is most sensitive as well as has a positive impact on the R^* and all the parameters are less sensitive to N^*.

10.7 Numerical Simulations

We perform the numerical simulations of both the continuous system (10.2.6)–(10.2.9) and discrete system (10.4.6)–(10.4.7) to justify our analytic findings. We take the parameters $m = 2.3$, $\tilde{\theta} = 0.01$, $\tilde{\gamma} = 0.05$, $\tilde{\delta} = 0.01$, $\tilde{\mu} = 0.02$ as fixed and vary only $\tilde{\beta}$. We systematically discuss the following cases:

Case 1: When $\tilde{\beta} = 0.075$ then $R_0 = 0.9375 < 1$ and the DFE of the system (10.2.6)–(10.2.9) is locally asymptotically stable as shown in Figure 10.4, which is in accordance with the results stated in Theorem 10.3.2. The effect of m on the fraction of infectious population is shown in Figure 10.6 with different values of m and we observed that the endemic equilibrium state is influenced by media coefficient m for $R_0 = 0.9375 < 1$.

Case 2: When $\tilde{\beta} = 0.1$ then $R_0 = 1.25 > 1$ and it follows that the EE of the system (10.2.6)–(10.2.9) is locally asymptotically stable as shown in Figure 10.5, which is in accordance with the results stated in Theorem 10.3.3. The effect of m on the fraction of infectious population is shown in Figure 10.7 with different values of m and it is observed that in the endemic equilibrium state disease level is reduced by media coefficient m for $R_0 = 1.25 > 1$.

Case 3: We draw the bifurcation diagram of the model (10.4.6)–(10.4.7) taking $\tilde{\beta} = 1.5$. We see that from the fixed point (0.10522, 0.31278), flip bifurcation appears at $h = 0.188987$. From the Figure 10.8(a), it is observed that the fixed point of the system (10.4.6)–(10.4.7) is stable for $h < 0.188987$, give up its stability at $h = 0.188987$ and there appears period doubling bifurcation for $h > 0.188987$. In this

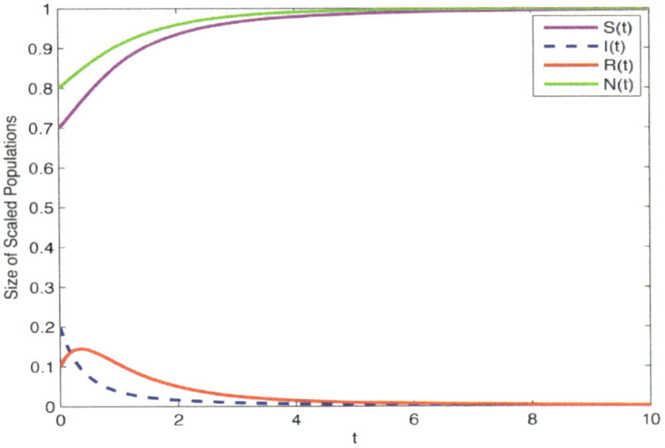

FIGURE 10.4 The variation of scaled population in scaled time for parametric values $\tilde{\beta} = 0.075$, $m = 2.3$, $\tilde{\theta} = 0.01$, $\tilde{\gamma} = 0.05$, $\tilde{\delta} = 0.01$, $\tilde{\mu} = 0.02$, $R_0 = 0.9375 < 1$.

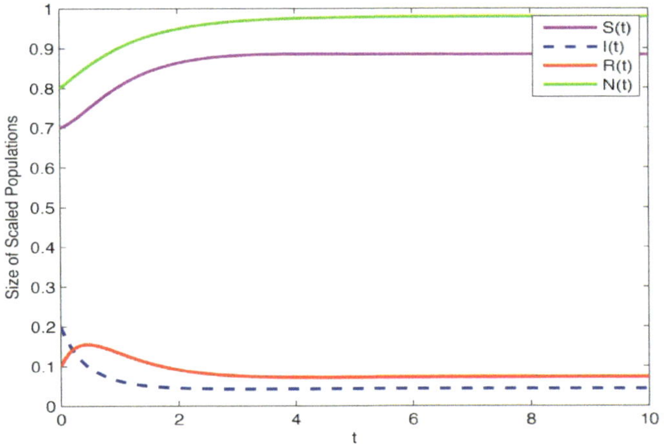

FIGURE 10.5 The variation of scaled population in scaled time for parametric values $\tilde{\beta} = 0.1$, $m = 2.3$, $\tilde{\theta} = 0.01$, $\tilde{\gamma} = 0.05$, $\tilde{\delta} = 0.01$, $\tilde{\mu} = 0.02$, $R_0 = 1.25 > 1$.

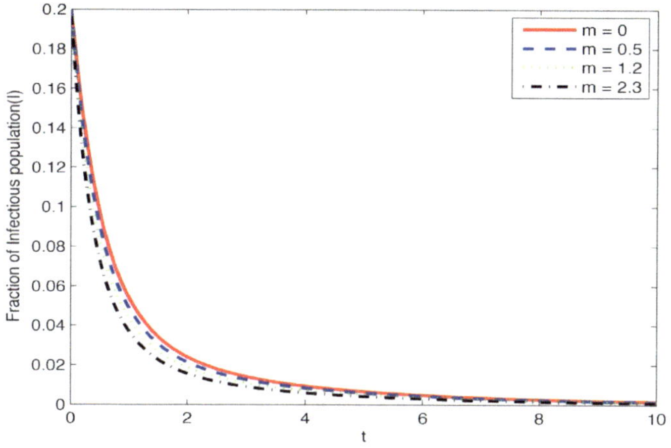

FIGURE 10.6 The effect of m on I for parametric values $\tilde{\beta} = 0.075$, $\tilde{\theta} = 0.01$, $\tilde{\gamma} = 0.05$, $\tilde{\delta} = 0.01$, $\tilde{\mu} = 0.02$, $R_0 = 0.9375 < 1$.

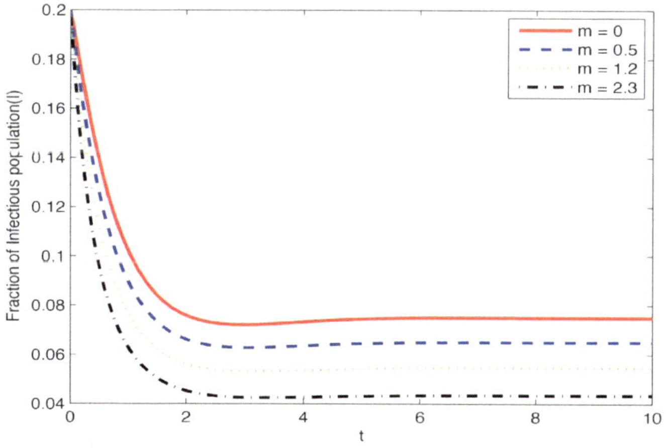

FIGURE 10.7 The effect of m on I for parametric values $\tilde{\beta} = 0.1$, $\tilde{\theta} = 0.01$, $\tilde{\gamma} = 0.05$, $\tilde{\delta} = 0.01$, $\tilde{\mu} = 0.02$, $R_0 = 1.25 > 1$.

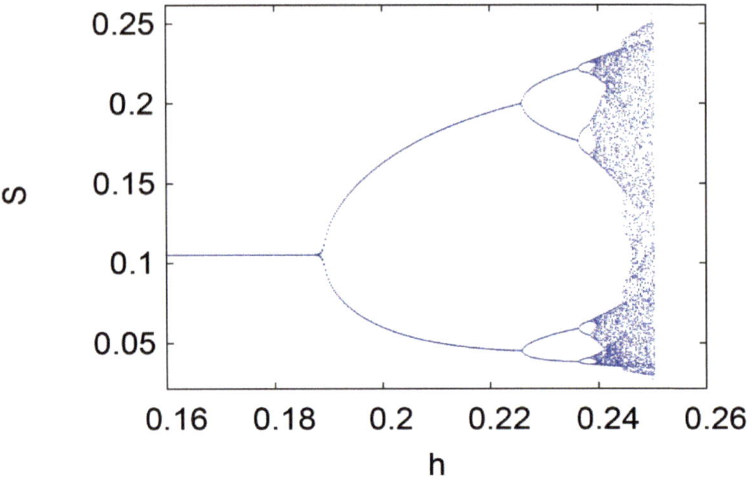

(a)

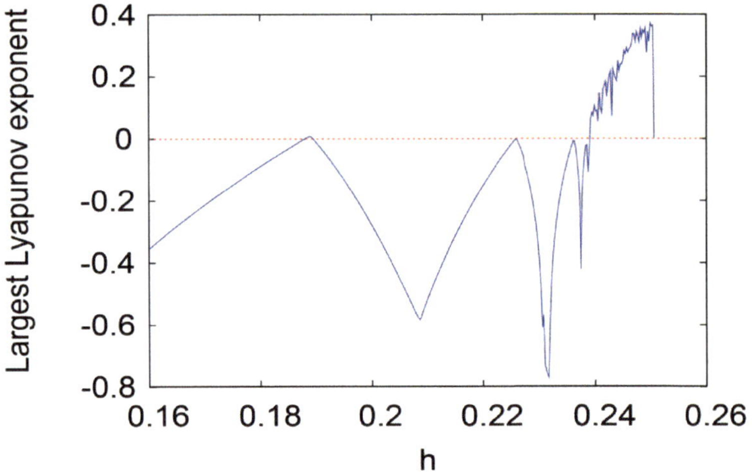

(b)

FIGURE 10.8 (a) Bifurcation diagram of system (10.4.6)–(10.4.7) for $\tilde{\beta} = 1.5$, $m = 2.3$, $\tilde{\theta} = 0.01$, $\tilde{\gamma} = 0.05$, $\tilde{\delta} = 0.01$, $\tilde{\mu} = 0.02$ with the initial value of $(S,I) = (0.1, 0.3)$ and h covering [0.16, 0.26]. (b) Largest Lyapunov exponents related to (a).

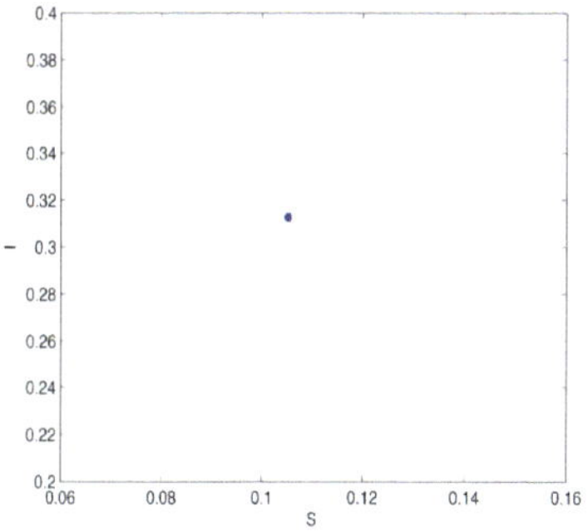

(a) $h = 0.185$

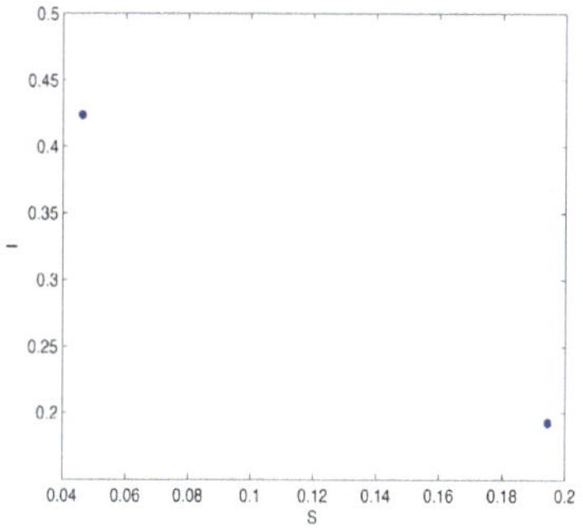

(b) $h = 0.22$

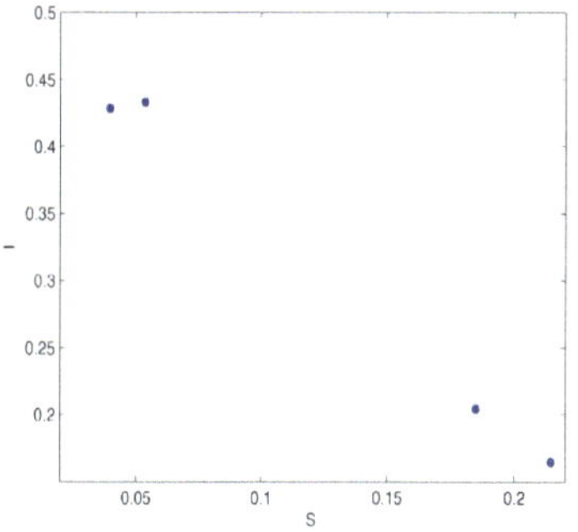

(c) $h = 0.23$

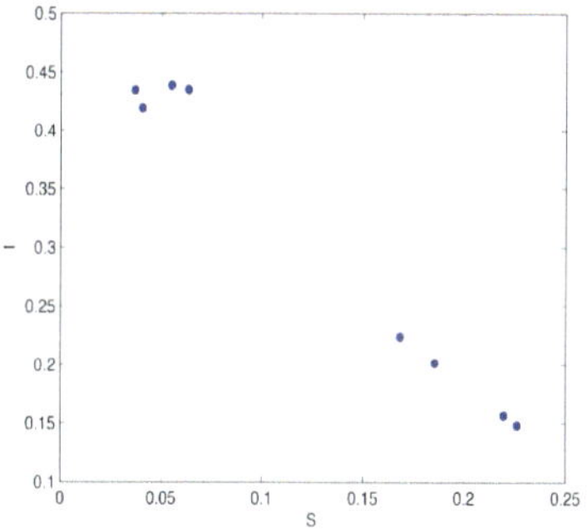

(d) $h = 0.238$

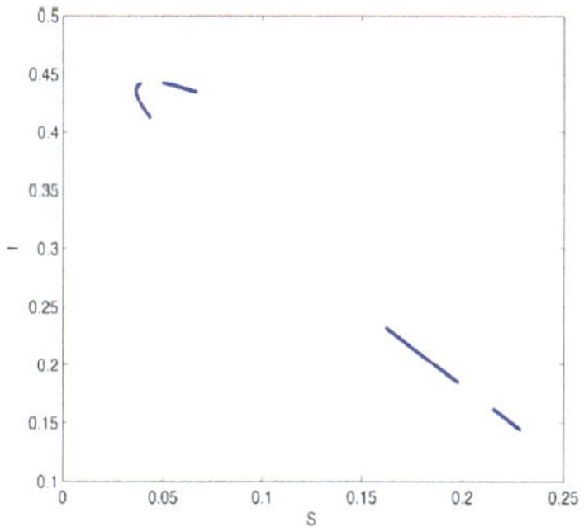

(e) $h = 0.24$

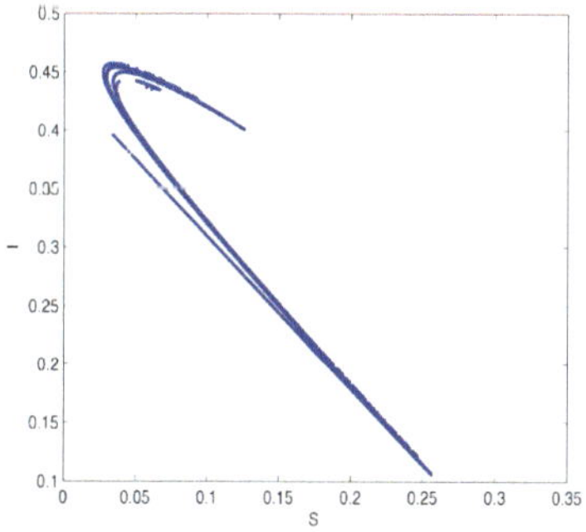

(f) $h = 0.25$

FIGURE 10.9 Phase portraits for several values of h from 0.185 to 0.25 related to Fig. 10.8 (a).

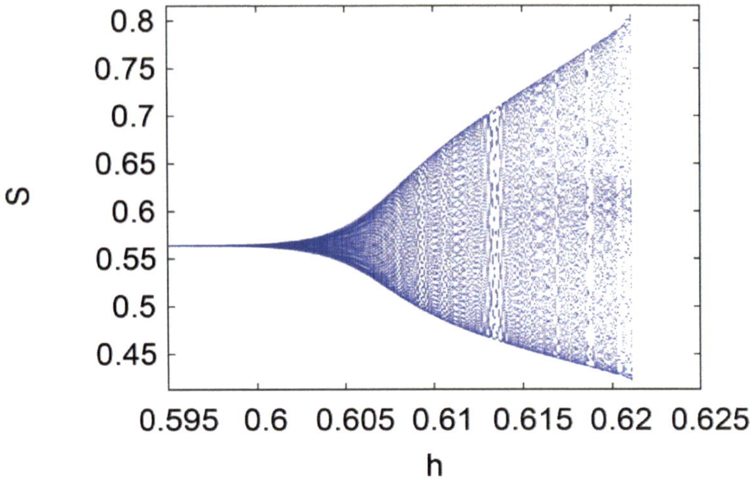

(a)

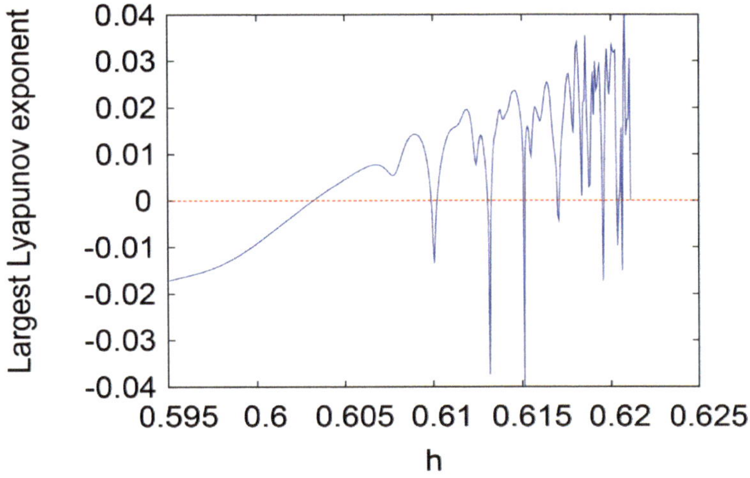

(b)

FIGURE 10.10 (a) Bifurcation diagram of system (10.4.6)–(10.4.7) for $\tilde{\beta} = 0.2$, $m = 2.3$, $\tilde{\theta} = 0.01$, $\tilde{\gamma} = 0.05$, $\tilde{\delta} = 0.01$, $\tilde{\mu} = 0.02$ with the initial value of $(S, I) = (0.5, 0.2)$ and h covering [0.595, 0.625]. (b) Largest Lyapunov exponents related to (a).

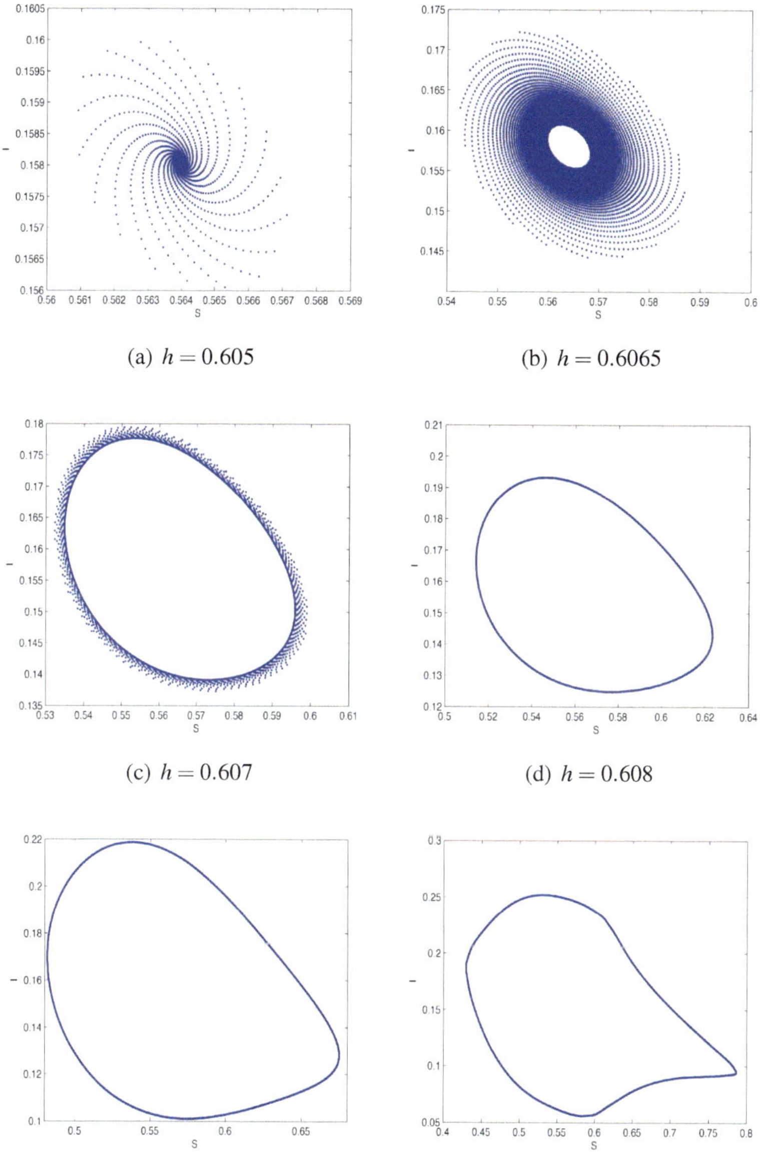

(a) $h = 0.605$

(b) $h = 0.6065$

(c) $h = 0.607$

(d) $h = 0.608$

(e) $h = 0.611$

(f) $h = 0.62$

FIGURE 10.11 Phase portraits for several values of h from 0.605 to 0.62 related to Figure 10.10 (a).

case $\gamma_1 = -12.6611$, $\gamma_2 = 7.14924$ which shows that the Theorem 10.5.3 holds good. Further, the phase portraits show that there are orbits of period 2, 4 and 8 at $h = 0.22$, $h = 0.23$ and $h = 0.238$ respectively, and chaotic sets at $h = 0.24$ and 0.25 (see Figure 10.9). Moreover, the Largest Lypunov exponents corresponding to $h = 0.24$ and 0.25 are positive that confirm the chaotic sets (see Figure 10.8(b)).

Case 4: We draw the bifurcation diagram of the model (10.4.6)–(10.4.7) taking $\tilde{\beta} = 0.2$. We see that from the fixed point (0.5639, 0.15802), Hopf bifurcation appears at $h = 0.60654$. From the Figure 10.10(a), we examine that the fixed point of the model (10.4.6)–(10.4.7) is stable for $h < 0.60654$, drops its stability at $h = 0.60654$ and an invariant circle exists for $h > 0.60654$. Here $s = -5.9564$ which shows that the Theorem 10.5.4 is true. Moreover, the phase portraits in Figure 10.11 show that a smooth invariant circle bifurcates from the fixed point and its radius increases with increase of h.

10.8 Summary

In this chapter, we proposed a SIRS epidemic model incorporating media awareness and investigate the asymptotic stability of the model in both disease-free equilibrium and endemic equilibrium states. The disease-free state is locally asymptotically stable for basic reproduction number $R_0 < 1$, a transcritical bifurcation occurs at $R_0 = 1$ and a locally asymptotically stable endemic equilibrium exists for $R_0 > 1$. We observed that the coefficient of media awareness m does not effect R_0, but the endemic equilibrium state is well influenced by media coefficient. In the limiting case, we reduced the SIRS system to the discrete-time SI system and also investigated the existence of bifurcation for discrete-time system in the closed first quadrant R^2_+. The map undergoes flip bifurcation and Hopf bifurcation at the fixed points of the discrete system under specific conditions when the step size h alters in the deleted neighborhood of F_{B1} or F_{B2} and H_B.

We calculate sensitivity indices of the reproduction number and endemic equilibrium to various model parameters and identified respective sensitive parameters. Numerical simulations of the discrete system display cascade of period-doubling bifurcation in the orbits of period 2, 4, 8 and chaotic orbits in case of flip bifurcation; and smooth invariant circles in case of Hopf bifurcation. It means that the infected population coexists with the susceptible population in the period-n orbits or smooth invariant circle. These results show that the discrete system has a rich and complex dynamical behavior.

Chapter 11

Dynamics of SEIRVS Epidemic Model with Temporary Disease Induced Immunity and Media Awareness

11.1 Introduction

The vaccine stimulates an individual's immune system to develop adaptive immunity against the pathogens which is known as vaccine induced immunity. Quite often, the vaccine-induced immunity requires boosting after some period of time, as the vaccine effectiveness wanes due to absence of exposure to the disease. Vaccination reduces the portion of susceptible populations, therefore, the spread of the diseases can be controlled by the effective vaccination program. One of the examples is the successful elimination of smallpox in all over the world with the vaccination. Although vaccines are already developed for various infectious diseases, but still, there are many infectious diseases for which no effective vaccines exist. Further, most of the pharmaceutical interventions, such as vaccines and anti-viral medications to prevent the disease are too expensive, may not be available in many areas of the world in sufficient quantities to make a significant contribution toward reducing deaths [130–132]. Therefore, to control the spread of epidemics, it is

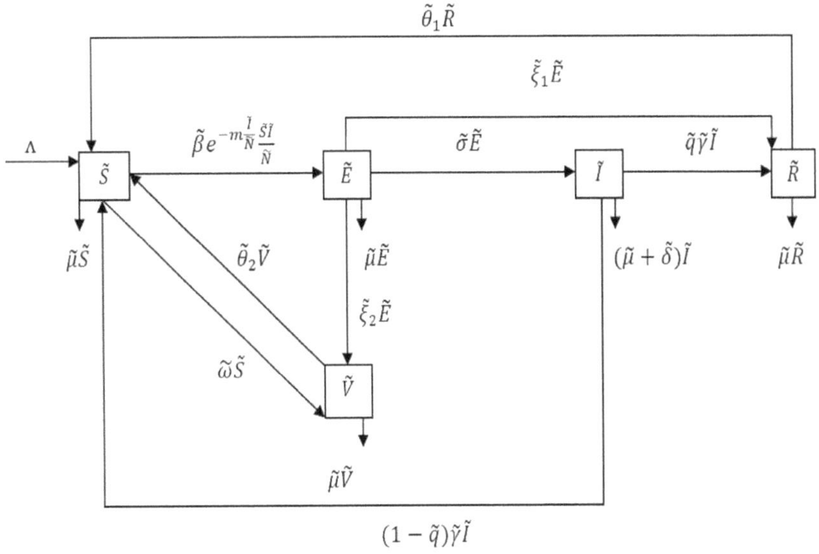

FIGURE 11.1 The schematic diagram of the model.

very important to carry out studies on the disease models with pharmaceutical as well as non-pharmaceutical interventions.

This chapter is organized as follows. In Section 11.2, formulation of a SEIRVS epidemic model incorporating media awareness is presented. In Section 11.3, the dynamical behavior of the system is studied and obtained the conditions for locally asymptotically stability in case of disease-free equilibrium and endemic equilibrium. In Section 11.4, the sensitivity analysis of the effective reproduction number and endemic steady state with respect to model parameters is performed. In Section 11.5, we presented some numerical simulations to support our analytical findings and finally a brief conclusion is given in the last section.

11.2 Formulation of Mathematical Model

We proposed a SEIRVS epidemic model with awareness through media and with the assumptions (ii)–(v) of the model proposed in Chapter 9 including the following new assumptions:

(i) The population $\tilde{N}(\tilde{t})$ at ant time $\tilde{t}$ is divided into various mutually exclusive compartments, namely, susceptible($\tilde{S}$), exposed($\tilde{E}$), infected($\tilde{I}$), recovered($\tilde{R}$) and vaccinated($\tilde{V}$).

(ii) Media induced effective transmission rate is proposed as $\beta(\tilde{I}) = \beta e^{-\frac{m\tilde{I}}{\tilde{N}}}$.

(iii) Due to pre-existing immunity, a fraction of exposed population instead of being infected, develops disease acquired temporary immunity and joins at a constant rate ($\tilde{\xi}_1$) to the recovered class [136].

(iv) Exposed individuals are vaccinated at a constant rate $\tilde{\xi}_2$.

(v) Due to the disease induces polarized temporary immunity, a fraction ($\tilde{q}$) immunized individuals join the recovered class and the remaining (1 – $\tilde{q}$) fraction rejoin the susceptible class [190–192].

(vi) The immunized individuals acquires temporary immunity against the disease and the acquired immunity wanes with time (disease-induced immunity wanes at rate θ_1 and vaccine-induced immunity wanes at rate θ_2). Hence the immunized individuals rejoins the susceptible class after the weaning period [190, 191].

(vii) The movement of the population is instantaneous from one compartment to another.

The proposed SEIRVS epidemic system with a media induced transmission rate is of the form:

$$\frac{d\tilde{S}}{d\tilde{t}} = \Lambda - \tilde{\beta} e^{-m\frac{I}{N}} \frac{\tilde{S}\tilde{I}}{\tilde{N}} - \tilde{\mu}\tilde{S} - \tilde{\omega}\tilde{S} + \tilde{\theta}_1\tilde{R} + \tilde{\theta}_2\tilde{V} + (1-\tilde{q})\tilde{\gamma}\tilde{I}, \quad (11.2.1)$$

$$\frac{d\tilde{E}}{d\tilde{t}} = \tilde{\beta} e^{-m\frac{I}{N}} \frac{\tilde{S}\tilde{I}}{\tilde{N}} - \tilde{\mu}\tilde{E} - \tilde{\sigma}\tilde{E} - \tilde{\xi}_1\tilde{E} - \tilde{\xi}_2\tilde{E}, \quad (11.2.2)$$

$$\frac{d\tilde{I}}{d\tilde{t}} = \tilde{\sigma}\tilde{E} - \tilde{\gamma}\tilde{I} - \tilde{\delta}\tilde{I} - \tilde{\mu}\tilde{I}, \quad (11.2.3)$$

$$\frac{d\tilde{R}}{d\tilde{t}} = \tilde{\xi}_1\tilde{E} + \tilde{q}\tilde{\gamma}\tilde{I} - \tilde{\theta}_1\tilde{R} - \tilde{\mu}\tilde{R}, \quad (11.2.4)$$

$$\frac{d\tilde{V}}{d\tilde{t}} = \tilde{\omega}\tilde{S} + \tilde{\xi}_2\tilde{E} - \tilde{\mu}\tilde{V} - \tilde{\theta}_2\tilde{V}, \quad (11.2.5)$$

with initial conditions:

$$\tilde{S}(0) = \tilde{S}_0 > 0, \tilde{E}(0) = \tilde{E}_0 > 0, \tilde{I}(0) = \tilde{I}_0 > 0, \tilde{R}(0) = \tilde{R}_0, \tilde{V}(0) = \tilde{V}_0 > 0 \tag{11.2.6}$$

and the detail of the parameters of the proposed model is described in Table 11.1.

Also $\tilde{N}(\tilde{t}) = \tilde{S}(\tilde{t}) + \tilde{E}(\tilde{t}) + \tilde{I}(\tilde{t}) + \tilde{R}(\tilde{t}) + \tilde{V}(\tilde{t})$. Therefore

$$\frac{d\tilde{N}}{d\tilde{t}} = \Lambda - \tilde{\mu}\tilde{N} - \tilde{\delta}\tilde{I}.$$

Consider the region:

$$\Gamma = \left\{ (\tilde{S}, \tilde{E}, \tilde{I}, \tilde{R}, \tilde{V}) : 0 \leq \tilde{S}, \tilde{E}, \tilde{I}, \tilde{R}, \tilde{V} \leq \frac{\Lambda}{\tilde{\mu}} \right\}.$$

Proposition 11.2.1. *All the solution trajectories of the system (11.2.1)–(11.2.6) initiating inside* Γ*, will stay within the interior of* Γ.

Proof. Let $R^5_+ = \left\{ (\tilde{S}, \tilde{E}, \tilde{I}, \tilde{R}, \tilde{V}) \in R^5 : \tilde{S}, \tilde{E}, \tilde{I}, \tilde{R}, \tilde{V} \geq 0 \right\}$ be the five dimensional space. From the system (11.2.1)–(11.2.6), we observe that

$$\frac{d\tilde{S}}{d\tilde{t}}\Big|_{\tilde{S}=0} = \Lambda + \tilde{\theta}_1\tilde{R} + \tilde{\theta}_2\tilde{V} + (1 - \tilde{q})\tilde{\gamma}\tilde{I} > 0,$$

$$\frac{d\tilde{E}}{d\tilde{t}}\Big|_{\tilde{E}=0} = \tilde{\beta} e^{-m\frac{I}{N}} \frac{\tilde{S}\tilde{I}}{\tilde{N}} > 0,$$

$$\frac{d\tilde{I}}{d\tilde{t}}\Big|_{\tilde{I}=0} = \tilde{\sigma}\tilde{E} > 0,$$

$$\frac{d\tilde{R}}{d\tilde{t}}\Big|_{\tilde{R}=0} = \tilde{\xi}_1\tilde{E} + \tilde{q}\tilde{\gamma}\tilde{I} > 0,$$

$$\frac{d\tilde{V}}{d\tilde{t}}\Big|_{\tilde{V}=0} = \tilde{\omega}\tilde{S} + \tilde{\xi}_2\tilde{E} > 0,$$

and $\tilde{S}(\tilde{t}), \tilde{E}(\tilde{t}), \tilde{I}(\tilde{t}), \tilde{R}(\tilde{t}), \tilde{V}(\tilde{t})$ are continuous function of $\tilde{t}$. Thus the vector field initiating in R^5_+ will remain inside R^5_+ for all the time. Also the total population $\tilde{N}(\tilde{t}) = \tilde{S}(\tilde{t}) + \tilde{E}(\tilde{t}) + \tilde{I}(\tilde{t}) + \tilde{R}(\tilde{t}) + \tilde{V}(\tilde{t})$ satisfies $\frac{d\tilde{N}}{dt} = \Lambda - \tilde{\mu}\tilde{N} - \tilde{\delta}\tilde{I}$. Then $\frac{d\tilde{N}}{dt} < \Lambda - \tilde{\mu}\tilde{N}$ as $\tilde{t} \to \infty$ implies that $0 \leq \tilde{N}(\tilde{t}) \leq \frac{\Lambda}{\tilde{\mu}} = \tilde{N}^0$. Therefore the system (11.2.1)–(11.2.6) is bounded and any solution of the system originates from Γ remains in Γ. □

TABLE 11.1 Description of Parameters for the System (11.2.1)–(11.2.6)

Parameter	Description	Unit
Λ	Recruitment rate of susceptible	days^{-1}
$1/\tilde{\mu}$	Average life-span	days
$\tilde{\beta}$	Transmission rate of exposed individuals (in the absence of NPIs through media awareness)	days^{-1}
$1/\tilde{\sigma}$	Average time-span of infected individuals in exposed class	days
$\tilde{\delta}$	Disease-induced death rate	days^{-1}
$1/\tilde{\gamma}$	Average length of infection of the infected individual	days
$\tilde{\omega}$	Rate at which susceptible individuals are vaccinated	days^{-1}
$\tilde{q}$	Fraction of immunized individuals getting disease acquired immunity	–
m	Coefficient of media awareness	–
$\tilde{\theta}_1$	Rate at which disease-induced immunity wanes	days^{-1}
$\tilde{\theta}_2$	Rate at which vaccine-induced immunity wanes	days^{-1}
$\tilde{\xi}_1$	Rate of recovery from exposed class due to preexisting immunity or natural immunity	days^{-1}
$\tilde{\xi}_2$	Rate at which exposed individuals are vaccinated	days^{-1}

We non-dimensionalize the above system using

$$S=\frac{\tilde{S}}{\tilde{N}},E=\frac{\tilde{E}}{\tilde{N}},I=\frac{\tilde{I}}{\tilde{N}},R=\frac{\tilde{R}}{\tilde{N}},V=\frac{\tilde{V}}{\tilde{N}},N=\frac{\tilde{N}}{\tilde{N^0}},\tilde{N^0}=\frac{\Lambda}{\tilde{\mu}},t=\tilde{\mu}\tilde{t}.$$

Since $S=1-(E+I+R+V)$, dropping the equation

$$\frac{dS}{dt}=\frac{1}{N}-\beta e^{-mI}SI-\omega S+\theta_1 R+\theta_2 V-\frac{S}{N}+\delta SI+(1-aq)\gamma I,$$

the equivalent non-dimensional system is given by

$$\frac{dE}{dt} = \beta e^{-mI}SI-(\sigma+\xi_1+\xi_2)E-\frac{E}{N}+\delta EI:=f_1, \quad (11.2.7)$$

$$\frac{dI}{dt} = \sigma E-(\gamma+\delta)I-\frac{I}{N}+\delta I^2:=f_2, \quad (11.2.8)$$

$$\frac{dR}{dt} = \xi_1 E+aq\gamma I-\theta_1 R-\frac{R}{N}+\delta RI:=f_3, \quad (11.2.9)$$

$$\frac{dV}{dt} = \omega S+\xi_2 E-\theta_2 V-\frac{V}{N}+\delta VI:=f_4, \quad (11.2.10)$$

$$\frac{dN}{dt} = 1-N-\delta NI:=f_5, \quad (11.2.11)$$

where

$$\beta=\frac{\tilde{\beta}}{\tilde{\mu}},\omega=\frac{\tilde{\omega}}{\tilde{\mu}},\theta_1=\frac{\tilde{\theta_1}}{\tilde{\mu}},\theta_2=\frac{\tilde{\theta_2}}{\tilde{\mu}},$$

$$q=\frac{\tilde{q}}{\tilde{\mu}},\gamma=\frac{\tilde{\gamma}}{\tilde{\mu}},\xi_1=\frac{\tilde{\xi_1}}{\tilde{\mu}},\xi_2=\frac{\tilde{\xi_2}}{\tilde{\mu}},\sigma=\frac{\tilde{\sigma}}{\tilde{\mu}},\delta=\frac{\tilde{\delta}}{\tilde{\mu}},a=\tilde{\mu}$$

and with the initial conditions:

$$E(0)=E_0>0,I(0)=I_0>0,R(0)=R_0>0,V(0)=V_0>0,N(0)=N_0>0. \quad (11.2.12)$$

In the following section, we will study the dynamical behavior of the system (11.2.7)–(11.2.11) with the initial condition (11.2.12).

11.3 Dynamical Behavior of the System

Now, we will calculate the effective reproduction number, feasible steady states and analyze the local stability of the equilibria for the proposed system. The biological feasible region for the non-dimensional system is

$$\Omega = \{(E,I,R,V,N) : 0 \leq E,I,R,V,N \leq 1\}.$$

The system (11.2.7)–(11.2.12) has the disease free equilibrium (DFE) $E^0 = (0,0,0,\frac{\omega}{h},1)$, where $h = 1+\theta_2+\omega$. Now, we calculate the effective reproduction number R_V. Let $x = (E,I)$. Therefore

$$\frac{dx}{dt} = f - v,$$

where

$$f = \begin{pmatrix} \beta e^{-mI}(1-E-I-R-V)I \\ 0 \end{pmatrix}$$

and

$$v = \begin{pmatrix} (\sigma+\xi_1+\xi_2)E + \frac{E}{N} - \delta EI \\ -\sigma E + (\gamma+\delta)I + \frac{I}{N} - \delta I^2 \end{pmatrix}.$$

We have

$$F = Df|_{E^0} = \begin{pmatrix} 0 & \beta\left(\frac{1+\theta_2}{1+\theta_2+\omega}\right) \\ 0 & \beta \end{pmatrix}$$

and

$$V = Dv|_{E^0} = \begin{pmatrix} 1+\sigma+\xi_1+\xi_2 & 0 \\ -\sigma & 1+\delta+\gamma \end{pmatrix}.$$

The next generation matrix for the model is given by

$$K = FV^{-1} = \begin{pmatrix} \frac{\beta\sigma(1+\theta_2)}{(1+\theta_2+\omega)(1+\sigma+\xi_1+\xi_2)(1+\gamma+\delta)} & \frac{\beta(1+\theta_2)}{(1+\theta_2+\omega)(1+\gamma+\delta)} \\ 0 & 0 \end{pmatrix}.$$

The effective reproduction number of the model is given by $R_V = \rho(FV^{-1})$. Therefore

$$R_V = \frac{\beta\sigma(1+\theta_2)}{(1+\theta_2+\omega)(1+\sigma+\xi_1+\xi_2)(1+\gamma+\delta)}.$$

We know that in the absence of vaccination program ($\tilde{\omega} = 0,\ \tilde{\theta}_2 = 0,\ \tilde{\xi}_2 = 0$), the effective reproduction number R_V reduces to the basic reproduction number R_0, given by

$$R_0 = \frac{\beta\sigma}{(1+\sigma+\xi_1)(1+\gamma+\delta)}.$$

Here, due to the vaccination program the effective reproduction number R_V is less than basic reproduction number R_0. Further the system (11.2.7)–(11.2.12) also has endemic equilibrium (EE) given by

$$\bar{E} = (E^*, I^*, R^*, V^*, N^*),$$

where $E^* = \left(\frac{1+\gamma+\delta}{\sigma}\right) I^*$, $R^* = kI^*$, $V^* = \frac{lI^*+\omega}{h}$, $N^* = \frac{1}{1+\delta I^*}$, and the value I^* is given by

$$\frac{e^{mI^*}}{R_V} = 1 - uI^*,$$

and

$$k = \frac{1}{\sigma(1+\theta_1)}[\xi_1(1+\gamma+\delta) + aq\gamma\sigma],$$

$$l = \frac{(\xi_2 - \omega)(1+\gamma+\delta)}{\sigma} - \omega(1+k),$$

$$u = 1 + \frac{(1+\gamma+\delta)(1+\theta_2+\xi_2)}{\sigma(1+\theta_2)} + \frac{\xi_1(1+\gamma+\delta)}{\sigma(1+\theta_1)} + \frac{aq\gamma}{(1+\theta_1)}.$$

If there is no media effect, i.e. $m = 0$, then

$$I^* = \frac{1 - \frac{1}{R_V}}{u}.$$

Clearly, in the absence of media effect, I^* exists if and only if $R_V > 1$.

Remark: For a particular set of parameters, the EE exists when $R_0 > 1$ in the absence of vaccination program (see Figure 11.2). In the case of vaccination program with same set of parametrs, the EE does not exist, since $R_V < 1$ even if $R_0 > 1$ (see Figure 11.3), otherwise the EE exists for $R_V > 1$ shown in Figure 11.4. In the Figure 11.2, the red curve represents $\frac{e^{mI^*}}{R_0}$, and, in Figures 11.3 and 11.4, the red curve represents $\frac{e^{mI^*}}{R_V}$. In the all three figures, blue dotted curve represents $1 - uI^*$.

Theorem 11.3.1. *The system (11.2.7)–(11.2.12) has*

(i) the disease free equilibrium (DFE) $E^0 = (0, 0, 0, \frac{\omega}{1+\theta_2+\omega}, 1)$ that exists for all the parameter values;

(ii) no endemic equilibrium (EE), if $R_V \leq 1$;

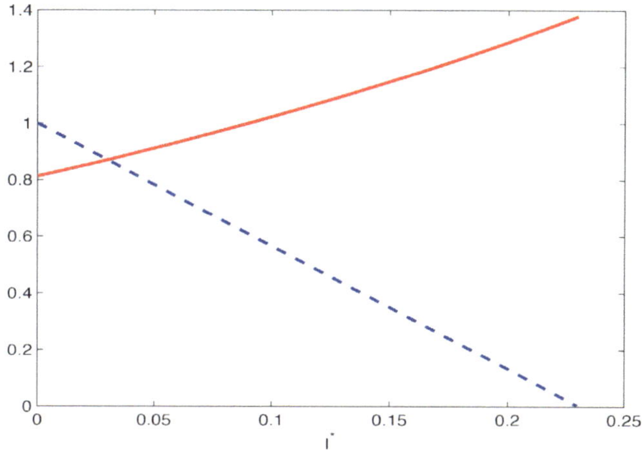

FIGURE 11.2 Existence of endemic equilibrium for the parametric values $\tilde{\beta} = 0.4$, $m = 2.3$, $\tilde{\omega} = 0$, $\tilde{\theta}_1 = 0.01$, $\tilde{\theta}_2 = 0$, $\tilde{q} = 0.8$, $\tilde{\gamma} = 0.1$, $\tilde{\xi}_1 = 0.01$, $\tilde{\xi}_2 = 0$, $\tilde{\sigma} = 0.02$, $\tilde{\delta} = 0.01$, $\tilde{\mu} = 0.02$ and $R_0 = 1.2308 > 1$. Here the red curve represents $\frac{e^{mI^*}}{R_0}$ and blue dotted curve represents $1 - uI^*$.

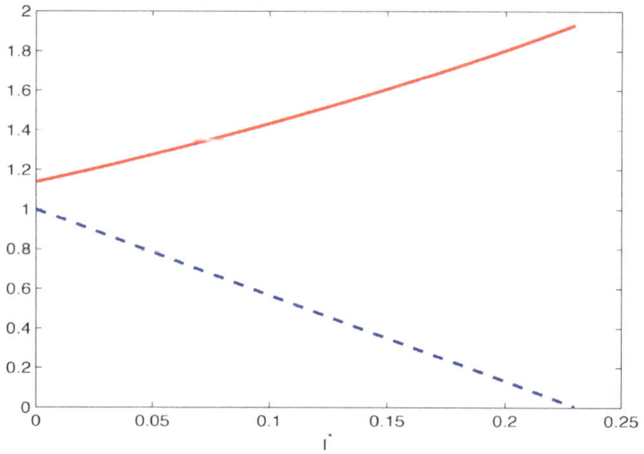

FIGURE 11.3 Non-existence of endemic equilibrium for the parametric values $\tilde{\beta} = 0.4$, $m = 2.3$, $\tilde{\omega} = 0.02$, $\tilde{\theta}_1 = 0.01$, $\tilde{\theta}_2 = 0.1$, $\tilde{q} = 0.8$, $\tilde{\gamma} = 0.1$, $\tilde{\xi}_1 = 0.01$, $\tilde{\xi}_2 = 0.01$, $\tilde{\sigma} = 0.02$, $\tilde{\delta} = 0.01$, $\tilde{\mu} = 0.02$, $R_0 = 1.2308 > 1$ and $R_V = 0.87912 < 1$. Here the red curve represents $\frac{e^{mI^*}}{R_V}$ and blue dotted curve represents $1 - uI^*$.

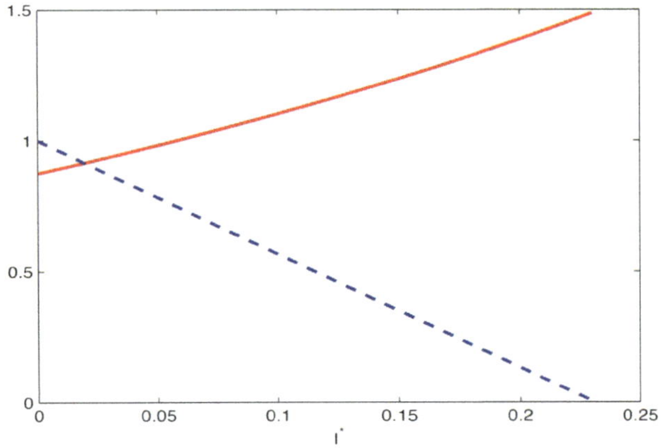

FIGURE 11.4 Existence of endemic equilibrium for parametric values $\tilde{\beta} = 0.52$, $m = 2.3$, $\tilde{\omega} = 0.02$, $\tilde{\theta}_1 = 0.01$, $\tilde{\theta}_2 = 0.1$, $\tilde{q} = 0.8$, $\tilde{\gamma} = 0.1$, $\tilde{\xi}_1 = 0.01$, $\tilde{\xi}_2 = 0.01$, $\tilde{\sigma} = 0.02$, $\tilde{\delta} = 0.01$, $\tilde{\mu} = 0.02$ and $R_V = 1.1429 > 1$. Here the red curve represents $\frac{e^{mI^*}}{R_V}$ and blue dotted curve represents $1 - uI^*$.

(iii) unique endemic equilibrium if $R_V > 1$.

Theorem 11.3.2. *The disease free equilibrium (DFE)* E^0 *is*

(i) locally asymptotically stable, if $R_V < 1$ *and*

(ii) unstable, if $R_V > 1$.

Proof. The variational matrix at the DFE is given by

$$J_0 = \begin{pmatrix} -1-\sigma-\xi_1-\xi_2 & \frac{\beta(1+\theta_2)}{(1+\theta_2+\omega)} & 0 & 0 & 0 \\ \sigma & -1-\gamma-\delta & 0 & 0 & 0 \\ \xi_1 & aq\gamma & -1-\theta_1 & 0 & 0 \\ \xi_2-\omega & -\omega+\frac{\delta\omega}{1+\theta_2+\omega} & -\omega & -1-\theta_2-\omega & \frac{\omega}{1+\theta_2+\omega} \\ 0 & -\delta & 0 & 0 & -1 \end{pmatrix}.$$

The characteristic equation of J_0 is given by

$$(\lambda+1)(\lambda+\theta_1+1)(\lambda+\theta_2+\omega+1)[\lambda^2+(2+b+c)\lambda+(1+b)(1+c)(R_V-1)]=0,$$

where $b = \sigma+\xi_1+\xi_2$ and $c = \gamma+\delta$.

If $R_V < 1$, then all the eigen values of J_0 have negative real parts. If $R_V > 1$, then one eigen value of J_0 has positive real part. Therefore disease free equilibrium is locally asymptotically stable, if $R_V < 1$ and unstable, if $R_V > 1$. □

Theorem 11.3.3. *The endemic equilibrium (EE) is locally asymptotically stable for $R_V > 1$, but close to $R_V = 1$.*

Proof. Here, we use the method based on central manifold theory to establish the local stability of endemic equilibrium taking β as bifurcation parameter. The critical value of the bifurcation parameter at $R_V = 1$ is $\beta^* = \frac{(1+b)(1+c)(1+\theta_2+\omega)}{\sigma(1+\theta_2)}$. It can be easily verified that the jacobian J_0 at $\beta = \beta^*$ has right eigen vector given by $W = (w_1, w_2, w_3, w_4, w_5)^T$ such that $J_0 W = 0$, where

$$w_1 = 1+\gamma+\delta, \quad w_2 = \sigma, \quad w_3 = \frac{\xi_1(1+\gamma+\delta)+aq\gamma\sigma}{1+\theta_1}, \quad w_5 = -\delta\sigma$$

and

$$w_4 = \frac{(\xi_2-\omega)(1+c)}{h} - \frac{\omega\sigma(h-\delta)}{h^2} - \frac{\omega\delta\sigma}{h^2} - \frac{\omega[\xi_1(1+c)+aq\gamma\sigma]}{h(1+\theta_1)}.$$

The left eigen vector is given by $V = (v_1, v_2, v_3, v_4, v_5)$ which satisfy $V.J_0 = 0$ and $V.W = 1$, where

$$v_1 = \frac{1}{b+c+2}, \quad v_2 = \frac{1+b}{\sigma(b+c+2)}, \quad v_3 = 0, \quad v_4 = 0, \quad v_5 = 0.$$

The associated non-zero partial derivatives of $F = (f_1, f_2, f_3, f_4, f_5)^T$ at the DFE and $\beta = \beta^*$ are given by

$$\frac{\partial^2 f_1}{\partial E \partial I} = -\beta+\delta, \quad \frac{\partial^2 f_1}{\partial E \partial N} = 1, \quad \frac{\partial^2 f_1}{\partial I^2} = -2\beta - \frac{2\beta m(1+\theta_2)}{(1+\theta_2+\omega)},$$

$$\frac{\partial^2 f_1}{\partial I \partial R} = -\beta, \quad \frac{\partial^2 f_1}{\partial I \partial V} = -\beta, \quad \frac{\partial^2 f_2}{\partial I^2} = 2\delta, \quad \frac{\partial^2 f_2}{\partial I \partial N} = 1, \quad \frac{\partial^2 f_3}{\partial I \partial R} = \delta,$$

$$\frac{\partial^2 f_3}{\partial R \partial N} = 1, \quad \frac{\partial^2 f_4}{\partial I \partial V} = \delta, \quad \frac{\partial^2 f_4}{\partial V \partial N} = 1, \quad \frac{\partial^2 f_4}{\partial N^2} = -\frac{2\omega}{1+\theta_2+\omega},$$

$$\frac{\partial^2 f_5}{\partial I \partial N} = -\delta, \quad \frac{\partial^2 f_1}{\partial I \partial \beta} = \frac{1+\theta_2}{1+\theta_2+\omega}.$$

TABLE 11.2 Parametric Values Used for Simulation of the System (11.2.7)–(11.2.12)

Parameter	Value	Reference
Λ	5.0	[136, 138]
$\tilde{\mu}$	0.02	[136, 138]
$\tilde{\beta}$	[0.5,0.8]	variable
$\tilde{\sigma}$	0.04	assumed
$\tilde{\delta}$	0.01	[136, 138]
$\tilde{\gamma}$	0.05	[136, 138]
$\tilde{\omega}$	[0.3,0.7]	[136
$\tilde{q}$	0.8	Assumed
m	[0,3]	Variable
$\tilde{\theta}_1$	0.01	[136, 138]
$\tilde{\theta}_2$	0.15	[136, 138]
$\tilde{\xi}_1$	0.01	Assumed
$\tilde{\xi}_2$	0.02	Assumed

Here we use notations $x_1 = E, x_2 = I, x_3 = R, x_4 = V, x_5 = N$. We have

$$A = \sum_{k,i,j=1}^{5} v_k w_i w_j \frac{\partial^2 f_k}{\partial x_i \partial x_j}$$

and

$$B = \sum_{k,i=1}^{5} v_k w_i \frac{\partial^2 f_k}{\partial x_i \partial \phi}.$$

By simple calculations we get

$$\begin{aligned} A = & -\frac{[(1+c)\beta-(1+b)\delta]\sigma}{b+c+2} - \frac{2\beta\sigma^2}{b+c+2} - \frac{2\beta\sigma^2 m(1+\theta_2)}{h} - \frac{\sigma\beta\xi_1(1+c)(1+\theta_2)}{h(b+c+2)(1+\theta_1)} \\ & -\frac{\sigma^2\beta aq\gamma}{(b+c+2)(\theta_1+1)} - \frac{\sigma\beta}{h(b+c+2)}\left[(\xi_2-\omega)(1+c)-\omega\sigma-\frac{\omega\sigma aq\gamma}{1+\theta_1}\right], \end{aligned}$$

and

$$B = \frac{\sigma(1+\theta_2)}{h(b+c+2)} > 0.$$

Now A is negative if $\beta > M_1$ and $\xi_2 > M_2$, which is one of the sufficient condition, where

$$M_1 = \frac{(1+b)\delta}{1+c}$$

and

$$M_2 = \frac{\omega}{(1+c)}\left[1+c+\sigma+\frac{\sigma a q \gamma}{1+\theta_1}\right].$$

Therefore, $A < 0$ and $B > 0$ at $\beta = \beta^*$ for $\beta > M_1$ and $\xi_2 > M_2$, which is one of the sufficient condition. Therefore, a transcritical bifurcation occurs at $R_V = 1$ and if $R_V > 1$, then the unique endemic equilibrium is locally asymptotically stable. □

11.4 Sensitivity Analysis

TABLE 11.3 The Sensitivity Indices $\gamma_{y_j}^{R_V} = \frac{\partial R_V}{\partial y_j} \times \frac{y_j}{R_V}$ of the Effective Reproduction Number R_V to the Parameters y_j for the Parameter Values Given in Table 11.2

Parameter (y_j)	Sensitivity index of R_V w.r.t. y_j $(\gamma_{y_j}^{R_V})$
β	1
σ	0.555556
δ	–0.125
γ	–0.625
ω	–0.701754
q	0
m	0
θ_1	0
θ_2	0.619195
ξ_1	–0.111111
ξ_2	–0.222222

In this section, we perform the sensitivity analysis of the effective reproduction number R_V (shown in Table 11.3) and endemic equilibrium (shown in Table 11.4) with respect to model parameters, for a particular

TABLE 11.4 The Sensitivity Indices $\gamma_{y_j}^{x_i} = \frac{\partial x_i}{\partial y_j} \times \frac{y_j}{x_i}$ of the State Variables to the Parameters y_j for the Parameter Values Given in Table 11.2

Parameter	$\gamma_{y_j}^{E^*}$	$\gamma_{y_j}^{I^*}$	$\gamma_{y_j}^{R^*}$	$\gamma_{y_j}^{V^*}$	$\gamma_{y_j}^{N^*}$
β	–5.545	–5.545	–5.545	–0.629	–0.073
σ	–3.711	–2.711	–3.044	–0.366	–0.035
δ	0.772	0.647	0.688	0.080	0.021
γ	3.690	3.065	3.940	0.415	0.040
ω	3.891	3.891	3.891	0.742	0.051
q	–0.169	–0.169	0.496	0.011	–0.002
m	1.202	–0.333	–0.248	–0.005	0.001
θ_1	–0.333	0.084	–0.248	–0.005	0.001
θ_2	0.084	–3.407	–3.407	–0.649	–0.045
ξ_1	–3.407	0.531	0.864	0.075	0.007
ξ_2	0.531	1.202	1.202	0.134	0.015

set of parameters is given in the Table 11.2. From the Table 11.3, we observe that β, σ, θ_2 has a positive impact on R_V and δ, γ, ω, ξ_1, ξ_2 have a negative impact on R_V. Moreover β and ω are most sensitive to R_V, hence we observe significant changes in R_V by small changes in these parameters.

From the Table 11.4, we observe that β, σ, q, θ_1, ξ_1 has a negative impact on the E^* and rest of the parameters have a positive impact. Moreover β, σ, γ, ω, ξ_1 are most sensitive parameter to E^*, hence we observe large change in E^* by a small change in these parameters. Similarly β, γ, ω, θ_2 are most sensitive parameter to I^*; β, σ, γ, ω, θ_2 are most sensitive parameter to R^*; and β, ω, θ_2 are most sensitive parameter to V^*. Further, all the parameters are less sensitive to N^*.

11.5 Numerical Simulations

We perform the numerical simulations of the model to justify the analytic findings. The parameter used for simulation of the system (11.2.7)–(11.2.12) are listed in Table 11.2 taking a time unit in days. We

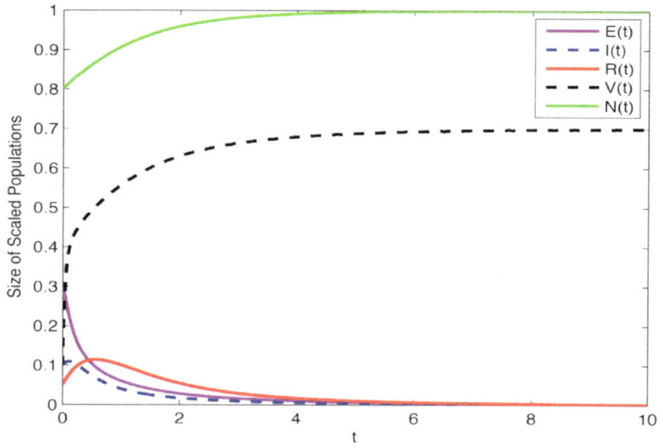

FIGURE 11.5 The variation of the scaled population in scaled time for parameter values $\tilde{\beta} = 0.5$, $m = 2.3$, $\tilde{\omega} = 0.4$, $\tilde{\theta}_1 = 0.01$, $\tilde{\theta}_2 = 0.15$, $\tilde{q} = 0.8$, $\tilde{\gamma} = 0.05$, $\tilde{\xi}_1 = 0.01$, $\tilde{\xi}_2 = 0.02$, $\tilde{\sigma} = 0.04$, $\tilde{\delta} = 0.01$, $\tilde{\mu} = 0.02$, $R_V = 0.82846 < 1$.

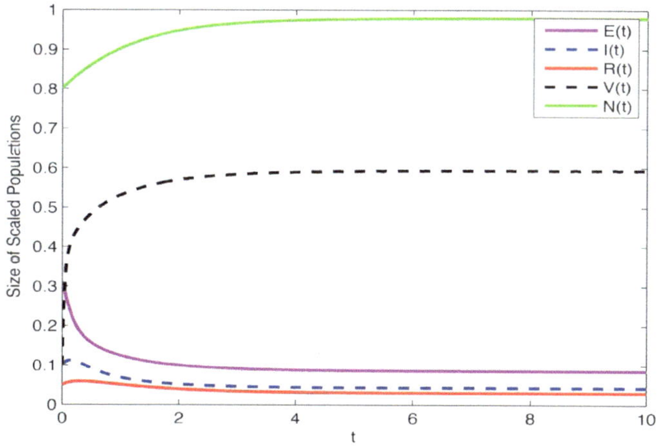

FIGURE 11.6 The variation of the scaled population in scaled time for parameter values $\tilde{\beta} = 0.8$, $m = 2.3$, $\tilde{\omega} = 0.4$, $\tilde{\theta}_1 = 0.01$, $\tilde{\theta}_2 = 0.15$, $\tilde{q} = 0.8$, $\tilde{\gamma} = 0.05$, $\tilde{\xi}_1 = 0.01$, $\tilde{\xi}_2 = 0.02$, $\tilde{\sigma} = 0.04$, $\tilde{\delta} = 0.01$, $\tilde{\mu} = 0.02$, $R_V = 1.3255 > 1$.

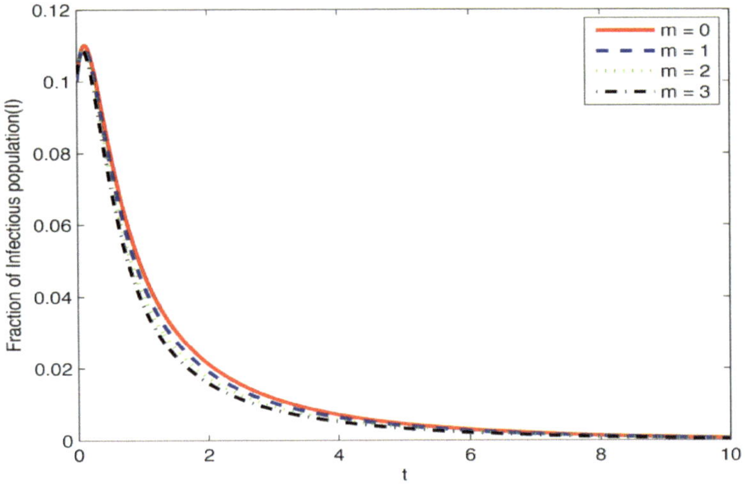

FIGURE 11.7 The effect of m on I for parametric value $R_V = 0.82846 < 1$.

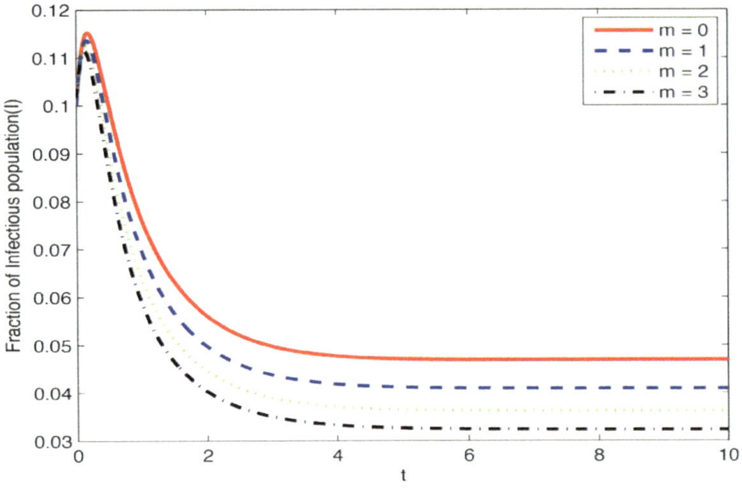

FIGURE 11.8 The effect of m on I for parametric value $R_V = 1.3255 > 1$.

use initial population sizes as $E_0 = 0.3$, $I_0 = 0.1$, $R_0 = 0.05$, $V_0 = 0.1$ and $N_0 = 0.8$. We discuss the following two cases by keeping the parameters $m = 2.3$, $\tilde{\omega} = 0.4$, $\tilde{\theta_1} = 0.01$, $\tilde{\theta_2} = 0.15$, $q = 0.8$, $\tilde{\gamma} = 0.05$, $\tilde{\xi_1} = 0.01$, $\tilde{\xi_2} = 0.02$, $\tilde{\sigma} = 0.04$, $\tilde{\delta} = 0.01$, $\tilde{\mu} = 0.02$ as fixed and varying $\tilde{\beta}$ only:

Case 1: When $\tilde{\beta} = 0.5$ then $R_V = 0.82846 < 1$ and the DFE is locally asymptotically stable as shown in Figure 11.5, which is in accordance with the results stated in Theorem 11.3.2.

Case 2: When $\tilde{\beta} = 0.8$ then $R_V = 1.3255 > 1$ and the EE is locally asymptotically stable as shown in Figure 11.6. Therefore, the results stated in Theorem 11.3.3 are true.

The effect of m on the fraction of infectious population is shown in Figures 11.7 and 11.8 with different values of m. We observe that the endemic equilibrium state is well influenced by media coefficient m as shown in Figure 11.8.

11.6 Summary

In this chapter, we proposed a SEIRVS epidemic model incorporating media awareness as an additional control strategy along with the vaccination and investigated the asymptotic stability behavior of the system at the equilibrium states. The disease-free state is locally asymptotically stable for effective reproduction number $R_V < 1$, a transcritical bifurcation appears at $R_V = 1$ and a locally asymptotically stable endemic equilibrium state exists for $R_V > 1$. Due to the vaccination program the effective reproduction number R_V is always less than the basic reproduction number R_0, which implies that we can achieve disease-free state with vaccination program even from the case of endemic state without some control strategy (see Figures 11.2 and 11.3). We observed that the coefficient of media awareness m does not effect R_V. We perform sensitivity analysis of the effective reproduction number and endemic equilibrium to various model parameters and identified respective sensitive parameters. Numerical simulations of the system justify the analytic findings and we also viewed that the endemic equilibrium state is largely affected by media coefficient m.

Bibliography

1. Murray, J. D., (2002). *Mathematical Biology-I: An Introduction, of Interdisciplinary Applied Mathematics,* vol. 17. New York: Springer.

2. White, G. C., (2000). *Modeling Population Dynamics, Ecology and Management of Mammals in North America.* New Jersey, USA: Prentice-Hall, Upper Saddle River, 84–107.

3. De Boer, R. J. (2010). *Modeling Population Dynamics: A Graphical Approach,* Utrecht University.

4. Newman, K., Buckland, S., Morgan, B., King, R., Borchers, D., Cole, D. J., Besbeas, P., Gimenez, O., & Thomas, L., (2014). *Modelling Population Dynamics,* Springer.

5. Kot, M., (2001). *Elements of Mathematical Ecology,* Cambridge University Press.

6. Lotka, A. J., (1925). *Elements of Physical Biology.* Bibliolife DBA of Bibilio Bazaar II LLC, (reprint on 2015).

7. Volterra, V., (1926). Fluctuations in the abundance of a species considered mathematically, *Nature, 118,* 558–560.

8. Berryman, A. A., (1992). The origins and evolution of predator-prey theory, *Ecology, 73*(5), 1530–1535.

9. May, R. M., (2001). *Stability and Complexity in Model Ecosystems,* Princeton University Press, vol. 6.

10. Freedman, H., (1987). *Deterministic Mathematical Models in Population Ecology*, HIFR Consulting Ltd., Edmonton, Alberta, Canada.
11. Robinson, C., (1998). *Dynamical Systems: Stability, Symbolic Dynamics, and Chaos*, CRC Press.
12. Burton, T. A., (2014). *Stability & Periodic Solutions of Ordinary & Functional Differential Equations*, Courier Corporation.
13. Dubey, B., (2007). A prey-predator model with a reserved area, *Nonlinear Analysis: Modelling and Control, 12*(4), 479–494.
14. Jeschke, J. M., Kopp, M., & Tollrian, R., (2002). Predator functional responses: discriminating between handling and digesting prey, *Ecological Monographs, 72*(1), 95–112.
15. Kooij, R. E., & Zegeling, A., (1996). A predator–prey model with Ivlev?s functional response, *Journal of Mathematical Analysis and Applications, 198*(2), 473–489.
16. Ma, W., & Takeuchi, Y., (1998). Stability analysis on a predator-prey system with distributed delays, *Journal of Computational and Applied Mathematics, 88*(1), 79–94.
17. Sen, M., Banerjee, M., & Morozov, A., (2012). Bifurcation analysis of a ratio-dependent prey–predator model with the Allee effect, *Ecological Complexity, 11*, 12–27.
18. Tripathi, J. P., Abbas, S., & Thakur, M., (2015). Dynamical analysis of a prey–predator model with Beddington–DeAngelis type function response incorporating a prey refuge, *Nonlinear Dynamics, 80*(1–2), 177–196.
19. Liu, X., (2010). A note on the existence of periodic solutions in discrete predator–prey models, *Applied Mathematical Modelling, 34*(9), 2477–2483.
20. Chen, F., (2006). Permanence and global attractivity of a discrete multispecies Lotka–Volterra competition predator–prey systems, *Applied Mathematics and Computation, 182*(1), 3–12.

21. Liao, X., Zhou, S., & Ouyang, Z., (2007). On a stoichiometric two predators on one prey discrete model, *Applied Mathematics Letters, 20*(3), 272–278.

22. Agarwal, R. P., (2000). *Difference Equations and Inequalities: Theory, Methods, and Applications,* CRC Press.

23. Agarwal, R. P., & Wong, P. J., (1997). *Advanced Topics in Difference Equations*, Springer.

24. Celik, C., & Duman, O., (2009). Allee effect in a discrete-time predator–prey system, *Chaos, Solitons & Fractals, 40*(4), 1956–1962.

25. Liu, X., & Xiao, D., (2007). Complex dynamic behaviors of a discrete-time predator–prey system, *Chaos, Solitons & Fractals, 32*(1), 80–94.

26. He, Z., & Lai, X., (2011). Bifurcation and chaotic behavior of a discrete-time predator–prey system, *Nonlinear Analysis: Real World Applications, 12*(1), 403–417.

27. Hu, Z., Teng, Z., & Zhang, L., (2011). Stability and bifurcation analysis of a discrete predator–prey model with non-monotonic functional response, *Nonlinear Analysis: Real World Applications, 12*(4), 2356–2377.

28. Jing, Z., & Yang, J., (2006). Bifurcation and chaos in discrete-time predator–prey system, *Chaos, Solitons & Fractals, 27*(1), 259–277.

29. Hu, Z., Teng, Z., & Zhang, L., (2014). Stability and bifurcation analysis in a discrete SIR epidemic model, *Mathematics and Computers in Simulation, 97,* 80–93.

30. Allen, L. J., (1983). Persistence and extinction in Lotka-Volterra reaction-diffusion equations, *Mathematical Biosciences, 65*(1), 1–12.

31. Angulo, J., & Linares, F., (1995). Global existence of solutions of a nonlinear dispersive model, *Journal of Mathematical Analysis and Applications, 195*(3), 797–808.

32. Capasso, V., (1978). Global solution for a diffusive nonlinear deterministic epidemic model, *SIAM Journal on Applied Mathematics, 35*(2), 274–284.

33. Casten, R. G., & Holland, C. J., (1978). Instability results for reaction diffusion equations with Neumann boundary conditions, *Journal of Differential Equations, 27*(2), 266–273.

34. Damgaard, C., (2003). Modeling plant competition along an environmental gradient, *Ecological Modelling, 170*(1), 45–53.

35. Dhar, J., (2003). Modelling and analysis: the effect of industrialization on diffusive forest resource biomass in closed habitat, *African Diaspora Journal of Math, 2*(1), 142–159.

36. Dobzhansky, T., & Wright, S., (1943). Genetics of natural populations. x. Dispersion rates in drosophila pseudoobscura, *Genetics, 28*(4), 304.

37. Dobzhansky, T., & Wright, S., (1947). Genetics of natural populations. xv. Rate of diffusion of a mutant gene through a population of drosophila pseudoobscura, *Genetics, 32*(3), 303.

38. Itô, Y., (1952). The growth form of populations in some aphids, with special reference to the relation between population density and the movements, *Researches on Population Ecology, 1*(1), 36–48.

39. Kono, T., (1952). Time-dispersion curve, *Researches on Population Ecology, 1*(1), 109–118.

40. Comins, H. N., & Blatt, D. W., (1974). Prey-predator models in spatially heterogeneous environments, *Journal of Theoretical Biology, 48*(1), 75–83.

41. Freedman, H., & Shukla, J., (1989). The effect of a predator resource on a diffusive predator-prey system, *Nat. Res. Model, 3*(3), 359–383.

42. Hsu, S. B., & Huang, T. W., (1995). Global stability for a class of predator-prey systems, *SIAM Journal on Applied Mathematics, 55*(3), 763–783.

43. McMurtrie, R., (1978). Persistence and stability of single-species and prey-predator systems in spatially heterogeneous environments, *Mathematical Biosciences, 39*(1–2), 11–51.

44. Okubo, A., (1980). Diffusion and ecological problems; *Mathematical Models, Tech. Rep.*

45. Fick, A., (1855). Poggendorff's flannel, *Physik, 94*(59), 297.

46. Fick, A., (1855). Ueber diffusion, *Annalen der Physik, 170*(1), 59–86.

47. Freedman, H., & Krisztin, T., (1992). Global stability in models of population dynamics with diffusion in patchy environments. *Proceedings of the Royal Society of Edinburgh: Section A Mathematics, 122*(1–2), 69–84.

48. Hastings, A., (1978). Global stability in Lotka-Volterra systems with diffusion, Jou*rnal of Mathematical Biology, 6*(2), 163–168.

49. Hastings, A., (1982). Dynamics of a single species in a spatially varying environment: the stabilizing role of high dispersal rates, *Journal of Mathematical Biology, 16*(1), 49–55.

50. Shigesada, N., & Roughgarden, J., (1982). The role of rapid dispersal in the population dynamics of competition, *Theoretical Population Biology, 21*(3), 353–372.

51. Kapur, J. N., (1985). *Mathematical Models in Biology and Medicine*, Affiliated East-West Press.

52. Freedman, H. I., (1980). *Deterministic Mathematical Models in Population Ecology*, Marcel Dekker, New York.

53. Freedman, H., (1987). Single species migration in two habitats: Persistence and extinction, *Mathematical Modelling, 8,* 778–780.

54. Freedman, H., Shukla, J., & Takeuchi, Y., (1989). Population diffusion in a two-patch environment, *Mathematical Biosciences, 95*(1), 111–123.

55. Freedman, H., & Wu, J., (1992). Steady-state analysis in a model for population diffusion in a multi-patch environment, *Nonlinear Analysis: Theory, Methods & Applications, 18*(6), 517–542.

56. Gopalsamy, K., (1977). Competition, dispersion and coexistence, *Mathematical Biosciences, 33*(1), 25–33.

57. Nallaswamy, R., & Shukla, J., (1982). Effects of convective and dispersive migration on the linear stability of a two species system with mutualistic interactions and functional response, *Bulletin of Mathematical Biology, 44*(2), 271–282.

58. Timm, U., & Okubo, A., (1992). Diffusion-driven instability in a predator-prey system with time-varying diffusivities, *Journal of Mathematical Biology, 30*(3), 307–320.

59. Cosner, C., & Lazer, A. C., (1984). Stable coexistence states in the Volterra–Lotka competition model with diffusion, *SIAM Journal on Applied Mathematics, 44*(6), 1112–1132.

60. Steele, J.H. (1976). Patchiness. In: The Ecology of the Sea, 98–115, Cushing, D. H. and Walsh, J. J. (eds.). W.B. Saunders Co., Philadelphia.

61. Volovskaia, M. L., (1990). *Epidemiology and Fundamentals of Infectious Diseases*, Mir Publishers.

62. Ahrens, W., & Pigeot, I., (2005). *Handbook of Epidemiology*, Springer.

63. Hui, J., & De Zhu, (2007). Dynamics of SEIS epidemic models with varying population size, *International Journal of Bifurcation and Chaos*, *17*(05), 1513–1529.

64. Liu, X., Liu, Y., Zhang, Y., Chen, Z., Tang, Z., Xu, Q., Wang, Y., Zhao, P., & Qi, Z., (2013). Pre-existing immunity with high neutralizing activity to 2009 pandemic H1N1 influenza virus in shanghai population, *PloS One, 8*(3), e58810.

65. Gao, R., Cao, B., Hu, Y., Feng, Z., Wang, D., Hu, W., Chen, J., Jie, Z., Qiu, H., Xu, K., et al., (2013). Human infection with a novel

avian-origin influenza A (h7n9) virus, *New England Journal of Medicine, 368*(20), 1888–1897.

66. Tharakaraman, K., Jayaraman, A., Raman, R., Viswanathan, K., Stebbins, N. W., Johnson, D., Shriver, Z., Sasisekharan, V., & Sasisekharan, R., (2013). Glycan receptor binding of the influenza A virus H7N9 hemagglutinin, *Cell, 153*(7), 1486–1493.

67. Chao, D. L., Bloom, J. D., Kochin, B. F., Antia, R., & Longini, I. M., (2012). The global spread of drug-resistant influenza, *Journal of The Royal Society Interface, 9*(69), 648–656.

68. Safi, M. A., & Gumel, A. B., (2013). Dynamics of a model with quarantine-adjusted incidence and quarantine of susceptible individuals, *Journal of Mathematical Analysis and Applications 399*(2), 565–575.

69. Zhou, X., & Cui, J., (2011). Analysis of stability and bifurcation for an SEIV epidemic model with vaccination and nonlinear incidence rate, *Nonlinear Dynamics, 63*(4), 639–653.

70. Hu, Z., Teng, Z., & Jiang, H., (2012). Stability analysis in a class of discrete sirs epidemic models, *Nonlinear Analysis: Real World Applications, 13*(5), 2017–2033.

71. Kaddar, A., Abta, A., & Alaoui, H., (2010). Stability analysis in a delayed SIR epidemic model with a saturated incidence rate, *Nonlinear Analysis: Modelling and Control, 15*(3), 299–306.

72. Zhang, T., Liu, J., & Teng, Z., (2009). Bifurcation analysis of a delayed sis epidemic model with stage structure, *Chaos, Solitons & Fractals, 40*(2), 563–576.

73. Samsuzzoha, M., Singh, M., & Lucy, D., (2013). Uncertainty and sensitivity analysis of the basic reproduction number of a vaccinated epidemic model of influenza, *Applied Mathematical Modelling, 37*(3), 903–915.

74. He, Y., Gao, S., & Xie, D., (2013). An SIR epidemic model with time-varying pulse control schemes and saturated infectious force, *Applied Mathematical Modelling, 37*(16), 8131–8140.

75. Buonomo, B., Lacitignola, D., & Vargas-De-León, C., (2014). Qualitative analysis and optimal control of an epidemic model with vaccination and treatment, *Mathematics and Computers in Simulation, 100,* 88–102.

76. Denphedtnong, A., Chinviriyasit, S., & Chinviriyasit, W., (2013). On the dynamics of SEIRS epidemic model with transport-related infection, *Mathematical Biosciences, 245*(2), 188–205.

77. Xu, R., & Ma, Z., (2010). Global stability of a delayed SEIRS epidemic model with saturation incidence rate, *Nonlinear Dynamics, 61*(1–2), 229–239.

78. Kang, H., & Fu, X., (2015). Epidemic spreading and global stability of an sis model with an infective vector on complex networks, *Communications in Nonlinear Science and Numerical Simulation, 27*(1), 30–39.

79. Jokinen, S., Osterlund, P., Julkunen, I., & Davidkin, I., (2007). Cellular immunity to mumps virus in young adults 21 years after measles-mumps-rubella vaccination, *The Journal of Infectious Diseases*, *196*(6), 861–867.

80. Dayan, G. H., Quinlisk, M. P., Parker, A. A., Barskey, A. E., Harris, M. L., Schwartz, J. M. H., Hunt, K., Finley, C. G., Leschinsky, D. P., O?Keefe, A. L., Clayton, J., Kightlinger, L. K., Dietle, E. G., Berg, J., Kenyon, C. L., Goldstein, S. T., Stokley, S. K., Redd, S. B., Rota, P. A., Rota, J., Bi, D., Roush, S. W., Bridges, C. B., Santibanez, T. A., Parashar, U., Bellini, W. J., & Seward, J. F., (2008). Recent resurgence of mumps in the United States, *The New England Journal of Medicine, 358*(15), 1580–1589.

81. Mathews, J. D., McCaw, C. T., McVernon, J., McBryde, E. S., & McCaw, J. M., (2007). A biological model for influenza transmission: pandemic planning implications of asymptomatic infection and immunity, *PLoS One, 2*(11), 1–6.

82. Alexander, M. E., & Moghadas, S. M., (2005). Bifurcation analysis of an SIRS epidemic model with generalized incidence, *SIAM Journal on Applied Mathematics, 65*(5), 1794–1816.

83. Brauer, F., (1990). Models for the spread of universally fatal diseases, *Journal of Mathematical Biology, 28*(4), 451–462.

84. Ciupe, S., De Bivort, B., Bortz, D., & Nelson, P., (2006). Estimates of kinetic parameters from HIV patient data during primary infection through the eyes of three different models, *Mathematical Biosciences, 200,* 1–27.

85. Del Valle, S., Hethcote, H., Hyman, J. M., & Castillo-Chavez, C., (2005). Effects of behavioral changes in a smallpox attack model, *Mathematical Biosciences, 195*(2), 228–251.

86. Upadhyay, R. K., & Roy, P., (2014). Spread of a disease and its effect on population dynamics in an eco-epidemiological system, *Communications in Nonlinear Science and Numerical Simulation, 19*(12), 4170–4184.

87. Liu, X., & Wang, C., (2010). Bifurcation of a predator–prey model with disease in the prey, *Nonlinear Dynamics, 62*(4), 841–850.

88. Hethcote, H. W., Wang, W., Han, L., & Ma, Z., (2004). A predator–prey model with infected prey, *Theoretical Population Biology, 66*(3), 259–268.

89. Sinha, S., Misra, O., & Dhar, J., (2010). Modelling a predator–prey system with infected prey in polluted environment, *Applied Mathematical Modelling, 34*(7), 1861–1872.

90. Mukhopadhyay, B., & Bhattacharyya, R., (2009). Role of predator switching in an eco-epidemiological model with disease in the prey, *Ecological Modelling, 220*(7), 931–939.

91. Reef, S. E., Frey, T. K., Theall, K., Abernathy, E., Burnett, C. L., Icenogle, J., McCauley, M. M., & Wharton, M., (2002). The changing epidemiology of rubella in the 1990s: on the verge of elimination and new challenges for control and prevention, *JAMA, 287*(4), 464–472.

92. Mansour-Ghanaei, F., Rahimi, H., Joukar, F., Bagherzadeh, A., Heidarzadeh, A., Rahbar, A., Rokhshad, H., Rezvani, S., Balou,

H., Sarshad, A., et al., (2008). Mass vaccination of measles and rubella (MR) in Guilan, Northern Iran: Evaluation of coverage and complications, *Iranian Red Crescent Medical Journal, 10*(3), 173–179.

93. Nisbet, R., Blythe, S., Gurney, W., & Metz, J., (1985). Stage-structure models of populations with distinct growth and development processes, *Mathematical Medicine and Biology, 2*(1), 57–68.

94. Dyson, J., Villella-Bressan, R., & Webb, G., (2000). A nonlinear age and maturity structured model of population dynamics: I. basic theory, *Journal of Mathematical Analysis and Applications, 242*(1), 93–104.

95. Calsina, A., et al., (1999). Asymptotic behavior of an age-structured population model and optimal maturation age, *Journal of Mathematical Analysis and Applications, 233*(2), 808–826.

96. Chen, Y., & Changming, S., (2008). Stability and Hopf bifurcation analysis in a prey–predator system with stage-structure for prey and time delay, *Chaos, Solitons & Fractals, 38*(4), 1104–1114.

97. Dhar, J., & Jatav, K. S., (2013). Mathematical analysis of a delayed stage- structured predator–prey model with impulsive diffusion between two predators territories, *Ecological Complexity, 16,* 59–67.

98. Kuang, Y., (1993). *Delay Differential Equations*: with applications in population dynamics, Academic Press.

99. Driver, R. D., (1977). Ordinary and delay differential equations, vol. 20, Springer-Verlag, New York.

100. Beretta, E., & Takeuchi, Y., (1995). Global stability of an SIR epidemic model with time delays, *Journal of Mathematical Biology, 33*(3), 250–260.

101. Jin, Z., & Ma, Z., (2006). The stability of an SIR epidemic model with time delays. *Mathematical Biosciences and Engineering: MBE, 3*(1), 101–109.

102. Gopalsamy, K., (1992). *Stability and Oscillations in Delay Differential Equations of Population Dynamics*, Springer.

103. Huo, H. F., & Li, W. T., (2004). Existence and global stability of periodic solutions of a discrete predator–prey system with delays, *Applied Mathematics and Computation, 153*(2), 337–351.

104. Fan, Y. H., & Li, W. T., (2004). Permanence for a delayed discrete ratio- dependent predator–prey system with holling type functional response, *Journal of Mathematical Analysis and Applications, 299*(2), 357–374.

105. Gakkhar, S., & Singh, A., (2012). Complex dynamics in a prey predator system with multiple delays, *Communications in Nonlinear Science and Numerical Simulation, 17*(2), 914–929.

106. Zhang, C. H., Yan, X. P., & Cui, G. H., (2010). Hopf bifurcations in a predator–prey system with a discrete delay and a distributed delay, *Nonlinear Analysis: Real World Applications, 11*(5), 4141–4153.

107. Cooke, K., Kuang, Y., & Li, B., (1998). Analysis of an antiviral immune response model with time delays, *The Canadian Applied Mathematics Quarterly, 6*(4), 321–354.

108. Cooke, K., Van den Driessche, P., & Zou, X., (1999). Interaction of maturation delay and nonlinear birth in population and epidemic models, *Journal of Mathematical Biology, 39*(4), 332–352.

109. Ma, W., Song, M., & Takeuchi, Y., (2004). Global stability of an SIR epidemic model with time delay, *Applied Mathematics Letters, 17*(10), 1141–1145.

110. Cañada, A., & Zertiti, A., (1994). Method of upper and lower solutions for nonlinear delay integral equations modelling

epidemics and population growth, *Mathematical Models and Methods in Applied Sciences, 4*(1), 107–119.

111. Forde, J. E., (2005). Delay differential equation models in mathematical biology, *PhD Thesis*, The University of Michigan.
112. White, L., Buttery, J., Cooper, B., Nokes, D., & Medley, G., (2008). Rotavirus within day care centers in Oxfordshire, UK: characterization of partial immunity, *Journal of Royal Society Interface, 5*, 1481–1490.
113. Hope-Simpson, R., (1992). *The Transmission of Epidemic Influenza*, Plenum Press, New York.
114. Van Baalen, M., (2002). Contact networks and the evolution of virulence. In: *Adaptive Dynamics of Infectious Diseases: In Pursuit of Virulence Management*, Cambridge University Press, Cambridge.
115. Park, K., (2007). *Park's Textbook of Preventive and Social Medicine*, India, Bhanot.
116. Tchuenche, J., Khamis, S., Agusto, F., & Mpeshe, S., (2011). Optimal control and sensitivity analysis of an influenza model with treatment and vaccination, *Acta Biotheoretica, 59*(1), 1–28.
117. Metchnikoff, E., (1905). *Immunity in Infective Diseases*, Cambridge: University Press.
118. Koch, R., (1876). The etiology of anthrax, based on the life history of *Bacillus anthracis*, *Beitr. Biol. Pflanz, 2,* 277–310.
119. Koch, R., (1982). The etiology of tuberculosis, *Review of Infectious Diseases, 4*(6), 1270–1274.
120. Beijerinck, M., (1898). Concerning a *Contagium Vium Fluidum* as cause of the spot disease of tobacco leaves.
121. Lu, C., Chiang, B., Chi, W., Chang, M., Ni, Y., Hsu, H., Twu, S., Su, I., Huang, L., & Lee, C., (2004). Waning immunity to plasma-derived hepatitis b vaccine and the need for boosters 15 years after neonatal vaccination, *Hepatology, 40*(6), 1415–1420.

122. Mossong, J., & Muller, C. P., (2003). Modelling measles re-emergence as a result of waning of immunity in vaccinated populations, *Vaccine, 21*(31), 4597–4603.

123. Leuridan, E., & Van Damme, P., (2007). Passive transmission and persistence of naturally acquired or vaccine-induced maternal antibodies against measles in newborns, *Vaccine, 25*(34), 6296–6304.

124. Zaman, G., Kang, Y. H., & Jung, I. H., (2008). Stability analysis and optimal vaccination of an SIR epidemic model, *BioSystems, 93*(3), 240–249.

125. Curtiss III, R., (2011). The impact of vaccines and vaccinations: Challenges and opportunities for modelers, *Mathematical Biosciences and Engineering, 8*(1), 77–93.

126. Hazen, E., & Brown, R., (1950). Two antifungal agents produced by a soil actinomycete, *Science*, New York, *112*(2911), 423–423.

127. Duran-Reynals, M. L. D. A., et al., (1946). *Fever Bark Tree*, New York: Doubleday.

128. Prusiner, P., & Sundaralingam, M., (1973). A new class of synthetic nucleoside analogues with broad-spectrum antiviral properties, *Nature*, *244*(134), 116–118.

129. Glasser, J. W., Hupert, N., McCauley, M. M., & Hatchett, R., (2011). Modeling and public health emergency responses: lessons from SARS, *Epidemics, 3*(1), 32–37.

130. Sun, C., Yang, W., Arino, J., & Khan, K., (2011). Effect of media-induced social distancing on disease transmission in a two patch setting, *Mathematical Biosciences, 230*(2), 87–95.

131. Blendon, R. J., Benson, J. M., DesRoches, C. M., Raleigh, E., & Taylor-Clark, K., (2004). The public's response to severe acute respiratory syndrome in Toronto and the United States, *Clinical Infectious Diseases, 38*(7), 925–931.

132. Kaper, J., Rappuoli, R., & Buckley, M., (2005). Vaccine Development: Current Status and Future Needs. *American Academy of Microbiology.*

133. Pang, J., & Cui, I. A., (2009). An SIRS epidemiological model with nonlinear incidence rate incorporating media coverage, in: *Second International Conference on Information and Computing Science, IEEE*, pp. 116–119.

134. Mushayabasa, S., Bhunu, C. P., & Smith, R. J., (2012). Assessing the impact of educational campaigns on controlling HCV among women in prison settings, *Communications in Nonlinear Science and Numerical Simulation, 17*(4), 1714–1724.

135. Tracht, S. M., Del Valle, S. Y., & Hyman, J. M., (2010). Mathematical modeling of the effectiveness of facemasks in reducing the spread of novel influenza A (H1N1), *PLoS One, 5*(2), e9018.

136. Tchuenche, J. M., Dube, N., Bhunu, C. P., Smith, R. J., & Bauch, C. T., (2011). The impact of media coverage on the transmission dynamics of human influenza, *BMC Public Health, 11,* S5.

137. Liu, R., Wu, J., & Zhu, H., (2007). Media/psychological impact on multiple outbreaks of emerging infectious diseases, *Computational and Mathematical Methods in Medicine, 8*(3), 153–164.

138. Liu, Y., & Cui, J., (2008). The impact of media coverage on the dynamics of infectious disease, *International Journal of Biomathematics, 1*(1), 65–74.

139. Cui, J., Sun, Y., & Zhu, H., (2008). The impact of media on the control of infectious diseases, *Journal of Dynamics and Differential Equations, 20*(1), 31–53.

140. Cui, J., Tao, X., & Zhu, H., (2008). An SIS infection model incorporating media coverage, *Journal of Mathematics, 38*(5), 1323–1334.

141. Funk, S., Gilad, E., Watkins, C., & Jansen, V. A., (2009). The spread of aware- ness and its impact on epidemic outbreaks,

Proceedings of the National Academy of Sciences, 106(16), 6872–6877.

142. Liu, W., & Zheng, Q., (2015). A stochastic sis epidemic model incorporating media coverage in a two patch setting, *Applied Mathematics and Computation, 262,* 160–168.

143. Grewal, B. S., & Grewal, J., (2003). *Higher Engineering Mathematics*, vol. 39, Khanna Publishers.

144. Ahmad, S., & Rao, M. R. M., (1999). *Theory of Ordinary Differential Equations: With Applications of Biology and Engineering,* Affiliated East-West Private Ltd.

145. Wiggins, S., (2003). *Introduction to Applied Nonlinear Dynamical Systems and Chaos*, Springer.

146. Castillo-Chavez, C., & Song, B., (2004). Dynamical models of tuberculosis and their applications, *Mathematical Biosciences and Engineering, 1*(2), 361–404.

147. Tu, P. N., (2012). Dynamical systems: an introduction with applications in economics and biology, Springer Science & Business Media.

148. Bali, N., & Goyal, M., (2011). *A Textbook of Engineering Mathematics*, (UP Technical University, Lucknow) Sem-II, Laxmi Publications.

149. Guckenheimer, J., & Holmes, P., (1990). *Non-Linear Oscillations, Dynamical Systems, and Bifurcations of Vector Fields*, Springer-Verlag.

150. Diekmann, O., Heesterbeek, J., & Metz, J. A., (1990). On the definition and the computation of the basic reproduction ratio *R*0 in models for infectious diseases in heterogeneous populations, *Journal of Mathematical Biology, 28*(4), 365–382.

151. Driessche, P. V. D., Watmough, J., & Van den Driessche, P., (2002). Reproduction numbers and sub-threshold endemic equilibria for compart- mental models of disease transmission, *Mathematical Biosciences, 180,* 29–48.

152. Chitnis, N., Hyman, J. M., & Cushing, J. M., (2008). Determining important parameters in the spread of malaria through the sensitivity analysis of a mathematical model, *Bulletin of Mathematical Biology, 70*(5), 1272–1296.

153. Bhunu, C. P., Mushayabasa, S., & Smith, R., (2011). Assessing the effects of poverty in tuberculosis transmission dynamics, *Applied Mathematical Modelling, 36*(9), 4173–4185.

154. Bhunu, C. P., & Mushayabasa, S., (2012). A theoretical analysis of smoking and alcoholism, *Journal of Mathematical Modelling and Algorithms, 11*(4), 387–408.

155. Bhunu, C. P., & Mushayabasa, S., (2013). Assessing the effects of drug misuse on HIV/AIDS prevalence, *Theory in Biosciences, 132*(2), 83–92.

156. Bhunu, C., (2014). Homelessness and drug misuse in developing countries: A mathematical approach, *Communications in Nonlinear Science and Numerical Simulation, 19*(6), 1908–1917.

157. Hassell, M. P., (1978). *The Dynamics of Arthropod Predator-Prey Systems*, Princeton University Press.

158. Peitgen, H. O., & Richter, P. H., (2013). The beauty of fractals: images of complex dynamical systems, *Springer Science & Business Media.*

159. Gumowski, I., & Mira, C., (1980). *Recurrences and Discrete Dynamic Systems*, Springer.

160. Leslie, P., (1948). Some further notes on the use of matrices in population mathematics, *Biometrika, 35*(3–4), 213–245.

161. Leslie, P., (1958). A stochastic model for studying the properties of certain biological systems by numerical methods, *Biometrika,* 16–31.

162. Freedman, H., Rai, B., & Waltman, P., (1986). Mathematical models of population interactions with dispersal. II: Differential

survival in a change of habitat, *Journal of Mathematical Analysis and Applications, 115*(1), 140–154.

163. Freedman, H., & Waltman, P., (1977). Mathematical models of population interactions with dispersal. I: stability of two habitats with and without a predator, *SIAM Journal on Applied Mathematics, 32*(3), 631–648.

164. Shukla, J., Freedman, H., Pal, V., Misra, O., Agarwal, M., & Shukla, A., (1989). Degradation and subsequent regeneration of a forestry resource: a mathematical model, *Ecological Modelling, 44*(3), 219–229.

165. Brown, W., (1981). *Burwash Uplands Caribou Herd: Distribution and Movement Studies*, Report prepared for Foothills Pipelines (Yukon) Ltd by Beak Consultants Ltd, Calgary, Alberta.

166. Rothe, F., & Shafer, D. S., (1984). *Lecture Notes in Mathematics.*

167. Bailey, P., Shampine, L., & Waltman, P., (1968). *Nonlinear Two-Point Boundary Value Problems.*

168. Bernfeld, S., & Lakshmikantham, V., (1974). *An Introduction to Nonlinear Boundary Value Problems.* New York: Academic Press.

169. Munn, R., & Fedorov, V., (1986). The environmental assessment, IIASA project report, *International Institute for Applied Systems Analysis*, vol. 1, Laxenburg, Austria.

170. Allen, L. J., (1983). Persistence and extinction in single-species reaction-diffusion models, *Bulletin of Mathematical Biology, 45*(2), 209–227.

171. Bansal, S., & Meyers, L. A., (2012). The impact of past epidemics on future disease dynamics, *Journal of Theoretical Biology, 309,* 176–184.

172. Hallam, T. G., (1979). A temporal study of diffusion effects on a population modelled by quadratic growth, *Nonlinear Analysis: Theory, Methods & Applications, 3*(1), 123–133.

173. Levin, S. A., (1986).Population models and community structure in heterogeneous environments, in: *Mathematical Ecology*, Springer, pp. 295–320.

174. Rothe, F., (1984). *Global Solutions of Reaction-Diffusion Systems*.

175. Shukla, J., & Verma, S., (1981). Effects of convective and dispersive inter- actions on the stability of two species, *Bulletin of Mathematical Biology, 43*(5), 593–610.

176. Shukla, V., Shukla, J., & Das, P., (1981). Environmental effects on the linear stability of a three species food chain model, *Mathematical Biosciences, 57*(1–2), 35–58.

177. Skellam, J. G., (1951). Random dispersal in theoretical populations, *Biometrika, 38*(1/2), 196–218.

178. Herbert, D., Elsworth, R., & Telling, R., (1956). The continuous culture of bacteria; a theoretical and experimental study, *Microbiology, 14*(3), 601–622.

179. Novick, A., & Szilard, L., (1950). Description of the chemostat, *Science, 112*(2920), 715–716.

180. Williams, F., (1971). Dynamics of microbial populations, *Systems Analysis and Simulation in Ecology, 1*, 147–267.

181. Gopalsamy, K., (1986). Convergence in a resource-based competition system, *Bulletin of Mathematical Biology, 48*(5–6), 681–699.

182. Hsu, S. B., (1982). On a resource based ecological competition model with interference, *Journal of Mathematical Biology, 12*(1), 45–52.

183. Mitra, D., Mukherjee, D., Roy, A., & Ray, S., (1992). Permanent coexistence in a resource-based competition system, *Ecological Modelling, 60*(1), 77–85.

184. Moore, J., et al., (2002). *Parasites and the Behavior of Animals*. Oxford, University Press.

185. Hadeler, K., & Freedman, H., (1989). Predator-prey populations with parasitic infection, *Journal of Mathematical Biology, 27*(6), 609–631.

186. Ruan, S., (2001). Absolute stability, conditional stability and bifurcation in Kolmogorov-type predator-prey systems with discrete delays, *Quarterly of Applied Mathematics, 59*(1), 159–174.

187. Song, Y., Han, M., & Wei, J., (2005). Stability and Hopf bifurcation analysis on a simplified bam neural network with delays, *Physica D: Nonlinear Phenomena, 200*(3), 185–204.

188. Sahu, G. P., & Dhar, J., (2012). Analysis of an SVEIS epidemic model with partial temporary immunity and saturation incidence rate, *Applied Mathematical Modelling, 36*(3), 908–923.

189. Khazeni, N., Hutton, D. W., Garber, A. M., Hupert, N., & Owens, D. K., (2009). Effectiveness and cost-effectiveness of vaccination against pandemic influenza (H1N1) 2009, *Annals of Internal Medicine, 151*(12), 829–839.

190. Hethcote, H., (2000). The mathematics of infectious diseases, *SIAM Review, 42*(4), 599–653.

191. Taylor, M. L., & Carr, T. W., (2009). An SIR epidemic model with partial temporary immunity modeled with delay, *Journal of Mathematical Biology, 59*(6), 841–880.

Index

N

O

P